Operative Standards *for* Cancer Surgery

Volume 1

Breast, Lung, Pancreas, Colon

PRESENTED BY THE AMERICAN COLLEGE OF SURGEONS
AND THE ALLIANCE FOR CLINICAL TRIALS IN ONCOLOGY

Operative Standards
for Cancer Surgery

Volume 1

Breast, Lung, Pancreas, Colon

PRESENTED BY THE AMERICAN COLLEGE OF SURGEONS
AND THE ALLIANCE FOR CLINICAL TRIALS IN ONCOLOGY

EDITORIAL BOARD

HEIDI NELSON, MD, FACS
American College of Surgeons Clinical Research Program Director
Mayo Clinic
Rochester, Minnesota

KELLY K. HUNT, MD, FACS
American College of Surgeons Clinical Research Program Director
MD Anderson Cancer Center
Houston, Texas

NIRMAL VEERAMACHANENI, MD, FACS
ACS CRP Cancer Care Standards Development Committee, Vice-Chair
Lung Team Chair
University of Kansas
Kansas City, Kansas

SARAH BLAIR, MD, FACS
Breast Team Chair
University of California at San Diego
San Diego, California

GEORGE J. CHANG, MD, MS, FACS, FASCRS
Colon Team Chair
MD Anderson Cancer Center
Houston, Texas

AMY HALVERSON, MD, FACS, FASCRS, CO-CHAIR
Colon Team Co-Chair
Northwestern University
Chicago, Illinois

MATTHEW H. G. KATZ, MD, FACS
ACS CRP Cancer Care Standards Development Committee, Chair
Pancreas Team Co-Chair
MD Anderson Cancer Center
Houston, Texas

MITCHELL C. POSNER, MD, FACS
Pancreas Team Co-Chair
University of Chicago
Chicago, Illinois

This manual was prepared and published through the support of the American College of Surgeons.

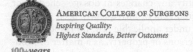

AMERICAN COLLEGE OF SURGEONS
Inspiring Quality:
Highest Standards, Better Outcomes

100+years

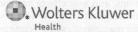

. Wolters Kluwer

Health

Philadelphia • Baltimore • New York • London
Buenos Aires • Hong Kong • Sydney • Tokyo

ALLIANCE
FOR CLINICAL TRIALS IN ONCOLOGY

Acquisitions Editor: Keith Donnellan
Product Development Editor: Brendan Huffman
Production Project Manager: David Saltzberg
Design Coordinator: Stephen Druding
Senior Manufacturing Manager: Beth Welsh
Marketing Manager: Dan Dressler
Production Service: Absolute Service, Inc.

9 8 7 6 5

Printed in the United States of America

Library of Congress Cataloging-in-Publication Data

Operative standards for cancer surgery / presented by the American College
of Surgeons and the Alliance for Clinical Trials in Oncology ; editorial
board Heidi Nelson, Kelly K. Hunt, Nirmal Veeramachaneni, Sarah Blair,
George Chang, Amy Halverson, Matthew Katz, Mitchell Posner.
    p. ; cm.
Includes bibliographical references.
ISBN 978-1-4511-9475-3
I. Nelson, Heidi, editor. II. American College of Surgeons, issuing body.
III. Alliance for Clinical Trials in Oncology, issuing body.
[DNLM: 1. Neoplasms--surgery. 2. Surgical Procedures,
Operative--standards. QZ 268]
RD651
616.99'4059--dc23
                              2015011470

Dedicated to the memory of
Keith Amos, MD.

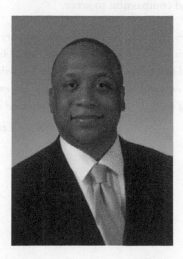

American surgery lost a rising star in June 2013. Dr. Keith Dave Amos was a loving husband to his wife, Ahaji Amos; a loving father to his three daughters, Hunter, Logan, and Daryn; and a caring friend, mentor, and surgeon. This work is dedicated to him.

Keith's career in academic surgery was an illustrious one marked by numerous honors and distinctions. A native of Minden, Louisiana, Keith matriculated at Xavier University in New Orleans, where he became interested in biomedical research as a Minority Access to Research Careers Scholar.

After graduating from Xavier, Keith attended Harvard Medical School and was selected as a Howard Hughes Medical Institute Cloister Fellow. He completed his surgery residency at Washington University in St. Louis and a surgical oncology fellowship at The University of Texas MD Anderson Cancer Center in Houston. He joined the faculty at the University of North Carolina in 2007 and dedicated his career to treating breast cancer and melanoma patients. At the time of his death, Keith was serving as the American College of Surgeons Claude H. Organ Traveling Fellow.

Keith served as an editor for the breast chapter of this book. Besides being a skilled surgeon, Keith was an example of the clinician–investigator. He contributed to numerous publications on topics ranging from preoperative staging of breast cancer patients to education techniques to foster the skills set of graduating medical students. He was very active in the American College of Surgeons and a number of cooperative groups to address issues facing patients with breast cancer and melanoma.

Keith had a positive impact on countless individuals, one too great to adequately describe in this brief remembrance. His untimely death has left multiple charitable organizations, professional societies, and patient advocacy groups without a dedicated friend and supporter. He is deeply missed by his friends, family, students, and patients.

Following Keith's death, the University of North Carolina established a remembrance Web site in his honor. The following entry, typical of the hundreds posted, is a testament to Keith's good character and compassion to serve.

"I didn't know Dr. Amos very well, and he didn't know me very well, either. But that didn't stop him from giving time from his very busy life to guide and advise me along with many of my classmates. Dr. Amos touched our whole community with his unhesitating generosity with his time and attention, while still enjoying a family life that was the envy of his colleagues. Had he never scrubbed in, picked up a scalpel, or sewn a stitch, he would still have been a great man."

—University of North Carolina, Senior Medical Student

FOUNDING ORGANIZATIONS
American College of Surgeons
Alliance for Clinical Trials in Oncology

SPONSORING ORGANIZATIONS
American College of Surgeons
Alliance for Clinical Trials in Oncology

LIAISON ORGANIZATIONS
American Association for Thoracic Surgery (AATS)
American Society of Breast Surgeons (ASBrS)
American Society of Colon and Rectal Surgery (ASCRS)
Eastern Cooperative Oncology Group (ECOG)/
American College of Radiology Imaging Network (ACRIN)
General Thoracic Surgical Club (GTSC)
National Accreditation Program for Breast Centers (NAPBC)
National Cancer Institute of Canada (NCIC)
NRG Oncology
Society for Surgery of the Alimentary Tract (SSAT)
Society of American Gastrointestinal and Endoscopic Surgeons (SAGES)
Society of Surgical Oncology (SSO)
Society of Thoracic Surgeons (STS)
Southwest Oncology Group (SWOG)
The Cardiothoracic Surgery Network (CTSNet)

EXECUTIVE OFFICE
American College of Surgeons
Executive Office
633 North Saint Clair Street
Chicago, IL 60611-3211

BREAST

Rebecca Aft, MD, PhD, FACS,
Lymphadenectomy Workgroup Leader
Professor of Surgery
Washington University
St. Louis, Missouri

Lisa Bailey, MD, FACS
Bay Area Breast Surgeons
Medical Director, Carol Ann Read Breast
Health Center
Alta Bates Summit Medical Center
Oakland, California

Nancy Baxter, MD, PhD, FRCSC, FACS,
Methodologist
Chief, Division of General Surgery
St. Michael's Hospital
Toronto, Ontario, Canada

Sarah Blair, MD, FACS
Chair, Partial Mastectomy Workgroup Leader
Professor of Surgery
Breast Team Chair
Surgical Oncology
University of California
San Diego, California

Aaron Bleznak, MD, MBA, FACS
Vice President and Senior Medical Director
Sentara Medical Group
Assistant Professor of Clinical Surgery
Eastern Virginia Medical School
Norfolk, Virginia

Peter W. Blumencranz, MD, FACS
Medical Director
The Comprehensive Breast Care Center of
Tampa Bay
Clearwater, Florida

Judy C. Boughey, MB, BChir, FACS
Vice-Chair for Research, Department of Surgery
Professor of Surgery
Program Director–Multidisciplinary Breast
Surgery Fellowship
Mayo Clinic College of Medicine
Rochester, Minnesota

Kai Chen, MD
Clinical Research Fellow
Department of Surgery
Johns Hopkins Hospital
Baltimore, Maryland

Carol S. Connor, MD, FACS
Professor of Surgery
Chief, Division of Breast Surgery
Department of Surgery
University of Kansas
Kansas City, Kansas
Representing ASBrS

Lisa Curcio, MD, FACS
Medical Director, Surgical Services
Breastlink
Laguna Hills, California
Representing ASBrS

Diana Dickson-Witmer, MD, FACS
Breast Team Art/Illustration Editor
Medical Director, Christiana Care Breast Center
Director, Christiana Care Breast Program
Helen F Graham Cancer Center and Research
Institute
Newark, Delaware
Clinical Assistant Professor of Surgery
Sidney Kimmel College of Medicine
Thomas Jefferson University
Philadelphia, Pennsylvania

Mahmoud El Tamer, MD, FACS
Attending Surgeon, Breast Service
Department of Surgery
Memorial Sloan Kettering Cancer Center
Professor of Surgery
Weill Cornell Medical College
New York, New York

Erin Garvey, MD
General Surgery Resident
Mayo Clinic
Phoenix, Arizona

Richard J. Gray, MD, FACS
Consultant, Section of Surgical Oncology
Co-Director, Multidisciplinary Breast Clinic
Associate Professor of Surgery
Mayo Clinic
Scottsdale, Arizona

E. Shelley Hwang, MD, MPH, FACS
Total Mastectomy Workgroup Leader
Professor of Surgery
Chief Breast Surgical Oncology
Duke University Medical Center
Charlotte, North Carolina

Lisa Jacobs, MD, FACS
Associate Professor of Surgery
Johns Hopkins University
Baltimore, Maryland

Thomas B. Julian, MD, FACS
Director, Breast Surgical Oncology
Allegheny Health Network
Senior Surgical Director, Medical Affairs
National Surgical Adjuvant Breast and Bowel
Project
Professor of Surgery
Temple University School of Medicine
Professor of Surgery
Drexel University College of Medicine
Pittsburgh, Pennsylvania

Seema A. Khan, MD, FACS
Professor of Surgery
Bluhm Family Professor of Cancer Research
Co-Leader Breast Cancer Program
Robert H. Lurie Comprehensive Cancer Center
Northwestern University
Chicago, Illinois
Representing ECOG

Henry Kuerer, MD, PhD, FACS
Professor of Surgical Oncology
Director, Breast Surgical Oncology Training
Program
Medical Director, Clinical Expansion
MD Anderson Cancer Center
Houston, Texas

Swati A. Kulkarni, MD, FACS
Associate Professor of Surgery Section of
General Surgery
The University of Chicago Medicine &
Biological Sciences
Chicago, Illinois

Scott H. Kurtzman, MD, FACS
Chairman of Surgery and Program Director
Waterbury Hospital
General Surgery Residency Program Director
Professor of Surgery
University of Connecticut School of Medicine
Waterbury, Connecticut

Christine A. Lee, MD, FACS
Surgical Representative, SWOG Breast
Committee
Swedish Cancer Institute
Swedish Medical Center
Seattle, Washington
Representing SWOG

Sarah McLaughlin, MD
Associate Professor of Surgery
Section of Surgical Oncology
Program Director General Surgery Residency
Mayo Clinic
Jacksonville, Florida

Barbara A. Pockaj, MD, FACS
Chair, Section of Surgical Oncology
Michael M. Eisenberg Professor of Surgery
Mayo Clinic
Phoenix, Arizona

Susan Pories, MD, FACS
Co-Director, Hoffman Breast Center
Mount Auburn Hospital
Associate Professor of Surgery
Harvard Medical School
Cambridge, Massachusetts

Julieta Robin, MD
Surgical Breast Fellow
Allegheny General Hospital
Pittsburgh, Pennsylvania

Lisa M. Sclafani, MD, FACS
Attending Surgeon
Breast Surgery Service
Memorial Sloan Kettering Cancer Center
Professor of Clinical Surgery
Weill Cornell Medical College
New York, New York

Amelia Tower, DO
Surgical Breast Fellow
Allegheny General Hospital
Pittsburgh, Pennsylvania

Gary W. Unzeitig, MD, FACS
Laredo Breast Care
Laredo, Texas

Jamie L. Wagner, DO, FACOS
Assistant Professor of Surgery
Department of Surgery
University of Kansas School of Medicine
University of Kansas Cancer Center
Kansas City, Kansas

Lee Gravatt Wilke, MD, FACS
Sentinel Node Workgroup Leader
Professor of Surgery
Director, University of Wisconsin Breast Center
UW Health/UW School of Medicine and Public
Health
Madison, Wisconsin

COLON

Ovunc Bardakcioglu, MD, FACS, FASCRS
Associate Professor of Surgery
Chief Division of Colon and Rectal Surgery
University of Nevada School of Medicine
Las Vegas, Nevada

Don Buie, MD
Clinical Assistant Professor of Surgery
Alberta Provincial Health System
Calgary, Alberta, Canada
Representing ASCRS Standards Committee

George J. Chang, MD, MS, FACS, FASCRS
Colon Team Chair
Associate Professor of Surgical Oncology
Chief, Colon and Rectal Surgery
Associate Medical Director, Colorectal Center
Director of Clinical Operations, Minimally
Invasive and New Technologies
in Oncologic Surgery Program
MD Anderson Cancer Center
The University of Texas
Houston, Texas

Conor P. Delaney, MCh, PhD, FACS
Professor of Surgery, Chief of Colorectal
Surgery, Vice-Chair of Surgery
University Hospitals Case Medical Center
Cleveland, Ohio

David Dietz, MD, FACS
Colon Team Art/Illustration Editor
Vice-Chairman, Residency Program Director,
and Thomas C. and Sandra S. Sullivan Family
Endowed Chair
Department of Colorectal Surgery
Digestive Disease Institute
Cleveland Clinic
Cleveland, Ohio

Alessandro Fichera, MD, FACS, FASCRS
Professor and Section Chief Gastrointestinal
Surgery
Division of General Surgery, Department of
Surgery
University of Washington Medical Center
Seattle, Washington

James W. Fleshman, MD, FACS, FASCRS
Seeger Professor and Chairman, Department of
Surgery
Professor of Surgery, Texas A&M Health
Science Center
Baylor University Medical Center
Dallas, Texas
Representing SSO and SSAT

Amy L. Halverson, MD, FACS, FASCRS
Colon Team Co-Chair
Associate Professor of Surgery
Chief, Section of Colon and Rectal Surgery
Northwestern University Feinberg School of
Medicine
Chicago, Illinois

Steven Hochwald, MD, FACS
Vice-Chair and Chief of Gastrointestinal
Surgery
Professor of Oncology
Department of Surgical Oncology
Roswell Park Cancer Institute
Buffalo, New York

David W. Larson, MD, MBA, FACS, FASCRS
Chair of Colorectal Surgery
Director of Enterprise Cancer Quality
Mayo Clinic
Rochester, Minnesota

Robert D. Madoff, MD, FACS, FASCRS,
FRCSEd (Hon)
Professor of Surgery
Chief, Division of Colon and Rectal Surgery
Stanley M. Goldberg, MD Chair in Colon
and Rectal Surgery
Department of Surgery
University of Minnesota
Minneapolis, Minnesota
ASCRS/DCR Editor

Jorge Marcet, MD, FACS
Professor, Department of Oncologic Sciences
Program Director, Colorectal Surgery
Fellowship
Division Director, Colon and Rectal Surgery,
Morsani College of Medicine
University of South Florida
Tampa, Florida

David A. Margolin, MD, FACS
Professor and Director, Colon and Rectal
Surgical Research
The Ochsner Clinic Foundation
The University of Queensland School of Medi-
cine, Ochsner Clinical School
New Orleans, Louisiana

John R. T. Monson, MD, FRCS (Ire, Eng, Ed,
Glas [Hon]), FASCRS, FACS
Professor of Surgery and Oncology
Chief, Division of Colorectal Surgery and
Vice-Chairman of Surgery
Vice-Chairman of Quality and Outcomes
Director, Surgical Health Outcomes and
Research Enterprise (SHORE)
University of Rochester Medical Center
Rochester, New York

Ian M. Paquette, MD, FACS
Assistant Professor of Surgery
Division of Colon and Rectal Surgery
University of Cincinnati College of Medicine
Cincinnati, Ohio

Timothy M. Pawlik, MD, MPH, PhD, FACS
Professor of Surgery and Oncology
John L. Cameron, MD, Professor of
Alimentary Tract Diseases
Chief, Division of Surgical Oncology
Program Director, Surgical Oncology
Fellowship
Director, Johns Hopkins Medicine Liver
Tumor Center Multi-Disciplinary Clinic
Johns Hopkins Hospital
Baltimore, Maryland

Walter Peters, MD, MBA, FACS, FASCRS
University of Missouri
Boone Hospital Center
Columbia, Missouri
Representing the Alliance Community
Oncology Committee

Miguel A. Rodriguez-Bigas, MD, FACS
Professor of Surgery
Department of Surgical Oncology
MD Anderson Cancer Center
The University of Texas
Houston, Texas

Elin R. Sigurdson, MD, PhD, FACS, FRCS (C)
Professor
Chief, Division of General Surgical Oncology
Associate Chief of Academic Affairs
Fox Chase Cancer Center
Philadelphia, Pennsylvania
Representing ECOG/ACRIN

Luca Stocchi, MD, FACS
Colon Team Art/Illustration Editor
The Story-Garschina Chair in Colorectal
Surgery
Department of Colorectal Surgery
Digestive Disease Institute
Cleveland Clinic
Cleveland, Ohio

Alexander Stojadinovic, MD, FACS, Col (Ret)
United States Army, Medical Corps
Professor of Surgery, Uniformed Services
University
Professor of Medicine, Uniformed Services
University
Bethesda, Maryland
Medical Director, Bon Secours Cancer Institute
Richmond, Virginia

Steven D. Wexner, MD, PhD (Hon), FACS,
FRCS, FRCS (Ed)
Director, Digestive Disease Center and Chair
Department of Colorectal Surgery
Cleveland Clinic
Weston, Florida
Affiliate Professor of Clinical Biomedical
Science and Associate Dean for Academic
Affairs
Charles E. Schmidt College of Medicine
Florida Atlantic University
Boca Raton, Florida
Clinical Professor, Herbert Wertheim College
of Medicine
Florida International University
Miami, Florida
Representing SAGES

Neal Wilkinson, MD, FACS
Surgical Oncology
Kalispell Regional Medical Center
Kalispell, Montana
Representing NRG Oncology

LUNG

Khalid Amer, FRCS (C Th)
Thoracic Surgeon
University Hospital Southampton
Southampton, United Kingdom

Frank A. Baciewicz Jr, MD, FACS
Professor
Division of Cardiothoracic Surgery
Wayne State University
Chief, Thoracic Oncology
Karmanos Cancer Institute
Detroit, Michigan

Thomas L. Bauer II, MD, FACS
Medical Director, Thoracic Oncology Program
Director, Thoracic Surgery
Meridian Health
Jersey Shore University Medical Center
Neptune, New Jersey

Mark F. Berry, MD, MHS
Associate Professor
Department of Cardiothoracic Surgery
Stanford University
Stanford, California

Matthew Blum, MD, FACS
Director of Thoracic Surgery
Memorial Hospital-University of Colorado
Health
Colorado Springs, Colorado
Representing STS

Raphael Bueno, MD, FACS
Professor of Surgery
Harvard Medical School
Brigham and Women's Hospital
Boston, Massachusetts
Representing AATS

Lucian R. Chirieac, MD
Brigham and Women's Hospital,
Harvard Medical School
Boston, Massachusetts

Traves Crabtree, MD, FACS
Workgroup Co-Leader
Associate Professor, Surgery
Division of Cardiothoracic Surgery
Washington University
St. Louis, Missouri

Malcolm M. DeCamp, MD, FACS
Fowler McCormick Professor of Surgery
Northwestern University Feinberg School of
Medicine
Chief, Division of Thoracic Surgery
Northwestern Memorial Hospital
Chicago, Illinois
Representing GTSC and AATS

Todd L. Demmy, MD, FACS
Lung Team Art/Illustration Editor
Professor of Oncology and Chair, Thoracic
Surgery
Roswell Park Cancer Institute
Professor of Surgery, State University of New
York at Buffalo
Buffalo, New York

Marc de Perrot, MD, MSc
Associate Professor of Surgery, University of Toronto
Division of Thoracic Surgery
Princess Margaret Cancer Centre and Toronto General Hospital
University Health Network
Toronto, Ontario, Canada
Representing STS

Jean Deslauriers, MD
Professor of Surgery, Laval University
Thoracic Surgery, Institut Universitaire de Cardiologie et de Pneumologie de Québec
Québec City, Québec, Canada
Representing National Cancer Institute of Canada

Frank Detterbeck, MD, FACS, FCCP
Workgroup Co-Leader
Professor of Surgery, Section of Thoracic Surgery
Chief, Thoracic Surgery
Surgical Director, Thoracic Oncology
Clinical Program Leader,
Thoracic Oncology Program
Smilow Cancer Hospital
Yale School of Medicine
New Haven, Connecticut
Representing AATS

Jessica Donington, MD, FACS
Lung Team Art/Illustration Editor
Sublobal Resection Workgroup Leader
NYU Langone Medical Center
New York, New York
Representing GTSC, RTOG

Matthew A. Facktor, MD, FACS
Lobe/Bilobectomy Workgroup Leader
Director, Thoracic Surgery
Geisinger Medical Center
Danville, Pennsylvania

Mark K. Ferguson, MD, FACS
Professor, Department of Surgery and
The Cancer Research Center
Head, Thoracic Surgery Service
Director, Residency Program in Cardiothoracic Surgery
University of Chicago
Chicago, Illinois
Representing CTSNet

Felix G. Fernandez, MD, FACS
Assistant Professor of Surgery
General Thoracic Surgery
Emory University School of Medicine
Atlanta, Georgia

Sean C. Grondin, MD, MPH, FRCSC
University of Calgary
Foothills Medical Centre
Calgary, Canada

Mark Hennon, MD
Assistant Professor of Oncology
Roswell Park Cancer Institute
Assistant Professor of Surgery
State University of New York at Buffalo
Buffalo, New York

Rodney J. Landreneau, MD, FACS
Division Director, General Thoracic Surgery
System Director, Thoracic Oncology
Co-Director, Esophageal and Lung Institute
Allegheny Health Network
Pittsburgh, Pennsylvania

Michael Lanuti, MD, FACS
Lobe/Bilobectomy Workgroup Co-Leader
Director of Thoracic Oncology, Division of Thoracic Surgery
Associate Professor of Surgery
Harvard Medical School
Massachusetts General Hospital
Boston, Massachusetts

Moishe Liberman, MD, PhD
Director—CHUM Endoscopic
Tracheobronchial and Oesophageal Center
Associate Professor of Surgery Division of Thoracic Surgery
University of Montreal
Montreal, Quebec, Canada

Jules Lin, MD, FACS
Assistant Professor
Surgical Director, Lung Transplant
Section of Thoracic Surgery
University of Michigan
Ann Arbor, Michigan

Linda W. Martin, MD, MPH, FCCP, FACS
Lung Team Art/Illustration Editor
Assistant Professor, Department of Surgery
University of Maryland School of Medicine
Chief, Thoracic Surgery
Upper Chesapeake Medical Center
Bel Air, Maryland

Bryan Meyers, MD, MPH, FACS
Patrick and Joy Williamson Professor of
Surgery
Division of Cardiothoracic Surgery
Chief, Thoracic Surgery
Washington University
St. Louis, Missouri
Representing Alliance Respiratory Committee

Sudish C. Murthy, MD, PhD, FACS, FCCP
Section Head, General Thoracic Surgery
Surgical Director, Center of Major Airway
Disease
Thoracic and Cardiovascular Surgery
Cleveland Clinic
Cleveland, Ohio
Representing AATS

Basil Nasir, MBBCh
Thoracic Surgeon
Vancouver General Hospital
University of British Columbia
Gordon and Leslie Diamond Health Care Center
Vancouver, Canada

Varun Puri, MD, MSCI, FACS
Methodologist
Assistant Professor, Surgery
Division of Cardiothoracic Surgery
Washington University
St. Louis, Missouri

Joe B. Putnam Jr, MD, FACS
Ingram Professor of Surgery and Chair
Department of Thoracic Surgery
Professor of Biomedical Informatics
Program Director, Thoracic Surgery
Vanderbilt University Medical Center
Nashville, Tennessee

Rishindra M. Reddy, MD, FACS·
Assistant Clerkship Director, Department of
Surgery
Assistant Professor, Thoracic Surgery
University of Michigan
Ann Arbor, Michigan

Stacey Su, MD, FACS
Fox Chase Cancer Center
Philadelphia, Pennsylvania
Representing ECOG

Betty C. Tong, MD, MHS, FACS
Pneumonectomy Workgroup Leader
Assistant Professor
Division of Cardiovascular and Thoracic
Surgery
Duke University Medical Center
Durham, North Carolina
Representing STS

Nirmal Veeramachaneni, MD, FACS
Chair, Nodal Staging Workgroup Leader
Lung Team Chair
General Thoracic Surgeon
Clinical Associate Professor
University of Kansas
Kansas City, Kansas

Dennis Wigle, MD, PhD, FACS
Associate Professor of Surgery
Department of Thoracic Surgery
Mayo Clinic
Rochester, Minnesota
Representing GTSC and Alliance Respiratory
Committee

Douglas E. Wood, MD, FACS, FRCSEd (ad hom)
Professor and Chief
Division of Cardiothoracic Surgery
Vice-Chair, Department of Surgery
Endowed Chair in Lung Cancer Research
University of Washington
Seattle, Washington
Representing CTSNet

Kazuhiro Yasufuku, MD, PhD
Director, Interventional Thoracic Surgery
Program
Associate Professor of Surgery, University of
Toronto
Division of Thoracic Surgery, Toronto General
Hospital
University Health Network
Toronto, Ontario, Canada
Representing National Cancer Institute of
Canada

PANCREAS

Syed Arif Ahmad, MD
Professor of Surgery
Associate Director, University of Cincinnati
Cancer Institute
Program Leader, Gastrointestinal Oncology
and Head Pancreas Disease Center
The University of Cincinnati Medical Center
Cincinnati, Ohio

Peter Allen, MD, FACS
Memorial Sloan Kettering Cancer Center
New York, New York

Waddah B. Al-Refaie, MD, FACS
Chief of Surgical Oncology
MedStar Georgetown University Hospital
Department of Surgery
Surgeon in Chief
Lombardi Comprehensive Cancer Center
Washington, DC

M. Mura Assifi, MD
Fellow, Surgical Oncology
University of Pittsburgh Medical Center
Pittsburgh, Pennsylvania

Adam C. Berger, MD, FACS
Professor
Chief, Section of Surgical Oncology
Department of Surgery
Thomas Jefferson University
Philadelphia, Pennsylvania

Mitchell Chorost, MD, FACS
Associate Professor of Clinical Surgery
Weill Cornell Medical College
Director, Surgical Oncology
St. Francis Hospital
Roslyn, New York

Yun Shin Chun, MD, FACS
Director, Hepato-Pancreato-Biliary Programs
Virginia Piper Cancer Institute
Minneapolis, Minnesota

W. Charles Conway II, MD, FACS
Oschner Health System
New Orleans, Louisiana

Kristopher P. Croome, MD
Assistant Professor—Senior Associate
Consultant
Division of Transplantation Surgery
Mayo Clinic College of Medicine
Jacksonville, Florida

Wendy L. Frankel, MD
Kurtz Chair and Distinguished Professor
Vice-Chair and Director of Anatomic
Pathology
Director of GI Pathology
Department of Pathology
The Ohio State University
Columbus, Ohio

Paul Hansen, MD, FACS
Director of Surgical Oncology
Medical Director, Providence Hepatobiliary
and Pancreatic Cancer Program
Providence Cancer Center
Portland, Oregon

John P. Hoffman, MD, FACS
Fox Chase Cancer Center
Philadelphia, Pennsylvania

Matthew H. G. Katz, MD, FACS
Pancreas Team Co-Chair
Assistant Professor of Surgical Oncology
The University of Texas
MD Anderson Cancer Center
Houston, Texas

Kaitlyn Kelly, MD
Assistant Professor of Surgery
Division of Surgical Oncology
University of California, San Diego
La Jolla, California

Michael L. Kendrick, MD, FACS
Chair, Division of Subspecialty General Surgery
Professor of Surgery
Mayo Clinic College of Medicine
Rochester, Minnesota

Andrew M. Lowy, MD, FACS
Professor of Surgery
Chief, Division of Surgical Oncology
Moores Cancer Center
University of California at San Diego
La Jolla, California

Nipun Merchant, MD, FACS
Alan S. Livingstone Professor of Surgery
Vice-Chair of Surgical Oncology Services
Vice-Chair of Academic Affairs
Chief Surgical Officer, Sylvester Comprehensive
Cancer Center
University of Miami Medical Center
Miami, Florida

William H. Nealon, MD
Professor of Surgery
Yale University School of Medicine
New Haven, Connecticut

Timothy M. Pawlik, MD, MPH, PhD, FACS
Professor of Surgery and Oncology
John L. Cameron, MD, Professor of Alimentary
Tract Diseases
Chief, Division of Surgical Oncology
Program Director, Surgical Oncology
Fellowship
Director, Johns Hopkins Medicine Liver Tumor
Center Multi-Disciplinary Clinic
Johns Hopkins Hospital
Baltimore, Maryland

Peter W. T. Pisters, MD, MHCM, FACS
Professor of Surgery
University of Toronto
President and CEO
University Health Network
Toronto, Ontario, Canada

Mitchell C. Posner, MD, FACS
Pancreas Team Co-Chair
Thomas D. Jones Professor of Surgery and
Vice-Chairman
Chief, Section of General Surgery and Surgical
Oncology
Professor, Radiation and Cellular Oncology
University of Chicago Medicine
Chicago, Illinois

Aaron R. Sasson, MD, FACS
Professor of Surgery
Chief of GI Surgical Oncology
University of Nebraska Medical Center
Omaha, Nebraska

Roderich E. Schwarz, MD, PhD, FACS
Medical Director
IU Health Goshen Center for Cancer Care
Professor of Surgery
Indiana University School of Medicine,
South Bend
Goshen, Indiana

Brett C. Sheppard, MD, MS, FACS
Professor
Vice-Chair of Clinical Affairs
Oregon Health and Science University
Portland, Oregon

Mark J. Truty, MD, MSc
Assistant Professor—Consultant
Section Head—Hepatobiliary and Pancreatic
Surgery
Division of Subspecialty General Surgery
Department of Surgery
Mayo Clinic College of Medicine
Rochester, Minnesota

Susan Tsai, MD, MHS
Assistant Professor, Surgical Oncology
Medical College of Wisconsin
Milwaukee, Wisconsin

Jennifer F. Tseng, MD, MPH
Chief, Division of Surgical Oncology
Clinical Co-Director for Surgery
Beth Israel Deaconess Medical Center
Associate Professor
Harvard Medical School
Boston, Massachusetts

Caroline Verbeke, MD, PhD, FRCPath
Division of Pathology
Department of Laboratory Medicine
Karolinska Institute
Stockholm, Sweden

Charles Vollmer, MD, FACS
Pancreas Team Art/Illustration Editor
Director of Pancreatic Surgery
University of Pennsylvania
Philadelphia, Pennsylvania

Sharon M. Weber, MD, FACS
Tim and MaryAnn McKenzie Chair of
Surgical Oncology
Medical Director of Surgical Oncology
Carbone Cancer Center
Vice-Chair of Academic Affairs, General Surgery
University of Wisconsin
Madison, Wisconsin

Emily Winslow, MD, FACS
Assistant Professor of Surgery
University of Wisconsin
Madison, Wisconsin

Ronald Wolf, MD, FACS
Liver and Pancreas Surgeon
Gastrointestinal and Minimally Invasive
Surgery (GMIS)
The Oregon Clinic
Program Co-Director, Hepatobiliary and
Pancreatic Surgery
Providence Portland Cancer Center
Portland, Oregon

Nicholas J. Zyromski, MD, FACS
Associate Professor
Department of Surgery
Indiana University School of Medicine
Indianapolis, Indiana

LIST OF METHODOLOGISTS

Nancy Baxter, MD, PhD, FRCSC, FACRS
Chief, Division of General Surgery
St. Michael's Hospital
Toronto, Ontario, Canada

George J. Chang, MD, MS, FACS, FASCRS
Associate Professor of Surgical Oncology
Associate Medical Director, Colorectal Center
Director of Clinical Operations, Minimally
Invasive and New Technologies in Oncologic
Surgery Program
MD Anderson Cancer Center
The University of Texas
Houston, Texas

Timothy M. Pawlik, MD, MPH, PhD, FACS
Professor of Surgery and Oncology
John L. Cameron, MD, Professor of
Alimentary Tract Diseases
Chief, Division of Surgical Oncology
Program Director, Surgical Oncology
Fellowship
Director, Johns Hopkins Medicine Liver
Tumor Center Multi-Disciplinary Clinic
Johns Hopkins Hospital
Baltimore, Maryland

Varun Puri, MD, FACS
Assistant Professor, Surgery
Division of Cardiothoracic Surgery
Washington University
St. Louis, Missouri

It is a great pleasure to recognize the first edition of *Operative Standards for Cancer Surgery*, produced through cooperation between the American College of Surgeons and the Alliance for Clinical Trials in Oncology. This represents a unique benefit of the decade-long relationship between the ACS and National Cancer Institute cooperative groups and is in line with the hundred-year history of our commitment to quality.

As with any component of the care of patients, there is evidence of what is effective and there is accompanying variability in the actual practice. Much of clinical surgery is based on principles of ablation, correction of anatomic deficits, and reconstruction. The effectiveness of cancer operations has generally followed the principle of surgical removal. The technical elements that are critical to the proper conduct of a cancer operation ensure the best practice in optimal long-term outcomes. When evidence and experience demonstrate a technique that is essential for optimal outcomes, it is essential to teach that technique with precision and put it forth as an evidence-based standard.

This manual, using both text and illustrations, focuses on describing technical elements critical to proper conduct of cancer operations where best practice can be demonstrated. The authors have attempted to use the best evidence available, and this evidence represents the opinions of diverse and representative groups who care for cancer patients.

Defining those critical elements of each operation that are essential for surgical success is the purpose of *Operative Standards for Cancer Surgery*, and the areas covered have achieved this noble goal. Drs. Heidi Nelson and Kelly Hunt, along with the other surgeons that led disease site groups, are to be congratulated for the work they have done in producing this landmark approach to surgical care. This effort will become the standard by which cancer care is judged going forward and should be a standard for how all of surgical care is taught.

David B. Hoyt, MD, FACS
Executive Director
American College of Surgeons

xix

"It is part of your job to get out of your rut and see how others are doing things, what steps are being taken at the frontiers of your science or art, and bring those ideas home."

Francis D. Moore, MD

"People never improve unless they look to some standard or example higher or better than themselves."

Tyron Edwards
American Theologian
1809–1894

Surgery is an art, not a science. All surgeons know that the specifics of surgery for an individual patient, with all of their special anatomical and biologic features, cannot be reduced to a formula. As a result, surgery cannot be learned from a textbook; it must be learned in the operating room, in the clinic, on the wards, and during morbidity and mortality conferences. Surgery is learned by watching other surgeons and by adapting their examples to one's own style. Dr. John Mannick, the Chair of Surgery during my own training, famously stated, "Every surgery training program should have at least one really bad surgeon so that residents learn what not to do." We all knew that he was joking because bad surgery was not tolerated, but we also knew that learning from mistakes was a powerful source of education. Another favorite expression, attributed to Dr. Francis D. Moore, was, "Good surgical judgment comes from experience, and experience comes from having poor judgment."

Although it is an art, surgery at its best is informed by science—by objective data that guide optimal practice. During my own training, the "no touch" procedure for cancer surgery was advocated by some practitioners. These surgeons believed that meticulously ligating each vessel surrounding a tumor before manipulating it in any way could prevent metastatic spread by limiting the number of cells that broke free into the circulation. Although it is true that tumor cells are introduced into circulation at increased numbers during the conduct of surgery, we now have data showing that no clinical benefit is derived from extraordinary methods to prevent this. Other new surgical techniques have been added based on data from clinical studies. For example, total mesorectal excision is now a proven method of reducing mortality for rectal cancer, and the management of regional lymph nodes for breast cancer and melanoma has changed dramatically following results from clinical trials. Changes in surgical approaches continue to occur as a result of new instrumentation facilitating minimally invasive surgery and in response to improvements in chemotherapy and radiation therapy.

This publication represents an outstanding collaboration among many leaders in surgical oncology. It provides a detailed roadmap for optimal surgery as we know it today, and it therefore meets an important unmet need as an educational tool. Broad application of these standards to clinical practice will improve outcomes for many cancer patients. In addition, because data to guide optimal care can only be identified through standardization of techniques, this work provides an essential platform for developing further improvements. Fortunately, it is the nature of good surgeons to constantly refine their technique. We can therefore be confident that innovative surgeons will build upon this foundation in ways that will greatly benefit our patients.

Monica M. Bertagnolli, MD, FACS
Group Chair
Alliance for Clinical Trials in Oncology

It is with great pleasure that we introduce the first edition of *Operative Standards for Cancer Surgery*. This manual, presented by the American College of Surgeons (ACS) and the Alliance for Clinical Trials in Oncology, represents one of the unique benefits of the decade-long relationship between the ACS and the National Cancer Institute (NCI) Cooperative Groups. Since its inception 100 years ago, the ACS has demonstrated unwavering dedication to the creation and implementation of surgical standards. Standards were considered a founding principle of the ACS, and standards formed the basis for many of the programs that evolved within the ACS, including the Commission on Cancer, Committee on Trauma, the National Accreditation Program for Breast Centers, and the American Joint Committee on Cancer. For their part, the NCI Cooperative Groups, including the three legacy groups of the Alliance (the ACS Oncology Group, Cancer and Leukemia Group B, and North Central Cancer Treatment Group), have also provided much impetus over the years for surgeons to create standards for specific surgeries. Furthermore, clinical trials in cancer patients have often required that surgeons define the technical elements considered vital to cancer outcomes. In fact, trials whose study hypothesis focuses on a surgical question have required that surgery be performed according to a well-defined technical protocol complete with measures for quality assurance and control, as well as procedures for correlating surgical techniques with outcomes. The focus of the ACS and NCI Cooperative Groups on surgical standards and the emphasis clinical trials have placed on defining surgical techniques and correlating them with outcomes have brought us to a point at which we can provide, in this manual, the first comprehensive, evidence-based examination of cancer surgery techniques as standards.

In this manual, text and illustrations are used to describe the technical elements that are considered critical to the proper conduct of a cancer operation to ensure best practices and optimal oncologic outcomes. This manual is not a technical atlas, and its text and illustrations do not describe all aspects of a cancer operation; furthermore, it does not cover all perioperative standards, such as antibiotic use or prophylaxis for thromboembolic events, or even all intraoperative standards, such as the surgical pause or checklist, used in the surgical treatment of cancer patients. Instead, this manual focuses on the surgical activities that occur between skin incision and skin closure that directly affect cancer outcomes. It simply provides the best evidence available in the literature, as determined using state-of-the art methodologies, in support of specific surgical oncology techniques. This manual does not represent the expressed opinion of a single surgeon; rather, its authors were drawn from diverse and representational groups, including the ACS, the Alliance and NCI Cooperative Groups, and the Commission on Cancer, as well as national societies and organizations with an interest in the four cancer types covered herein.

We have tremendous respect for and are grateful to all the surgeons, leaders, and support staff who helped to create and shape this manual. First, we wish to thank the dozens of surgeons who spent nights, weekends, and holidays conducting searches, reviewing literature, debating key points, writing chapters, and selecting artwork and illustrations to assemble this manual. Without their volunteerism, this manual would never have been realized. Second, we wish to acknowledge the superb leadership skills of the surgeons who led the disease site groups (Drs. Blair, Chang, Katz, and Veeramachaneni). We would also like to acknowledge the art directors who gathered the illustrations and materials that bring visual clarity to the concepts described in this manual (Drs. Dickson-Witmer, Halverson, Martin, and Vollmer). Finally, we thank the dedicated and brilliant methodologists who walked us through the process of gathering and analyzing the evidence to produce the highest quality standards (Drs. Baxter, Chang, Pawlik, and Puri). We are also indebted to our publisher and colleagues (Keith Donnellan, acquisitions editor, Professional & Education, and Brendan Huffman, product manager–Editorial) for believing in this project and helping it take shape and form.

Of course, this project emerged because past ACS leadership saw the wisdom in engaging more surgeons in the NCI Cooperative Groups and because subsequent ACS and Alliance leadership preserved such engagement through the formation and support of the ACS Clinical Research Program. We therefore thank the ACS Board of Regents and Drs. Samuel Wells, Thomas Russell, David Hoyt, and Monica Bertagnolli. Finally, nothing of substance would have been accomplished without the steadfast dedication and logistical support of the ACS staff. Thank you, Carla Amato-Martz, for seeing this project through from start to finish.

We hope this first edition of *Operative Standards for Cancer Surgery* brings value to your practice as well as to your education and training programs. We also hope this manual inspires some readers to take an active role in creating an expanded second edition that includes additional cancer sites and/or challenge current standards and create new standards. If this manual helps surgeons, students, and/or trainees sharpen their focus on that which matters most during cancer surgery or improve the way in which they report and communicate their work, we will have fulfilled our ambitions.

Respectfully submitted,

Heidi Nelson, MD, FACS
Chair, Department of Surgery
Fred C. Andersen Professor of Surgery
Mayo Clinic
Rochester, New York

Kelly K. Hunt, MD, FACS
Hamill Foundation Distinguished Professor of Surgery in
Honor of Dr. Richard G. Martin Sr
Chief, Breast Surgical Oncology
Department of Surgical Oncology
The University of Texas
MD Anderson Cancer Center
Houston, Texas

Operative Standards for Cancer Surgery describes the essential intraoperative steps surgeons should follow to assure optimal oncologic outcomes. The first edition of this manual, a product of a collaborative effort between the Alliance and the Clinical Research Program of the American College of Surgeons, focuses on four common cancers, including breast, lung, pancreas, and colon.

Although adjuvant systemic therapy and radiation therapy play an important role in the management of these cancers, surgical resection remains the mainstay for any expectation for long-term cure. Accordingly, it is incumbent on the surgeon to perform the procedure in an organized, meticulous manner based on the best available evidence, putting aside any preconceived ideas that may have developed during training or prior experiences. Variations, no doubt, continue to exist. The mentality of "This is how I was trained to do it" or "This is the only correct way, my way, to do it" must shift to a willingness to adhere to the latest evidence-based technical information on the essential oncologic steps from incision to closure. This manual will be most effective when reviewed by both the managing surgeon and trainee preparing for a cancer resection in order to synchronize and understand the rationale for the essential steps. Imagine the undesirable situation where the trainee has studied the manual and the attending surgeon may not be quite up to date.

The manual will assist with standardization of surgical resection in patients who are enrolled in a clinical trial. Often, the criteria for an oncologic resection vary based on the principle investigator or the cooperative group. Future clinical trials should adopt the essential components of oncologic operations as described in this manual.

Operative Standards for Cancer Surgery is not just another surgical manual. It is unique for several reasons: (1) essential operative steps are evidence-based, (2) the strength or weakness of the evidence is cited, (3) it chronicles how an extensive literature search supports the recommended steps, (4) it poses controversial questions for each cancer site that could be answered best through a clinical trial, and (5) it makes the important distinction between the right and wrong thing to do during a cancer operation.

This beautifully illustrated and richly referenced manual is the culmination of expert input from a wide variety of surgeons with a special interest in cancer resections for these four sites. It is a seminal piece of work, a must-read for general surgeons, surgical oncologists, colorectal surgeons, thoracic surgeons, and surgical trainees caring for patients with cancers of the breast, lung, pancreas, and colon. Hopefully, future editions will expand the number of sites and be continuously updated.

David P. Winchester, MD, FACS
Medical Director, Cancer Programs
American College of Surgeons

Daniel P. McKellar, MD, FACS
Chair, Commission on Cancer
American College of Surgeons

INTRODUCTION

When the four disease sites were selected for the first edition of the manual, teams were developed to populate the disease site working groups. Representatives were sought from each of the NCI cooperative groups, the major professional societies for each of the disease sites, and the Commission on Cancer. The disease site working groups determined the operative procedures that would be included in the first edition and then assigned team members to each procedure, with a team leader responsible for organizing the team activities. Surgeons with expertise in health services research were assigned to each working group to serve as methodologists. The methodologists were responsible for developing a uniform process for the working groups to develop critical elements and key questions for each procedure.

METHODOLOGY FOR CRITICAL ELEMENTS

Critical elements for each procedure were developed by the working groups to include steps of the operative procedure that impact oncologic outcomes that occur from the time of skin incision to the time of skin closure. Once the list of critical elements was developed, surveys were used to rank order the elements by oncologic importance. The disease site working groups met by teleconference to choose the top four to five critical elements for each procedure for inclusion in the manual. Each step required consensus by all of the members of the disease site working groups. Literature reviews were performed for each critical element, and recommendations were made for each critical element to include the type of data available and the strength of the recommendation based on consensus of the experts populating the disease site working group.

METHODOLOGY FOR KEY QUESTIONS

Key questions were identified during the process of constructing critical elements for each procedure. Key questions were areas of controversy where consensus could not be assured in order to qualify as a critical element. The methodologists determined a process for systematic review of the literature and for summarizing the findings of the working groups. It was suggested that a professional librarian be involved in the literature search whenever possible. At least two individuals were assigned to perform the literature searches and to provide a critical appraisal of the literature.

The general framework was to include literature from the English language only using the PUBMED database to include literature published between 1990 and 2014. Randomized trials were preferred; however, when this type of data was not available, a literature review could include retrospective institutional studies with a minimum of 100 patients published after 1990 and cohort studies published after 1990.

Team members were asked to include all details of the literature review, including the date of search, a list of all search terms, a list of all abstracts reviewed (including total number reviewed), all inclusion and exclusion criteria, and all literature chosen for review in detail. Consort diagrams for workflow were developed for each key question to include the number of abstracts reviewed and number of manuscripts reviewed in detail. In some cases the GRADE system (see table below) was used to grade the level of evidence included in the detailed literature review. Summary tables were developed for each key question followed by recommendations based on the type of data and strength of available data. What follows is the process and workflow utilized by the disease site working group.

1. Identify key issues to address with literature review based on preliminary research and expert consensus regarding the key operative steps.
   a. Based on this preliminary review, identify key statements/questions for which detailed evidence review will be obtained.
      i. Question should include detail about the population, the intervention, and the outcome. For example, "*In patients with T4 colorectal cancer, does performing an en bloc resection reduce the risk of local recurrence?*"

2. Search strategy
   a. MeSH terms or keyword search of search engines: PUBMED, EMBASE, Cochrane
      i. Document search terms, total number of hits, number of abstracts reviewed, number of full papers reviewed.
   b. Previously published guidelines and consensus statements (e.g. National Guideline Clearinghouse: www.guideline.gov; relevant professional societies and organizations)
   c. Prior protocols from cooperative groups
      i. Obtain surgical specifications (if available) from prior cooperative group trials.
   d. Hand search of references, consultation with experts
   e. Limits
      i. e.g., Publication year 1990+
      ii. English language
      iii. Type of publication
   f. Documentation
      i. Search terms
      ii. Total number of hits
      iii. Number of abstracts reviewed
      iv. Number of full papers reviewed
      v. Number of papers included in the review

3. Data extraction
   a. Classify by study design (e.g. RCT, observational [cohort, case-control, case series], systematic reviews)
      i. Was there a stated objective or hypothesis?
      ii. Population

    iii. Retrospective/prospective
    iv. Intervention
    v. Comparison
    vi. Outcome
  b. Summarize key findings.
4. Appraisal of data quality
  a. APPRAISE.
    i. Did study include important elements?
    ii. Did the study clearly describe the inclusion and exclusion criteria? Were they justified?
    iii. Did the study identify and adjust for relevant covariates?
    iv. Did the study describe proportion of patients lost to follow-up? Was it <15%?
    v. Was the f/u duration sufficient for the reported outcome? Median f/u should be at least half as long as the time point being compared (e.g., at least 2.5 years f/u for 5-year survival data; ideally, median f/u is longer than that).
    vi. What is the risk of bias? Did the study identify potential sources of bias and address them?
      1. Risk is high, uncertain, or low.
    vii. Determine major limitations or criticisms.
  b. APPLY EXCLUSION.
    i. If the literature includes a large number of studies with similar results, it is reasonable to exclude poor studies from the review (e.g., sample size too small, conclusions not valid based on results, population too heterogenous to permit interpretation of the data, duplicate data as different study, significant bias to the results not addressed). A list of excluded studies should be provided with the corresponding reason for exclusion.
  c. ASSIGN GRADE OF THE EVIDENCE and PREPARE SUMMARY OF FINDINGS TABLE.

SUMMARY TABLE (for each key statement/question)
THE CLINICAL QUESTION
Population: T4b tumors
Intervention: en bloc resection
Comparison: margin + resection

DETERMINING QUALITY OF THE EVIDENCE:
++++   HIGH   Default for RCT
+++   MODERATE
++   LOW   Default for observational studies
+   VERY LOW

Quality is reduced by significant bias; inconsistency in the results; lack of good description of the population, intervention, control, and outcome of interest; imprecision (wide confidence intervals, may be associated with small sample sizes) and publication bias (tendency to publish only desired results).

Outcomes	Risk among control group	Corresponding risk among intervention (study) group	Relative effect	Sample size	GRADE of evidence	Comments	Risk of bias
Local recurrence	50%	20%	HR=0.4 (95% CI 0.25–0.6	40	++	Effect is strong and reproducible	Low

5. Recommendations

a. Assign overall strength of recommendation and quality of supportive evidence for each corresponding question.

b. Review GRADE based on evidence for group consensus.

   i. Group should review the document with the statements as presented by the primary reviewer(s) and ensure general agreement.

c. Compare recommendations to those of others.

	Description	Benefit vs. risk and burdens	Methodologic quality of supporting evidence	Implications
1A	Strong recommendation, high-quality evidence	Benefits clearly outweigh risk and burdens or vice versa	RCTs without important limitations or overwhelming evidence from observational studies	Strong recommendation, can apply to most patients in most circumstances without reservation
1B	Strong recommendation, moderate-quality evidence	Benefits clearly outweigh risk and burdens or vice versa	RCTs with important limitations (inconsistent results, methodologic flaws, indirect or imprecise) or exceptionally strong evidence from observational studies	Strong recommendation, can apply to most patients in most circumstances without reservation
1C	Strong recommendation, low- or very low quality evidence	Benefits clearly outweigh risk and burdens or vice versa	Observational studies or case series	Strong recommendation but may change when higher quality evidence becomes available
2A	Weak recommendation, high-quality evidence	Benefits closely balanced with risks and burdens	RCTs without important limitations or overwhelming evidence from observational studies	Weak recommendation, best action may differ depending on circumstances or patients' or societal values
2B	Weak recommendations, moderate-quality evidence	Benefits closely balanced with risks and burdens	RCTs with important limitations (inconsistent results, methodologic flaws, indirect or imprecise) or exceptionally strong evidence from observational studies	Weak recommendation, best action may differ depending on circumstances or patients' or societal values
2C	Weak recommendation, low- or very low quality evidence	Uncertainty in the estimates of benefits, risks, and burden; benefits, risk, and burden may be closely balanced	Observational studies or case series	Very weak recommendations; other alternatives may be equally reasonable

From Guyatt G, Gutterman D, Baumann MH, et al. Grading strength of recommendations and quality of evidence in clinical guidelines: report from an american college of chest physicians task force. *Chest* 2006;129(1):174–81

6. Overall themes
   a. Pragmatic approach recognizing that resources and time are limited
      i. Targeted, not exhaustive search of the literature but ensure balance
   b. Group members are an expert source for evaluating the validity of the recommendations.
   c. Expected in the reviews
      i. List of key statements/questions
      ii. Search strategy for each question
      iii. Documentation of search results for each question
      iv. List of excluded studies for each question
      v. Evidence summary tables for each question
      vi. Recommendation for each question

TABLE OF CONTENTS

SECTION I

BREAST

INTRODUCTION

Breast cancer treatment is rapidly changing, leaving clinicians unsure of best practices. Although surgical resection and staging remains the cornerstone of breast cancer treatment, it does not exist in a vacuum. The most effective way to cure patients is multidisciplinary care. Careful consideration must be given to the appropriate amount of tissue resected in the context of multimodality treatment. The surgeon must balance the aggressiveness of surgical resection to affect a cure, the cosmetic outcome, and the quality of life for the patient. These issues are important because the majority of patients will be long-term survivors and deserve good quality of life for many years. Clinical research in the surgical treatment of breast cancer has focused on less invasive procedures, providing patients with lower morbidity while maintaining the same overall survival. The purpose of this manual is to provide surgeons with what the group consensus believes is necessary to adequately resect breast tumors, maintain high overall survival rates, and at the same time provide patients with good cosmetic outcomes and quality of life. The manual will address the four major procedures in the surgical treatment of breast cancer, namely partial mastectomy, mastectomy, axillary node dissection, and sentinel node biopsy. These chapters will address the steps necessary to ensure oncologically safe resection of breast cancers based on the literature with grading of the evidence so the reader can decide the importance of each step. The partial mastectomy section outlines the evidence for each step necessary to decrease positive margin rates and prevent second operations, especially for nonpalpable breast cancers. In the mastectomy section, the most important technical aspects of mastectomy operation are outlined, including a discussion of the oncologic safety of skin-sparing and nipple-sparing mastectomy. The axillary dissection section reviews the evidence and steps needed to complete a level I and II dissection and when to consider a level III dissection. In addition, there is a review of the new literature on which patients still require axillary node dissection. In the sentinel node chapter, the best methods of identifying sentinel nodes with the lowest false negative rate are laid out step by step. These basic technical steps are necessary for surgeons who may be new trainees entering practice, surgeons who may not perform these operations often to make sure of good quality for patients, and to standardize practice for experts for clinical trials.

The main goal of surgery for breast cancer is to obtain locoregional control. Proper patient selection for the appropriate surgical procedure is critical to achieving such control; Clarke et al[1] predicted that for every four local recurrences at 5 years that are prevented, at least one death from breast cancer at 15 years is prevented. A large part of the challenge in providing optimal surgical treatment of breast cancer resides in the preoperative work-up and planning phase, during which the appropriate surgical therapy is determined. There are many safe avenues of treating patients, and surgeons must help their patients navigate a succession of complex decisions to achieve optimal, individualized treatment that incorporates the patients' desires. Some of the main factors that must be considered when determining the appropriate route of surgery for breast cancer include the patient's potential candidacy for breast-conserving surgery, the use of imaging studies to assess the patient's disease, the type of neoadjuvant therapy the patient has received, and the patient's BRCA mutation status. The main goal of this manual is to outline the most important technical decisions necessary during an operation, and that is the focus of each chapter. Preoperative factors, although important, are beyond the scope of the following chapters and are thus summarized here.

Breast-Conserving Surgery Candidacy

The appropriate selection of patients for breast-conserving surgery is important to the ultimate success of therapy. The goals of breast-conserving surgery are to achieve negative margins, obtain good to excellent cosmesis, and facilitate the delivery of appropriate radiation therapy. Consensus standards for breast-conserving surgery have been developed by the American College of Surgeons, the American College of Radiology, the College of American Pathologists, and the Society of Surgical Oncology.[2] Although cosmetic outcomes are an important part of the surgical treatment of breast cancer, the focus of this manual is to delineate the highest oncologic safety to prevent tumor recurrence, and thus oncoplastic techniques will not be reviewed here, as this manual focuses on oncologic safety.

Breast Imaging

Breast imaging is an ever increasing part of breast cancer screening and treatment planning. Mammography, the mainstay of breast imaging since the 1970s, is the only imaging modality that has been proven to reduce the breast cancer mortality rate. Therefore, mammography should always be included as part of the preoperative imaging of breast cancer patients.[3,4] Ultrasonography should also be considered for treatment planning. Breast ultrasonography is an inexpensive modality that can be used to further characterize mammographically identified lesions, identify clinically apparent but mammographically occult lesions, and localize lesions in areas not easily visualized with mammography.[5] Ultrasonography is also becoming more important in the axillary staging of patients with clinically suspicious axillary nodes and patients undergoing neoadjuvant systemic treatments.[6]

Another modality that is commonly used for the preoperative imaging of breast cancers is breast magnetic resonance imaging (MRI), which is undisputedly the most sensitive modality overall. The American College of Radiology recommends that all newly diagnosed breast cancer patients undergo breast MRI,[5] whereas the National Comprehensive Cancer Network suggests that breast MRI is optional for preoperative work-up but should be considered for patients with mammographically occult tumors.[7] However, the modality's high sensitivity contributes to its relatively high false positive rate, and some have expressed concerns about the utility of breast MRI for all newly diagnosed breast cancer patients. For example, randomized studies have not shown that breast MRI reduces positive margin rates or re-excision rates or improves local control rates in patients undergoing breast-conserving surgery.[8] Others question whether MRI has led to an increased mastectomy rate. Nevertheless, breast MRI is an excellent modality for monitoring tumor response to neoadjuvant treatment, and its findings may be used to identify candidates for breast-conserving surgery.[9] With the exception of those for patients with mammographically occult tumors, there are no standard guidelines for determining which patients would most benefit from the addition of MRI.

Neoadjuvant Therapy

Neoadjuvant therapy is the standard initial treatment for patients with inflammatory breast cancer or inoperable breast cancer.[10] Because neoadjuvant therapy can also downstage a primary breast cancer, making breast-conserving surgery a possibility in patients whose surgical options would otherwise be limited to mastectomy, it is also frequently used to initially treat patients with T2 or T3 tumors.[11] Several randomized trials have found no significant difference in survival between patients who undergo neoadjuvant therapy followed by surgery and those who undergo surgery followed by adjuvant systemic therapy.[12]

Pathologic Response to Neoadjuvant Chemotherapy

Tumor response to neoadjuvant chemotherapy depends on the original tumor biology and the type of systemic therapy.[13] The rate of pathologic complete response is lower in patients with low- to intermediate-grade estrogen receptor–positive cancers than in patients with cancers that have HER-2 overexpression or lack estrogen receptor, progesterone receptor, and HER-2 overexpression. The addition of targeted therapies for HER-2–overexpressing cancer has significantly increased the rate of pathologic complete response. Whether targeted therapies can downstage disease to provide patients with additional surgical options depends on the biology, size, and imaging characteristics of the original tumor and the type of systemic therapy.[14]

BRCA Mutation Status

Special attention should be given to the identification of women at risk for carrying a *BRCA1* or *BRCA2* mutation. The National Comprehensive Cancer Network and the U.S. Preventive Services Task Force have established guidelines for referring patients to genetic counselors for genetic testing for the *BRCA1* or *BRCA2* mutation.[7,15] On the basis of prevalence estimates, these guidelines suggest that genetic testing be offered to women with a 10% or greater probability of having a BRCA mutation. Interventions in women who carry a BRCA mutation include more frequent and/ or intensive surveillance, risk-reducing medications, and risk-reducing surgery. Risk-reducing surgical options include prophylactic bilateral mastectomy and prophylactic bilateral salpingo-oophorectomy. Patients with a BRCA mutation and a newly diagnosed breast cancer, who have a higher risk of contralateral breast cancer and local recurrence after breast-conserving therapy, should be counselled regarding their options for reducing this risk, with particular consideration of surgical prophylaxis.

REFERENCES

1. Clarke M, Collins R, Darby S, et al. Effects of radiotherapy and of differences in the extent of surgery for early breast cancer on local recurrence and 15-year survival: an overview of the randomised trials. *Lancet* 2005;366(9503):2087–2106.
2. Morrow M, Strom EA, Bassett LW, et al. Standard for breast conservation therapy in the management of invasive breast carcinoma. *CA Cancer J Clin* 2002;52(5):277–300.
3. Nelson HD, Tyne K, Naik A, et al. Screening for breast cancer: an update for the U.S. Preventive Services Task Force. *Ann Intern Med* 2009;151(10):727–737.
4. U.S. Preventive Services Task Force. Screening for breast cancer: U.S. Preventive Services Task Force recommendation statement. *Ann Intern Med* 2009;151(10):716–726.

5. Lee CH, Dershaw DD, Kopans D, et al. Breast cancer screening with imaging: recommendations from the Society of Breast Imaging and the ACR on the use of mammography, breast MRI, breast ultrasound, and other technologies for the detection of clinically occult breast cancer. *J Am Coll Radiol* 2010;7(1):18–27.
6. Houssami N, Ciatto S, Turner RM, et al. Preoperative ultrasound-guided needle biopsy of axillary nodes in invasive breast cancer: meta-analysis of its accuracy and utility in staging the axilla. *Ann Surg* 2011;254(2):243–251.
7. Gradishar WJ, Anderson BO, Blair SL, et al. Breast cancer version 3.2014. *J Natl Compr Canc Netw* 2014;12(4):542–590.
8. Houssami N, Turner R, Morrow M. Preoperative magnetic resonance imaging in breast cancer: meta-analysis of surgical outcomes. *Ann Surg* 2013;257(2):249–255.
9. Mukhtar RA, Yau C, Rosen M, et al. Clinically meaningful tumor reduction rates vary by prechemotherapy MRI phenotype and tumor subtype in the I-SPY 1 TRIAL (CALGB 150007/150012; ACRIN 6657). *Ann Surg Oncol* 2013;20(12):3823–3830.
10. Chia S, Swain SM, Byrd DR, et al. Locally advanced and inflammatory breast cancer. *J Clin Oncol* 2008;26(5):786–790.
11. Buchholz TA, Lehman CD, Harris JR, et al. Statement of the science concerning locoregional treatments after preoperative chemotherapy for breast cancer: a National Cancer Institute conference. *J Clin Oncol* 2008;26(5):791–797.
12. Wolmark N, Wang J, Mamounas E, et al. Preoperative chemotherapy in patients with operable breast cancer: nine-year results from National Surgical Adjuvant Breast and Bowel Project B-18. *J Natl Cancer Inst* 2001;(30):96–102.
13. Esserman LJ, Berry DA, DeMichele A, et al. Pathologic complete response predicts recurrence-free survival more effectively by cancer subset: results from the I-SPY 1 TRIAL—CALGB 150007/150012, ACRIN 6657. *J Clin Oncol* 2012;30(26):3242–3249.
14. Kaufmann M, von Minckwitz G, Mamounas EP, et al. Recommendations from an international consensus conference on the current status and future of neoadjuvant systemic therapy in primary breast cancer. *Ann Surg Oncol* 2012;19(5):1508–1516.
15. Moyer VA; U.S. Preventive Services Task Force. Risk assessment, genetic counseling, and genetic testing for BRCA-related cancer in women: U.S. Preventive Services Task Force recommendation statement. *Ann Intern Med* 2014;160(4):271–281.

CHAPTER 1

Partial Mastectomy

CRITICAL ELEMENTS

- Tumor Resection
- Tumor Localization
- Intraoperative Specimen Imaging
- Specimen Orientation
- Clip Placement for Radiation Targeting in Oncoplastic Cases

1. TUMOR RESECTION

Recommendation: The surgeon should aim to resect all gross disease with microscopically negative margins without violation of the tumor itself during the dissection (Fig. 1-1).

Type of Data: Period after trials.

Strength of Recommendation: The group strongly recommends performing partial mastectomy with the goal of resecting all gross disease with microscopically negative margins. This recommendation, which can be applied to most patients in most circumstances, is based on multiple randomized prospective studies demonstrating the benefits of the approach.

Rationale
In breast cancer patients undergoing partial mastectomy, surgical margins help determine future treatment. Because positive surgical margins are associated with an increased risk of local recurrence and, consequently, systemic disease, the primary goal of partial mastectomy is to remove the tumor with a negative microscopic margin. The primary goal of partial mastectomy in the operating room is to remove the cancer with an envelope of normal tissue around it to obtain negative margins (i.e., to achieve

6

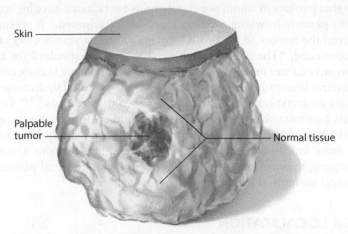

FIGURE 1-1 Wide local resection of gross disease. The palpable tumor in red is surrounded by normal breast tissue. Skin resection may be necessary when the tumor is approaching or directly involving the skin.

Labels on figure: Skin; Palpable tumor; Normal tissue

an R0 resection; see Fig. 1-1) while maintaining optimal breast cosmesis. In the operating room, surgeons must be cognizant of encompassing the tumor with normal tissue around it. For patients with tumors involving the skin and/or chest wall, en bloc resection that includes the overlying skin and/or underlying muscle should be performed. The oncologic safety of breast conservation has been proven over many years, multiple randomized studies having shown that local recurrence rates following lumpectomy with negative margins plus radiotherapy are significantly lower than those following lumpectomy with a positive margin plus radiotherapy.

The width of negative surgical margins necessary to minimize local recurrence in patients undergoing breast cancer surgery, including partial mastectomy, remain controversial. The National Surgical Adjuvant Breast and Bowel Project has long taken the position that unless tumor cells are immediately adjacent to the inked surface of the lumpectomy specimen, no further excision is needed. Long-term results of this approach and recurrence rates have been published.[1]

For example, the B-06 study, which randomized patients to lumpectomy alone versus lumpectomy plus radiation versus total mastectomy, has shown acceptable local recurrence rates with lumpectomy plus radiation compared to mastectomy with a greater than 20-year follow-up. Other randomized prospective trials from the National Cancer Institute, Veronesi et al, and the European Organization for Research and Treatment of Cancer (trial 10801) have shown similar results, reporting 5-year local recurrence rates of about 10% for patients who undergo lumpectomy with no tumor at the inked margin plus radiotherapy.[2–4] Unfortunately, these trials' findings are inconclusive, as the investigators did not know whether the surgeons resected additional tissue in cases involving "close" margins or "ink on tumor." Some thoughtful meta-analyses suggest that obtaining margins greater than 1 mm does not improve rates of local control.[5–7] Regardless, virtually all studies investigating surgical margins in breast cancer surgery have shown that patients in whom positive margins are retained have higher recurrence rates than do patients in whom negative margins are achieved.[8] A recent consensus statement from the Society of Surgical Oncology and American Society of Radiation Oncology concluded, "The use of no ink on tumor as the standard for an adequate margin in invasive cancer in the era of multidisciplinary therapy is associated with low rates of ipsilateral breast tumor recurrence and has the potential to decrease re-excision rates, improve cosmetic outcomes, and decrease health care costs."[9,10] Critics of this meta-analysis comment that the majority of the studies used were retrospective and details about adjuvant treatment were lacking, including radiation. Some surgeons still advocate a more individualized approach. When making decisions about treatment after lumpectomy, the care team should carefully consider the final pathologic assessment of surgical margins in a multidisciplinary fashion.[11]

2. TUMOR LOCALIZATION

Recommendation: Image-guided localization is necessary for nonpalpable lesions.

Type of Data: This recommendation is based on data from single-institution studies and small randomized controlled trials.

Strength of Recommendation: The group strongly recommends using image-guided tumor localization in patients with nonpalpable tumors.

Rationale

Most breast cancers, many of them nonpalpable, are detected by radiographic screening such as mammography. These nonpalpable lesions require image-guided localization to help maximize the likelihood that negative surgical margins will be achieved. Image-guided tumor localization is guided by the modality used to detect the tumor: mammography,[12] ultrasonography,[13] or magnetic resonance imaging[14] (Fig. 1-2). For lesions that span a large area (a large segment of malignant calcifications), bracketing the area by the use of wires or other markers to delineate the area improves the likelihood that the surgeon is able to completely remove the targeted lesions.[15]

The most commonly used modality for image-guided tumor localization is wire localization. Despite its very high success rate, wire localization has several drawbacks, including a high positive margin rate,[16] wire migration,[17] wire transection,[18] and surgery scheduling issues because it is performed on the same day, limiting the times and number of procedures performed per day. Alternatives to wire localization (see Fig. 1-2) include radioactive seed localization (RSL),[19] radioguided occult lesion localization (ROLL),[20] and intraoperative ultrasonography localization. Retrospective studies have shown that these techniques can decrease the volume of tissue excised and the rate of positive margins.[21] Single-center institutional series and small randomized trials have shown that, in experienced hands, these techniques can be used to delineate tumors with an accuracy similar to that of wire localization and may have positive margin rates that are lower than that of wire localization.[22–27] Regardless of the method of localization, the tumor targeted

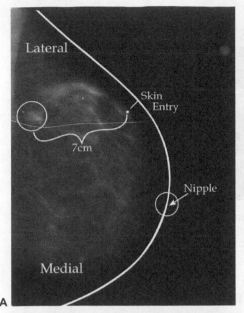

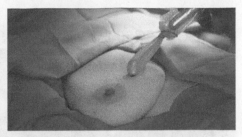

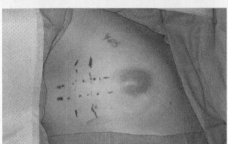

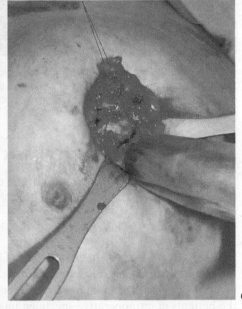

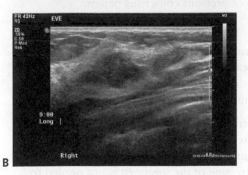

FIGURE 1-2 Tumor localization. This figure shows the three most common localization techniques. Part **A** is the gold standard wire localization. Part **B** demonstrates intraoperative ultrasound localization; upper panel shows marking of the skin and lower panel shows the ultrasound image of the tumor. Part **C** shows radioactive seed localization. The skin incision is placed over the skin with the highest counts by the gamma probe. For all techniques, a specimen radiograph is important to confirm the target is removed. (Photos and images courtesy of Barbara Pockaj, MD.)

for excision must be documented by specimen radiography[28,29] (see Fig. 1-3). Even for palpable lesions, where the surgeon's physical examination guides the location of the incision and the amount of tissue to be resected, the use of intraoperative ultrasonography has been shown to decrease the volume of tissue excised and the rate of positive margins.[30,31]

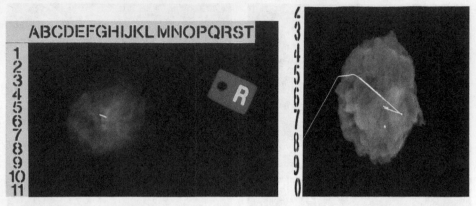

FIGURE 1-3 Intraoperative specimen radiography. The left picture depicts a specimen radiograph in a radioactive seed localized operation and the right picture is a specimen radiograph in a patient with a needle localized excision. Note confirmation of the marker clip is present in both. (Images courtesy of Barbara Pockaj, MD.)

3. INTRAOPERATIVE SPECIMEN IMAGING

Recommendation: Resection of the target lesion must be confirmed with intraoperative imaging studies.

Type of Data: This recommendation is based on data from retrospective studies.

Strength of Recommendation: The group strongly recommends performing intraoperative imaging studies to confirm the resection of the target area. This recommendation is based on data from retrospective studies, which have clearly shown that the benefits of intraoperative specimen imaging outweigh its risks to the patient, and is in agreement with the recommendations of previous consensus panels.

Rationale

The use of intraoperative imaging to confirm the resection of nonpalpable lesions has been the standard of care for the last 10 years. In 2001 (and again in both 2005 and 2009), the Image-Detected Breast Cancer: State-of-the-Art Diagnosis and Treatment Consensus Panel made the following recommendation:

> "Specimen radiography or specimen ultrasonography should be routinely performed for all excisions of image-detected abnormalities to help document the success of the procedure in finding the target. Specimen radiography should use two 90-degree orthogonal views. Compression of the specimen is not needed to obtain adequate images and should be avoided. Such compression can fracture the specimen and create false (artifactual) margins after inking."[32]

In addition, multiple retrospective studies have shown that the positive margin and re-excision rates of cases in which intraoperative imaging has been performed are lower than those of cases in which intraoperative imaging has not been performed.[33,34]

In addition, investigators who have examined the utility of the RSL technique have recommended that even in cases in which radioactive seeds have been utilized for tumor localization, specimen radiography is needed to confirm that the marker clip and seeds have been removed with the specimen.[35] Finally, the American Society of Breast Surgeons recommends that specimen radiography or specimen ultrasonography be performed routinely during the excision of abnormalities detected with imaging studies to document the removal of the target lesion.[36]

4. SPECIMEN ORIENTATION

Recommendation: During resection, specimen orientation should be achieved either by staining or painting the specimen or by marking the specimen with three sutures to facilitate margin assessment by the pathologist.

Type of Data: Small retrospective studies.

Strength of Recommendation: The procedure has a low burden of risk, but the data supporting its use, which are drawn from retrospective studies, are not strong. The group strongly recommends employing some form of specimen orientation to enable the pathologist to report surgical margins as accurately as possible. This information is important for planning any future surgery to excise remaining positive margins and for planning adjuvant radiotherapy.

Rationale

Specimen orientation at the time of excision enables the pathologist to replicate the specimen's anatomical position during pathologic evaluation. For consistency in reporting and communication, the surface of the lumpectomy specimen is commonly delineated into superficial, deep, superior, inferior, medial, and lateral sides. The orientation method that is least equivocal and most likely to minimize discordance between surgery and pathology settings appears to be intraoperatively marking each of the six sides of the specimen with inks or paints of different colors immediately following resection (Fig. 1-4).

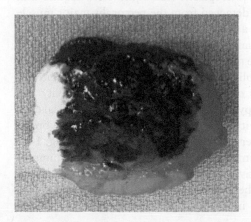

FIGURE 1-4 Partial mastectomy specimen orientation demonstrates multicolor inking intraoperatively for specimen orientation. (Photo courtesy of Christine Lee, MD.)

Another option for specimen orientation is to use three sutures to mark the anterior, lateral, and superior sides of the specimen. Specimen orientation with two sutures, which has been reported to result in high rates of discordance between surgery and pathology settings, is not recommended. The recommendation to use three rather than two sutures is primarily based on the findings of a limited prospective analysis of specimen disorientation using the two-suture technique and a retrospective analysis of intraoperative inking versus standard postoperative inking after initial orientation using the three-suture technique.[37] Most surgeons rely on the final postoperative pathologic evaluation for final margin assessment in order to decide whether additional tissue must be removed. Regardless of whether the pathologist examines the specimen during or after surgery, reliable specimen orientation is required to facilitate the decision to remove additional tissue of specific margins.[38,39]

5. CLIP PLACEMENT FOR RADIATION TARGETING IN ONCOPLASTIC CASES

Recommendation: In cases involving oncoplastic techniques, localization of the lumpectomy cavity with surgical clips is critical for the accurate planning of whole- or partial-breast irradiation.

Type of Data: This recommendation is based on observational studies only.

Strength of Recommendation: Placing surgical clips is a low-risk procedure, and it is not burdensome to the patient. The group strongly recommends marking the lumpectomy cavity with surgical clips to facilitate radiotherapy planning in cases involving oncoplastic tissue rearrangement.

Rationale
Clip placement in cases where oncoplastic techniques are utilized for immediate reconstruction is essential due to the uncertainty about the location of the excision cavity that can affect the targeting of breast irradiation, as well as the radiation boost delivered as part of whole-breast radiotherapy. Oncoplastic techniques often require that breast tissue adjacent to the tumor bed be detached from the pectoralis major muscle and mobilized to close the excision cavity and subsequently results in little or no seroma formation, making it difficult to visualize the lumpectomy cavity at the time of radiotherapy planning. In addition, because the breast tissue is rearranged, the position of the tumor bed may shift, further complicating radiotherapy planning.[39] Furthermore, the surgical scar is a poor indicator of the location of the excision cavity and cannot be reliably used to direct radiotherapy planning. The placement of surgical clips for the localization of the lumpectomy cavity after tumor resection and before breast reconstruction facilitates the accurate delivery of radiation to the tumor bed (Fig. 1-5).

Movement of the tumor bed owing to immediate breast remodeling after lumpectomy is not uncommon. In one retrospective study, the tumor bed, which had been marked with surgical clips, had extended beyond its original breast quadrant or had migrated completely to a different region in 8 (73%) of 11 patients at the time of

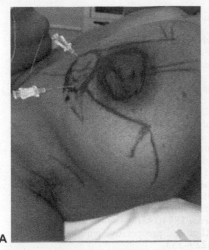
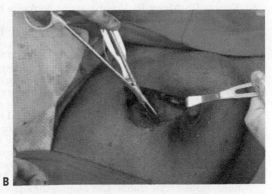

A   B

FIGURE 1-5 Clip placement for oncoplastic cases. Part **A** shows patient marked for bracketed needle localized lumpectomy with breast reduction. Part **B** shows intraoperative clip placement to allow for postoperative radiation planning. (Photo courtesy of Sarah Blair, MD.)

radiotherapy planning.[40] In another study evaluating 50 patients' radiation target field plans, which were based on surgical clip location, simulations revealed that the absence of surgical clips would have resulted in inadequate radiation doses in tangent fields in 4 (8%) patients and totally or marginally missed radiation boost targets in 23 (46%) patients.[41] Placing surgical clips provides a reliable means of delineating the tumor bed. In a study of 40 breast conservation patients, breast irradiation plans revealed that, compared with no surgical clip placement, the placement of surgical clips at the four cardinal points of the lumpectomy cavity resulted in a higher conformity index of tumor bed delineation and less interobserver variability among radiation oncologists.[42] Another study of 30 patients demonstrated that the relative positions of the implanted surgical clips remained consistent throughout the course of radiotherapy.[43]

REFERENCES

1. Fisher B, Anderson S, Bryant J, et al. Twenty-year follow-up of a randomized trial comparing total mastectomy, lumpectomy, and lumpectomy plus irradiation for the treatment of invasive breast cancer. *N Engl J Med* 2002;347(16):1233–1241.
2. van Tienhoven G, Voogd AC, Peterse JL, et al. Prognosis after treatment for loco-regional recurrence after mastectomy or breast conserving therapy in two randomised trials (EORTC 10801 and DBCG-82TM). EORTC Breast Cancer Cooperative Group and the Danish Breast Cancer Cooperative Group. *Eur J Cancer* 1999;35(1):32–38.
3. Jacobson JA, Danforth DN, Cowan KH, et al. Ten-year results of a comparison of conservation with mastectomy in the treatment of stage I and II breast cancer. *N Engl J Med* 1995;332(14): 907–911.
4. Veronesi U, Cascinelli N, Mariani L, et al. Twenty-year follow-up of a randomized study comparing breast-conserving surgery with radical mastectomy for early breast cancer. *N Engl J Med* 2002;347(16):1227–1232.
5. Morrow M, Harris JR, Schnitt SJ. Surgical margins in lumpectomy for breast cancer—bigger is not better. *N Engl J Med* 2012;367(1):79–82.

6. Revesz E, Kahn SA. What are safe margins of resection for invasive and in situ breast cancer? *Oncology (Williston Park)* 2011;25(10):890–895.
7. Singletary SE. Surgical margins in patients with early-stage breast cancer treated with breast conservation therapy. *Am J Surg* 2002;184(5):383–393.
8. Kopans DB, Meyer JE. Versatile spring hookwire breast lesion localizer. *AJR Am J Roentgenol* 1982;138(3):586–587.
9. Houssami N, Macaskill P, Marinovich ML, et al. The association of surgical margins and local recurrence in women with early-stage invasive breast cancer treated with breast-conserving therapy: a meta-analysis. *Ann Surg Oncol* 2014;21:717–730.
10. Moran MS, Schnitt SJ, Giuliano AE, et al. Society of Surgical Oncology-American Society for Radiation Oncology consensus guideline on margins for breast-conserving surgery with whole-breast irradiation in stages I and II invasive breast cancer. *J Clin Oncol* 2014;32:1507–1515.
11. Hunt KK, Sahin AA. Too much, too little, or just right? Tumor margins in women undergoing breast-conserving surgery. *J Clin Oncol* 2014;32:1401–1406.
12. Homer MJ, Pile-Spellman ER. Needle localization of occult breast lesions with a curved-end retractable wire: technique and pitfalls. *Radiology* 1986;161(2):547–548.
13. Kopans DB, Meyer JE, Lindfors KK, et al. Breast sonography to guide cyst aspiration and wire localization of occult solid lesions. *AJR Am J Roentgenol* 1984;143(3):489–492.
14. Landheer ML, Veltman J, van Eekeren R, et al. MRI-guided preoperative wire localization of nonpalpable breast lesions. *Clin Imaging* 2006;30(4):229–233.
15. Liberman L, Kaplan J, Van Zee KJ, et al. Bracketing wires for preoperative breast needle localization. *AJR Am J Roentgenol* 2001;177(3):565–572.
16. Kurniawan ED, Wong MH, Windle I, et al. Predictors of surgical margin status in breast-conserving surgery within a breast screening program. *Ann Surg Oncol* 2008;15(9):2542–2549.
17. Davis PS, Wechsler RJ, Feig SA, et al. Migration of breast biopsy localization wire. *AJR Am J Roentgenol* 1988;150(4):787–788.
18. Homer MJ. Transection of the localization hooked wire during breast biopsy. *AJR Am J Roentgenol* 1983;141(5):929–930.
19. McGhan LJ, McKeever SC, Pockaj BA, et al. Radioactive seed localization for nonpalpable breast lesions: review of 1,000 consecutive procedures at a single institution. *Ann Surg Oncol* 2011;18(11):3096–3101.
20. van der Ploeg IM, Hobbelink M, van den Bosch MA, et al. 'Radioguided occult lesion localisation' (ROLL) for non-palpable breast lesions: a review of the relevant literature. *Eur J Surg Oncol* 2008;34(1):1–5.
21. Barentsz MW, van Dalen T, Gobardhan PD, et al. Intraoperative ultrasound guidance for excision of non-palpable invasive breast cancer: a hospital-based series and an overview of the literature. *Breast Cancer Res Treat* 2012;135(1):209–219.
22. Fortunato L, Penteriani R, Farina M, et al. Intraoperative ultrasound is an effective and preferable technique to localize non-palpable breast tumors. *Eur J Surg Oncol* 2008;34(12):1289–1292.
23. Lovrics PJ, Cornacchi SD, Vora R, et al. Systematic review of radioguided surgery for non-palpable breast cancer. *Eur J Surg Oncol* 2011;37(5):388–397.
24. Lovrics PJ, Goldsmith CH, Hodgson N, et al. A multicentered, randomized, controlled trial comparing radioguided seed localization to standard wire localization for nonpalpable, invasive and in situ breast carcinomas. *Ann Surg Oncol* 2011;18(12):3407–3414.
25. Ngo C, Pollet AG, Laperrelle J, et al. Intraoperative ultrasound localization of nonpalpable breast cancers. *Ann Surg Oncol* 2007;14(9):2485–2489.
26. Olsha O, Shemesh D, Carmon M, et al. Resection margins in ultrasound-guided breast-conserving surgery. *Ann Surg Oncol* 2011;18(2):447–452.
27. Rahusen FD, Bremers AJ, Fabry HF, et al. Ultrasound-guided lumpectomy of nonpalpable breast cancer versus wire-guided resection: a randomized clinical trial. *Ann Surg Oncol* 2002;9(10):994–998.
28. Britton PD SL, Yamamoto AK, Koo B, et al. Breast surgical specimen radiographs: how reliable are they? *Eur J Radiol* 2011;79(2):245–2459.
29. Cox CE, Furman B, Stowell N, et al. Radioactive seed localization breast biopsy and lumpectomy: can specimen radiographs be eliminated? *Ann Surg Oncol* 2003;10(9):1039–1047.
30. Davis KM, Hsu CH, Bouton ME, et al. Intraoperative ultrasound can decrease the re-excision lumpectomy rate in patients with palpable breast cancers. *Am Surg* 2011;77(6):720–725.
31. Fisher CS, Mushawah FA, Cyr AE, et al. Ultrasound-guided lumpectomy for palpable breast cancers. *Ann Surg Oncol* 2011;18(11):3198–3203.
32. Silverstein MJ, Lagios MD, Recht A, et al. Image-detected breast cancer: state of the art diagnosis and treatment. *J Am Coll Surg* 2005;201(4):586–597.

33. Bathla L, Harris A, Davey M, et al. High resolution intra-operative two-dimensional specimen mammography and its impact on second operation for re-excision of positive margins at final pathology after breast conservation surgery. *Am J Surg* 2011;202(4):387–394.

34. Ciccarelli G, Di Virgilio MR, Menna S, et al. Radiography of the surgical specimen in early stage breast lesions: diagnostic reliability in the analysis of the resection margins. *Radiol Med* 2007;112(3):366–376.

35. Jakub JW, Gray RJ, Degnim AC, et al. Current status of radioactive seed for localization of non palpable breast lesions. *Am J Surg* 2010;199(4):522–528.

36. American Society of Breast Surgeons. Image confirmation of successful excision of image-localized breast lesion. https://www.breastsurgeons.org/new_layout/about/statements/QM/ASBrS_Image _confirmation_of_successful_excision_of_image-localized_breast_lesion.pdf. American Society of Breast Surgeons Web site. Accessed March 25, 2015.

37. Molina MA, Snell S, Franceschi D, et al. Breast specimen orientation. *Ann Surg Oncol* 2009;16(2):285–288.

38. Singh M, Singh G, Hogan KT, et al. The effect of intraoperative specimen inking on lumpectomy re-excision rates. *World J Surg Oncol* 2010;8:4.

39. Krawczyk JJ, Engel B. The importance of surgical clips for adequate tangential beam planning in breast conserving surgery and irradiation. *Int J Radiat Oncol Biol Phys* 1999;43(2):347–350.

40. Pezner RD, Tan MC, Clancy SL, et al. Radiation therapy for breast cancer patients who undergo oncoplastic surgery: localization of the tumor bed for the local boost. *Am J Clin Oncol* 2013;36(6):535–539.

41. Hunter MA, McFall TA, Hehr KA. Breast-conserving surgery for primary breast cancer: necessity for surgical clips to define the tumor bed for radiation planning. *Radiology* 1996;200(1): 281–282.

42. Dzhugashvili M, Tournay E, Pichenot C, et al. 3D-conformal accelerated partial breast irradiation treatment planning: the value of surgical clips in the delineation of the lumpectomy cavity. *Radiat Oncol* 2009;4:70.

43. Penninkhof J, Quint S, Boer H, et al. Surgical clips for position verification and correction of non-rigid breast tissue in simultaneously integrated boost (SIB) treatments. *Radiother Oncol* 2009;90(1):110–115.

Partial Mastectomy: Key Question

In patients undergoing breast conserving surgery, intraoperative margin assessment will reduce re-excision or positive margin rates compared to no intraoperative assessment.

INTRODUCTION

The management of breast margins remains important. Although the size of the preferred margin is controversial, what is clear is that positive margins of excision, even with varied definitions, are associated with higher rates of local recurrence. Thus the intraoperative management of breast margins is important in reducing the morbidity, cost, and inefficiency associated with reoperation for inadequate margins. In this chapter, we review the evidence for techniques of intraoperative management of breast cancer margins.

METHODOLOGY

A Medline search was made with the assistance of a professional medical librarian of multiple keywords involving breast neoplasms, breast operations, and intraoperative techniques, including all papers from 1995 through November 2013. Three hundred seventy-nine abstracts were identified. Ninety-nine of these were duplicates, leaving 280 abstracts for review. The first 50 abstracts were reviewed by four reviewers, who then met to ensure consistent inclusion criteria. The subsequent abstracts and manuscripts were reviewed by one of these four reviewers. Of the abstracts reviewed, 121 had a focus on intraoperative management or techniques that influence margins, including rates of local recurrence, reoperation, and/or inadequate margins of excision. Eighty-six papers were included after the elimination of 35 manuscripts that either had no English language version available, did not truly address intraoperative margin management with actionable data, had too small of a sample size to reach conclusions, or reported redundant data from other included manuscripts (Fig. 1-6).

FINDINGS

Intraoperative Use of Localization Methods: (1) Ultrasound

Ultrasound (US) use intraoperatively to guide excision and/or to evaluate the margin distance in the resected specimen has been associated with a reduced rate of positive margins in randomized and cohort trials (Table 1-1). Two randomized trials and several cohort studies suggest that US be used instead of palpation guidance for palpable tumors among surgeons who have or can develop good US skills (Grade 1B). US-guided excision may also be able to reduce the rate of positive margins compared to wire localization for surgeons skilled in its use,

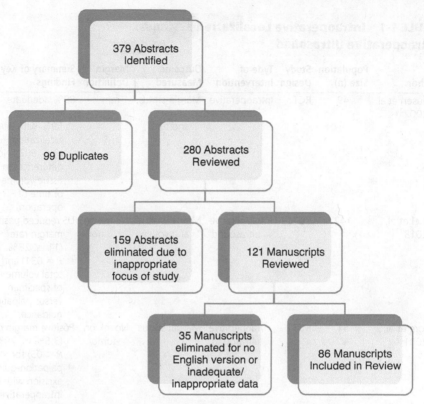

FIGURE 1-6 Flow diagram for selection of publications for inclusion.

but although one randomized trial found such a reduction in re-excision rates, a larger cohort study failed to demonstrate any difference. This combined with fewer studies of US versus wire localization leads us to a less certain recommendation that surgeons skilled in US consider its use as an alternative to wire localization (Grade 2B).

Intraoperative Use of Localization Methods: (2) Radioactive Seed Localization

Radioactive seed localization (RSL) has been consistently associated with lower rates of positive margins than wire localization (WL) in multiple cohort series, meta-analyses, and small randomized controlled trials (Table 1-2). In the largest available randomized trial, however, RSL and WL did not significantly differ in positive margin rates. This trial had an unusually low rate of positive margins in the WL group, and the RSL group had a significantly higher incidence of multifocal disease. The data suggest that the value of RSL as an alternative to wire localization is likely dependent on the rate of inadequate margins of excision with WL. If these rates are near 12% or

TABLE 1-1 Intraoperative Localization Methods: Intraoperative Ultrasound

Author	Population Size (n)	Study Design	Type of Intervention	Outcome Measured	Margin Definition	Summary of Key Findings
Rahusen et al, 2002[26]	49	RCT	Intraoperative ultrasound	Margin status, volume, and time	1 mm	89% adequate margins vs. 59% with wire localization ($P = .007$). No differences in tissue volume or time of operation.
Krekel et al, 2013[27]	142	RCT	Intraoperative ultrasound	Margin status and volume	No ink on tumor	US reduced positive margin rate (11 vs. 28%, $P = .031$) and total volume of specimen versus palpation guidance.
Moore et al, 2001[28]	51	RCT	Intraoperative ultrasound	Margin status	No ink on tumor	Positive margin rate (3.5% vs. 29%, $P < .05$) for palpation-guided excision with no intraoperative evaluation of margins

Additional studies: Davis et al, 2011[29]; Olsha et al, 2011[30]; Eichler et al, 2012[31]; Barentsz et al, 2012[32]; Harlow et al, 1999[33]; James et al, 2009.[34]
RCT, randomized controlled trial; US, ultrasound.

less, there is no advantage in considering RSL (Grade 1B). If these rates are 20% or greater, RSL should be considered as an alternative to WL (Grade 2B).

Intraoperative Use of Localization Methods: (3) Radioguided Occult Lesion Localization

Radioguided occult lesion localization (ROLL) is a technique utilized largely by European surgeons that has also been associated with lowered rates of positive margins compared to WL in most studies. However, as with RSL, the largest randomized trial failed to show a difference in positive margin rate, with the WL cohort having only a 12% rate of positive margins (Table 1-3). Thus, if the rates of inadequate margins are near 12% or less with WL, there is no advantage in considering ROLL (Grade 1B), but if these rates are 20% or greater, ROLL should be considered as an alternative to WL (Grade 2B). Only one trial compared RSL and ROLL, and this failed to demonstrate a difference in adequate margin rates between these two techniques.

TABLE 1-2   Intraoperative Localization Methods: Radioactive Seed Localization

Author	Population Size (n)	Study Design	Type of Intervention	Outcome Measured	Margin Definition	Summary of Key Findings	Comments
Gray et al, 2001[35]	97	RCT	RSL	Final margin status	1 mm	Initial specimen had lower rate of involved margins for RSL patients (26% vs. 57%, $P = .02$), despite the mean volume being similar (56 mL vs. 74 mL, $P = .48$).	Randomized vs. wire localization
Lovrics et al, 2011[36]	305	Multicenter RCT	RSL	Final margin status	No ink on tumor for positive and <1 mm for close	No significant difference in positive margin rates for RSL (11%) and WL (12%, $P = .99$) or for positive or close margins (RSL 19% and WL 22%; $P = .61$). Mean operative time (min) was shorter for RSL (19 vs. 22; $P < .001$). Specimen volume, weight, reoperation, and localization times were similar.	More cases of multifocal disease in the RSL group (15% vs. 6%; $P = .013$)
Ahmed et al, 2013[37]	8 studies	Meta-analysis	RSL	Final margin status and spec volume	Not stated	RSL had lower risk of positive margins (OR, 0.51; 95% CI, 0.36–0.72; $z = 3.88$; $P = .0001$); reoperation for margins (OR, 0.47; 95% CI, 0.33–0.69; $z = 3.96$; $P < .0001$) and shorter operative time	1 RCT and 7 cohort studies compared to wire localization

Additional studies: Cox et al, 2003[39]; Gobardhan et al, 2013[40]; Gray et al, 2004[41]; Hughes et al, 2008[42]; Murphy et al, 2013[43]; Donker et al, 2013.[44]
CI, confidence interval; OR, odds ratio; RCT, randomized controlled trial; RSL, radioactive seed localization; WL, wire localization.

TABLE 1-3   Intraoperative Localization Methods: Radioguided Occult Lesion Localization (ROLL)

Author	Population Size (n)	Study Design	Type of Intervention	Outcome Measured	Margin Definition	Summary of Key Findings	Comments
Postma et al, 2013[45]	314	RCT	ROLL	Final margin status, complication, and cost	No ink on tumor	Positive margins among 14% of ROLL patients vs. 12% of WL ($P = .644$). Total costs were similar for ROLL and WL (+26 per patient, 95% CI −250 to +311). The risk of complications was higher for ROLL than for WL (30% vs. 17%, $P = .006$).	
Medina-Franco et al, 2008[46]	16	RCT	ROLL	Final margin status	Not stated	Negative margins were achieved in 89% vs. 63% for WL ($P = .04$)	
Sajid et al, 2012[47]	449	Meta-analysis of 4 RCTs	ROLL	Final margin status, complication, and volume of tissue	Variable	Lower risk of positive margin with ROLL vs. WL (OR, 0.47; 95% CI, 0.22–0.99; $z = 1.99$; $P < .05$). Surgical time less with ROLL ($P < .00001$). The weight of the specimen is similar ($P = .27$).	

Additional studies: Audisio et al, 2005[48]; Belloni et al, 2011[49]; Duarte et al, 2007[50]; Lavoue et al, 2008[51]; Nadeem et al, 2005[52]; Zgajnar et al, 2005[53]; Donker et al, 2013.[44]
CI, confidence interval; OR, odds ratio; RCT, randomized controlled trial; ROLL, radioguided occult lesion localization; WL, wire localization.

Intraoperative Pathology

(1) Gross exam

There are only a few, relatively small studies of limited quality that examine the effect of gross pathologic examination of a specimen intraoperatively on positive margin rates.[1-3] The limited data available, however, suggests that gross pathology likely lowers the rate of reoperation for margins and should be considered where intraoperative pathology is available (Grade 2B). One trial showed that intraoperative inking of the specimen resulted in fewer reoperations when compared to postoperative inking,[4] but there is too little data to make a recommendation for this technique.

(2) Frozen section analysis

Most surgeons do not use frozen section analysis for margin management.[5] No randomized trial has been performed on frozen section analysis, but a large number of cohort trials have consistently shown that this technique is associated with a lower rate of reoperations for inadequate margins (Table 1-4). Because frozen section analysis involves added cost, its cost-effectiveness necessarily depends on the rate of positive margins (and therefore reoperations) without its use. Frozen section analysis has been shown to be cost-effective when positive margin rates are >25%. Based purely on the effect on margin management, frozen section analysis should be considered unless reoperation rates are already low (<15%) (Grade 2B).

(3) Imprint cytology

Few surgeons ultilize imprint cytology intraoperatively.[5] Like frozen section analysis, no randomized trial has shown this technique to improve the rates of positive margins, but a number of cohort trials have demonstrated that imprint cytology is associated with lower rates of positive margins and perhaps lower local recurrence risk (Table 1-4). Imprint cytology is dependent on the availability of cytology expertise. When such expertise is available, imprint cytology should be considered for intraoperative margin management (Grade 2C) and appears to be at least as reliable as intraoperative frozen section analysis (Grade 2C).

Cavity Shave Margins

Cavity shave margins is a technique of resecting an additional margin of tissue at each of the margins intraoperatively (or in some cases, selected margins) after excision of the main lumpectomy specimen for postoperative pathologic evaluation. Cavity shave margins have been associated with a lower rate of positive margins in multiple cohort studies, but many of these trials had a high rate of positive margins in the control group (Table 1-5). Cavity shave margins should be considered to reduce the rate of positive margins in breast-conserving surgery if the rate of positive margins is otherwise >25% (Grade 2C) and may be particularly valuable where intraoperative pathology is unavailable.

Specimen Radiography

The use of specimen radiography does not clearly improve the rates of reoperation for margins.[3,6-12] Specimen radiography may be helpful in judging the adequacy of

TABLE 1-4 Intraoperative Pathology Methods and Margins

Author	Study Design	Population Size (n)	Type of Intervention	Outcome Measured	Margin Definition	Summary of Key Findings	Comments
Esbona et al, 2012[54]	Systematic review	37 cohort studies; 10,489 tumors	Frozen section analysis and imprint cytology vs. permanent histology	Margin status	Not defined	The reoperation rate for margins with frozen section analysis (10 ± 6%) was significantly lower than with permanent histology only (35 ± 3%, P = .0001). The final re-excision rate of IC (11 ± 4%) was also significantly lower than control (35 ± 3%, P = .001).	No difference in reoperation rate, sensitivity, or specificity of frozen section vs. imprint cytology
Osborn et al, 2011[55]	Mathematical modeling	N/A	Frozen section analysis	Cost of frozen section analysis strategy	Not stated	The cost to the provider is less by doing intraoperative frozen section analysis when the reoperation rate was >36% without frozen section. The cost to the payer was less when the re-excision rate was >26%.	Compared to permanent histology only
Camp et al, 2005[56]	Case series	257	Frozen section analysis of shave margins	Margin status and LR	2 mm	Reoperation rate for margins 5.8% vs. 33% without frozen section of shave margins (P = .001). No difference in LR rates.	

Additional studies: Caruso et al, 2011[63]; Cendan et al, 2005[64]; Chen et al, 2012[65]; Noguchi et al, 1995[66]; Riedl et al, 2009[67]; Weber et al, 1997[68]; Cox et al, 1997[69]; Creager et al, 2002[70]; Mannell, 2005[71]; Valdes et al, 2007.[72] IC, imprint cytology; LR, local recurrence.

TABLE 1-5   Intraoperative Cavity Shave Margins

Author	Population Size (n)	Study Design	Type of Intervention	Outcome Measured	Margin Definition	Summary of Key Findings	Comments
Fukamachi et al, 2010[73]	122	Case series	Cavity shave margins with frozen section	Final margin status	5 mm	Decreased positive margin rate from 27% to 10% ($P < .001$). Frozen section sensitivity 78.6%, specificity 100%, PPV 100%, NPV 94%, 0% LR rate over 61.4 months.	Time of process was mean of 53 minutes.
Janes et al, 2006[74]	217	Case series	Superior and inferior cavity shave margins	Final margin status	5 mm = close	Close margins reduced: OR 0.17 (95% CI 0.08–0.48, $P = .001$).	Compared to group with cavity shaves based on specimen radiograph
Hequet et al, 2013[75]	294	Multicenter cohort	Cavity shave margins	Final margin status	2 mm	25% rate of reoperation for margins. Cavity shaving avoided the need for re-excision in 25%. LR rate 3.7% after follow-up range of 4–9 years.	
Hewes et al, 2009[76]	957	Case series	Cavity shave margins	Final margin status, LR, and OS	1 mm	Concordance between original resection margins and cavity biopsy was only 32%; a negative margin carried an 11% risk of residual disease. Positive cavity biopsy associated with reduced OS and DSS. LR rate was 1.8% 5 years.	

(continued)

TABLE 1-5 Intraoperative Cavity Shave Margins (Continued)

Author	Population Size (n)	Study Design	Type of Intervention	Outcome Measured	Margin Definition	Summary of Key Findings	Comments
Kobbermann et al, 2011[78]	533	Matched cohort	Cavity shave margins	Final margin status	2 mm	Reoperation rate for margins was 22% for cavity shave margin patients vs. 42.0% in a match cohort ($P = .011$).	
Malik et al, 1999[79]	543	Case series	Cavity shave margins	Final margin status	No ink on tumor	Shave margins positive in 37%. Reoperation needed in 15%. LR rate 2% at median 53 months.	
Rizzo et al, 2010[80]	320	Case series	Cavity shave margins	Final margin status and LR	1 mm	Negative margin rate was 85% with addition of cavity shave margins vs. 57% for patients that did not ($P < .05$).	
Tengher-Barna et al, 2009[81]	107	Case series	Cavity shave margins	Final margin status	3 mm	Shave margins positive in 35% and prevented reoperation in 20%. 30% reoperation rate for margins.	

CI, confidence interval; LR, Local recurrence; NPV, negative predictive value; OS, overall survival; PPV, positive predictive value.

margins of excision for lesions associated with microcalcifications. The addition of specimen radiography for the purpose of improving the rates of inadequate margins of excision cannot currently be recommended based on the available evidence (Grade 2C) but remains important for documenting removal of the targeted lesion.

MISCELLANEOUS TECHNIQUES

Individual trials have investigated the use of intraoperative magnetic resonance imaging and cryo-assisted localization,[13,14] and there are several reports in the literature of emerging technologies to assess margins in a more comprehensive or automated fashion.[15-23] The Marginprobe device was recently approved for use in the United States, and although it did not reduce overall reoperation rates (including mastectomy), its use significantly reduced lumpectomy re-excision rates with a larger effect in nonpalpable tumors.[24,25] There is insufficient evidence to make recommendations regarding these techniques and devices.

CONCLUSIONS

Surgeons have many intraoperative tools available to help lower the rates of positive margins of excision among breast cancer patients. Although the available literature for these tools is often not of the highest quality, the accumulated evidence provides substantial guidance as to which techniques are best applied and will have the most impact on a given surgeon's breast cancer practice. This evidence is especially helpful in devising alternative or adjuvant strategies that can be applied and should be considered if reoperation rates are significant (i.e., ≥20%).

REFERENCES

1. Balch GC, Mithani SK, Simpson JF, et al. Accuracy of intraoperative gross examination of surgical margin status in women undergoing partial mastectomy for breast malignancy. *Am Surg* 2005;71(1):22–27; discussion 27–28.
2. Fleming FJ, Hill AD, McDermott EW, et al. Intraoperative margin assessment and re-excision rate in breast conserving surgery. *Eur J Surg Oncol* 2004;30(3):233–237.
3. Cabioglu N, Hunt KK, Sahin AA, et al. Role for intraoperative margin assessment in patients undergoing breast-conserving surgery. *Ann Surg Oncol* 2007;14(4):1458–1471.
4. Singh M, Singh G, Hogan KT, et al. The effect of intraoperative specimen inking on lumpectomy re-excision rates. *World J Surg Oncol* 2010;8:4.
5. Blair SL, Thompson K, Rococco J, et al. Attaining negative margins in breast-conservation operations: is there a consensus among breast surgeons? *J Am Coll Surg* 2009;209(5):608–613.
6. Bathla L, Harris A, Davey M, et al. High resolution intra-operative two-dimensional specimen mammography and its impact on second operation for re-excision of positive margins at final pathology after breast conservation surgery. *Am J Surg* 2011;202(4):387–394.
7. Chagpar A, Yen T, Sahin A, et al. Intraoperative margin assessment reduces reexcision rates in patients with ductal carcinoma in situ treated with breast-conserving surgery. *Am J Surg* 2003;186(4):371–377.
8. Ciccarelli G, Di Virgilio MR, Menna S, et al. Radiography of the surgical specimen in early stage breast lesions: diagnostic reliability in the analysis of the resection margins. *Radiol Med* 2007;112(3):366–376.
9. Kim SH, Cornacchi SD, Heller B, et al. An evaluation of intraoperative digital specimen mammography versus conventional specimen radiography for the excision of nonpalpable breast lesions. *Am J Surg* 2013;205(6):703–710.
10. Layfield DM, May DJ, Cutress RI, et al. The effect of introducing an in-theatre intra-operative specimen radiography (IOSR) system on the management of palpable breast cancer within a single unit. *Breast* 2012;21(4):459–463.

11. McCormick JT, Keleher AJ, Tikhomirov VB, et al. Analysis of the use of specimen mammography in breast conservation therapy. *Am J Surg* 2004;188(4):433–436.
12. Carmichael AR, Ninkovic G, Boparai R. The impact of intra-operative specimen radiographs on specimen weights for wide local excision of breast cancer. *Breast* 2004;13(4):325–328.
13. Hirose M, Kacher DF, Smith DN, et al. Feasibility of MR imaging-guided breast lumpectomy for malignant tumors in a 0.5-T open-configuration MR imaging system. *Acad Radiol* 2002;9(8):933–941.
14. Tafra L, Fine R, Whitworth P, et al. Prospective randomized study comparing cryo-assisted and needle-wire localization of ultrasound-visible breast tumors. *Am J Surg* 2006;192(4):462–470.
15. Haka AS, Volynskaya Z, Gardecki JA, et al. In vivo margin assessment during partial mastectomy breast surgery using Raman spectroscopy. *Cancer Res* 2006;66(6):3317–3322.
16. Fine RE, Schwalke MA, Pellicane JV, et al. A novel ultrasound-guided electrosurgical loop device for intra-operative excision of breast lesions; an improvement in surgical technique. *Am J Surg* 2009;198(2):283–286.
17. Cortes-Mateos MJ, Martin D, Sandoval S, et al. Automated microscopy to evaluate surgical specimens via touch prep in breast cancer. *Ann Surg Oncol* 2009;16(3):709–720.
18. Blair SL, Wang-Rodriguez J, Cortes-Mateos MJ, et al. Enhanced touch preps improve the ease of interpretation of intraoperative breast cancer margins. *Am Surg* 2007;73(10):973–976.
19. Cuntz MC, Levine EA, O'Dorisio TM, et al. Intraoperative gamma detection of 125I-lanreotide in women with primary breast cancer. *Ann Surg Oncol* 1999;6(4):367–372.
20. Keller MD, Majumder SK, Kelley MC, et al. Autofluorescence and diffuse reflectance spectroscopy and spectral imaging for breast surgical margin analysis. *Lasers Surg Med* 2010;42(1):15–23.
21. Keller MD, Vargis E, de Matos Granja N, et al. Development of a spatially offset Raman spectroscopy probe for breast tumor surgical margin evaluation. *J Biomed Opt* 2011;16(7):077006.
22. Martin DT, Sandoval S, Ta CN, et al. Quantitative automated image analysis system with automated debris filtering for the detection of breast carcinoma cells. *Acta Cytologica* 2011;55(3):271–280.
23. Nguyen FT, Zysk AM, Chaney EJ, et al. Intraoperative evaluation of breast tumor margins with optical coherence tomography. *Cancer Res* 2009;69(22):8790–8796.
24. Allweis TM, Kaufman Z, Lelcuk S, et al. A prospective, randomized, controlled, multicenter study of a real-time, intraoperative probe for positive margin detection in breast-conserving surgery. *Am J Surg* 2008;196(4):483–489.
25. Karni T, Pappo I, Sandbank J, et al. A device for real-time, intraoperative margin assessment in breast-conservation surgery. *Am J Surg* 2007;194(4):467–473.
26. Rahusen FD, Bremers AJA, Fabry HFJ, et al. Ultrasound-guided lumpectomy of nonpalpable breast cancer versus wire-guided resection: a randomized clinical trial. *Ann Surg Oncol* 2002;9(10):994–998.
27. Krekel NM, Haloua MH, Lopes Cardozo AMF, et al. Intraoperative ultrasound guidance for palpable breast cancer excision (COBALT trial): a multicentre, randomised controlled trial. *Lancet Oncol* 2013;14(1):48–54.
28. Moore MM, Whitney LA, Cerilli L, et al. Intraoperative ultrasound is associated with clear lumpectomy margins for palpable infiltrating ductal breast cancer. *Ann Surg* 2001;233(6):761–768.
29. Davis KM, Hsu CH, Bouton ME, et al. Intraoperative ultrasound can decrease the re-excision lumpectomy rate in patients with palpable breast cancers. *Am Surg* 2011;77(6):720–725.
30. Olsha O, Shemesh D, Carmon M, et al. Resection margins in ultrasound-guided breast-conserving surgery. *Ann Surg Oncol* 2011;18(2):447–452.
31. Eichler C, Hübbel A, Zarghooni V, et al. Intraoperative ultrasound: improved resection rates in breast-conserving surgery. *Anticancer Res* 2012;32(3):1051–1056.
32. Barentsz MW, van Dalen T, Gobardhan PD, et al. Intraoperative ultrasound guidance for excision of non-palpable invasive breast cancer: a hospital-based series and an overview of the literature. *Breast Cancer Res Treat* 2012;135(1):209–219.
33. Harlow SP, Krag DN, Ames SE, et al. Intraoperative ultrasound localization to guide surgical excision of nonpalpable breast carcinoma. *J Am Coll Surg* 1999;189(3):241–246.
34. Jakub JW, Gray RJ, Degnim AC, et al. Current status of radioactive seed for localization of non palpable breast lesions. *Am J Surg* 2010;199(4):522–528.
35. Gray RJ, Salud C, Nguyen K, et al. Randomized prospective evaluation of a novel technique for biopsy or lumpectomy of nonpalpable breast lesions: radioactive seed versus wire localization. *Ann Surg Oncol* 2001;8(9):711–715.

36. Lovrics PJ, Goldsmith CH, Hodgson N, et al. A multicentered, randomized, controlled trial comparing radioguided seed localization to standard wire localization for nonpalpable, invasive and in situ breast carcinomas. *Ann Surg Oncol* 2011;18(12):3407–3414.
37. Ahmed M, Douek M. Radioactive seed localisation (RSL) in the treatment of non-palpable breast cancers: systematic review and meta-analysis. *Breast* 2013;22(4):383–388.
38. Barentsz MW, van den Bosch MA, Veldhuis WB, et al. Radioactive seed localization for non-palpable breast cancer. *Br J Surg* 2013;100(5):582–588.
39. Cox CE, Furman B, Stowell N, et al. Radioactive seed localization breast biopsy and lumpectomy: can specimen radiographs be eliminated? *Ann Surg Oncol* 2003;10(9):1039–1047.
40. Gobardhan PD, de Wall LL, van der Laan L, et al. The role of radioactive iodine-125 seed localization in breast-conserving therapy following neoadjuvant chemotherapy. *Ann Oncol* 2013;24(3):668–673.
41. Gray RJ, Pockaj BA, Karstaedt PJ, et al. Radioactive seed localization of nonpalpable breast lesions is better than wire localization. *Am J Surg* 2004;188(4):377–380.
42. Hughes JH, Mason MC, Gray RJ, et al. A multi-site validation trial of radioactive seed localization as an alternative to wire localization. *Breast J* 2008;14(2):153–157.
43. Murphy JO, Moo TA, King TA, et al. Radioactive seed localization compared to wire localization in breast-conserving surgery: initial 6-month experience. *Ann Surg Oncol* 2013;20(13):4121–4127.
44. Donker M, Drukker CA, Valdés Olmos RA, et al. Guiding breast-conserving surgery in patients after neoadjuvant systemic therapy for breast cancer: a comparison of radioactive seed localization with the ROLL technique. *Ann Surg Oncol* 2013;20(8):2569–2575.
45. Postma EL, Koffijberg H, Verkooijen HM, et al. Cost-effectiveness of radioguided occult lesion localization (ROLL) versus wire-guided localization (WGL) in breast conserving surgery for nonpalpable breast cancer: results from a randomized controlled multicenter trial. *Ann Surg Oncol* 2013;20(7):2219–2226.
46. Medina-Franco H, Abarca-Pérez L, García-Alvarez MN, et al. Radioguided occult lesion localization (ROLL) versus wire-guided lumpectomy for non-palpable breast lesions: a randomized prospective evaluation. *J Surg Oncol* 2008;97(2):108–111.
47. Sajid MS, Parampalli U, Haider Z, et al. Comparison of radioguided occult lesion localization (ROLL) and wire localization for non-palpable breast cancers: a meta-analysis. *J Surg Oncol* 2012;105(8):852–858.
48. Audisio RA, Nadeem R, Harris O, et al. Radioguided occult lesion localisation (ROLL) is available in the UK for impalpable breast lesions. *Ann R Coll Surg Engl* 2005;87(2):92–95.
49. Belloni E, Canevari C, Panizza P, et al. Nonpalpable breast lesions: preoperative radiological guidance in radioguided occult lesion localisation (ROLL). *Radiol Med* 2011;116(4):564–574.
50. Duarte GM, Cabelloa C, Torresan RZ, et al. Radioguided Intraoperative Margins Evaluation (RIME): preliminary results of a new technique to aid breast cancer resection. *Eur J Surg Oncol* 2007;33(10):1150–1157.
51. Lavoue V, Nos C, Clough KB, et al. Simplified technique of radioguided occult lesion localization (ROLL) plus sentinel lymph node biopsy (SNOLL) in breast carcinoma. *Ann Surg Oncol* 2008;15(9):2556–2561.
52. Nadeem R, Chagla LS, Harris O, et al. Occult breast lesions: A comparison between radioguided occult lesion localisation (ROLL) vs. wire-guided lumpectomy (WGL). *Breast* 2005;14(4):283–289.
53. Zgajnar J, Hocevar M, Frkovic-Grazio S, et al. Radioguided occult lesion localization (ROLL) of the nonpalpable breast lesions. *Neoplasma* 2004;51(5):385–389.
54. Esbona K, Li Z, Wilke LG. Intraoperative imprint cytology and frozen section pathology for margin assessment in breast conservation surgery: a systematic review. *Ann Surg Oncol* 2012;19(10):3236–3245.
55. Osborn JB, Keeney GL, Jakub JW, et al. Cost-effectiveness analysis of routine frozen-section analysis of breast margins compared with reoperation for positive margins. *Ann Surg Oncol* 2011;18(11):3204–3209.
56. Camp ER, McAuliffe PF, Gilroy JS, et al. Minimizing local recurrence after breast conserving therapy using intraoperative shaved margins to determine pathologic tumor clearance. *J Am Coll Surg* 2005;201(6):855–861.
57. Jorns JM, Visscher D, Sabel M, et al. Intraoperative frozen section analysis of margins in breast conserving surgery significantly decreases reoperative rates: one-year experience at an ambulatory surgical center. *Am J Clin Pathol* 2012;138(5):657–669.
58. Sabel MS, Jorns JM, Wu A, et al. Development of an intraoperative pathology consultation service at a free-standing ambulatory surgical center: clinical and economic impact for patients undergoing breast cancer surgery. *Am J Surg* 2012;204(1):66–77.

59. Olson TP, Harter J, Muñoz A, et al. Frozen section analysis for intraoperative margin assessment during breast-conserving surgery results in low rates of re-excision and local recurrence. *Ann Surg Oncol* 2007;14(10):2953–2960.

60. Cox CE, Pendas S, Ku NN, et al. Local recurrence of breast cancer after cytological evaluation of lumpectomy margins. *Am Surg* 1998;64(6):533–537; discussion 537–538.

61. D'Halluin F, Tas P, Rouquette S, et al. Intra-operative touch preparation cytology following lumpectomy for breast cancer: a series of 400 procedures. *Breast* 2009;18(4):248–253.

62. Weinberg E, Cox C, Dupont E, et al. Local recurrence in lumpectomy patients after imprint cytology margin evaluation. *Am J Surg* 2004;188(4):349–354.

63. Caruso F, Ferrara M, Castiglione G, et al. Therapeutic mammaplasties: full local control of breast cancer in one surgical stage with frozen section. *Eur J Surg Oncol* 2011;37(10):871–875.

64. Cendan JC, Coco D, Copeland EM III. Accuracy of intraoperative frozen-section analysis of breast cancer lumpectomy-bed margins. *J Am Coll Surg* 2005;201(2):194–198.

65. Chen K, Zeng Y, Jia H, et al. Clinical outcomes of breast-conserving surgery in patients using a modified method for cavity margin assessment. *Ann Surg Oncol* 2012;19(11):3386–3394.

66. Noguchi M, Minami M, Earashi M, et al. Intraoperative histologic assessment of surgical margins and lymph node metastasis in breast-conserving surgery. *J Surg Oncol* 1995;60(3):185–190.

67. Riedl O, Fitzal F, Mader N, et al. Intraoperative frozen section analysis for breast-conserving therapy in 1016 patients with breast cancer. *Eur J Surg Oncol* 2009;35(3):264–270.

68. Weber S, Storm FK, Stitt J, et al. The role of frozen section analysis of margins during breast conservation surgery. *Cancer J Sci Am* 1997;3(5):273–277.

69. Cox CE, Hyacinthe M, Gonzalez RJ, et al. Cytologic evaluation of lumpectomy margins in patients with ductal carcinoma in situ: clinical outcome. *Ann Surg Oncol* 1997;4(8):644–649.

70. Creager AJ, Shaw JA, Young PR, et al. Intraoperative evaluation of lumpectomy margins by imprint cytology with histologic correlation: a community hospital experience. *Arch Pathol Lab Med* 2002;126(7):846–848.

71. Mannell A. Breast-conserving therapy in breast cancer patients: a 12-year experience. *S Afr J Surg* 2005;43(2):28–30.

72. Valdes EK, Boolbol SK, Ali I, et al. Intraoperative touch preparation cytology for margin assessment in breast-conservation surgery: does it work for lobular carcinoma? *Ann Surg Oncol* 2007;14(10):2940–2945.

73. Fukamachi K, Ishida T, Usami S, et al. Total-circumference intraoperative frozen section analysis reduces margin-positive rate in breast-conservation surgery. *Jpn J Clin Oncol* 2010;40(6):513–520.

74. Janes SEJ, Stankheb M, Singha S, et al. Systematic cavity shaves reduces close margins and re-excision rates in breast conserving surgery. *Breast* 2006;15(3):326–330.

75. Héquet D, Bricou A, Koual M, et al. Systemic cavity shaving: modifications of breast cancer management and long-term local recurrence, a multicentre study. *Eur J Surg Oncol* 2013;39(8):899–905.

76. Hewes JC, Imkampe A, Haji A, et al. Importance of routine cavity sampling in breast conservation surgery. *Br J Surg* 2009;96(1):47–53.

77. Keskek M, Kothari M, Ardehali B, et al. Factors predisposing to cavity margin positivity following conservation surgery for breast cancer. *Eur J Surg Oncol* 2004;30(10):1058–1064.

78. Kobbermann A, Unzeitig A, Xie XJ, et al. Impact of routine cavity shave margins on breast cancer re-excision rates. *Ann Surg Oncol* 2011;18(5):1349–1355.

79. Malik HZ, George WD, Mallon EA, et al. Margin assessment by cavity shaving after breast-conserving surgery: analysis and follow-up of 543 patients. *Eur J Surg Oncol* 1999;25(5):464–469.

80. Rizzo M, Iyengar R, Gabram SG, et al. The effects of additional tumor cavity sampling at the time of breast-conserving surgery on final margin status, volume of resection, and pathologist workload. *Ann Surg Oncol* 2010;17(1):228–234.

81. Tengher-Barna I, Hequet D, Reboul-Marty J, et al. Prevalence and predictive factors for the detection of carcinoma in cavity margin performed at the time of breast lumpectomy. *Mod Pathol* 2009;22(2):299–305.

Total Mastectomy

CRITICAL ELEMENTS

- Incision Placement
- Boundaries of Mastectomy
- Mastectomy Flap Elevation
- Excision of the Pectoralis Major Muscle
- Prevention of Seroma/Drain Placement

1. INCISION PLACEMENT

Recommendation: Incisions for total mastectomy should be placed to facilitate the removal of the preponderance of breast tissue to achieve local disease control and decrease the risk of recurrent breast cancer.

Type of Data: Retrospective case series.

Strength of Recommendation: The consensus of the group supports this guideline based on historic evidence.

Rationale

Incision placement for total mastectomy is dictated by whether immediate reconstruction of the affected breast will be performed. The type of total mastectomy planned—simple total mastectomy, skin-sparing mastectomy, or nipple-sparing mastectomy—also guides incision placement.

Mastectomy without Immediate Breast Reconstruction

In patients not undergoing immediate breast reconstruction, a simple total mastectomy is performed. In these cases, an elliptical incision that encompasses the nipple–areola complex (NAC) and removes enough skin to achieve a smooth, even chest wall

29

A

B

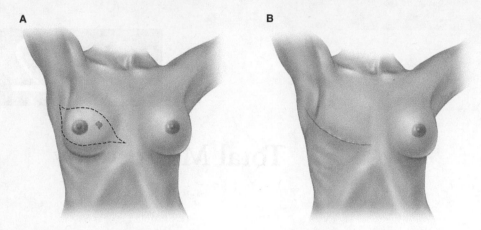

FIGURE 2-1   Standard mastectomy incisions if no immediate reconstruction is planned. Part **A** demonstrates removal of skin over tumor and prior core biopsy sites and part **B** demonstrates the appearance of the chest wall after closure of the skin.

without tension or redundant skin ("dog ears") is made (Fig. 2-1). Although no strong data support the excision of percutaneous core biopsy scars not incorporated within the planned mastectomy incision, the general consensus is that any scar resulting from previous open biopsy or lumpectomy should be removed at the time of mastectomy, ideally within the ellipse of removed skin. The removal of a remote scar caused by previous open biopsy or lumpectomy may necessitate a separate incision.

Special consideration must be given to patients with inflammatory breast cancer. These patients have a very high rate of local disease recurrence. They are most successfully treated with neoadjuvant chemotherapy followed by a modified radical mastectomy (i.e., a simple total mastectomy plus axillary lymph node dissection) and subsequently adjuvant therapy with irradiation of the chest wall and regional lymphatics. Modified radical mastectomy involves the resection of all involved skin, confirmation of negative surgical margins, and closure resulting in a flat chest wall without redundancy to facilitate the delivery of adjuvant radiotherapy. Any skin with evidence of residual disease following neoadjuvant chemotherapy must be resected to negative margins. A similar incision is made for modified radical mastectomies as total or simple mastectomies; however, for modified radical mastectomies, the surgeon may extend the incision more laterally to get a complete exposure of the axillary nodes. In simple mastectomies, many surgeons will have a small separate axillary incision for the sentinel node biopsy.

Mastectomy with Immediate Breast Reconstruction

Compared with mastectomy without immediate breast reconstruction, mastectomy with immediate breast reconstruction has more options for incision placement. In patients undergoing immediate breast reconstruction, a skin-sparing mastectomy is performed, and the surgical oncologist and reconstructive surgeon must work together to plan the mastectomy incision(s). In the case of a small or moderately sized breast,

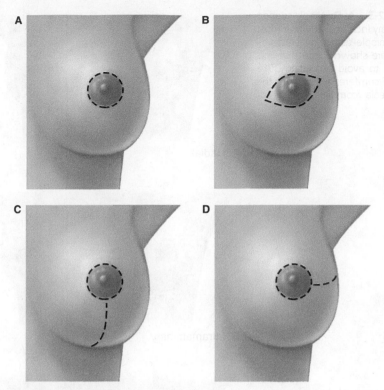

FIGURE 2-2 Incisions for skin-sparing mastectomy. **A:** Round periareolar, **(B)** small elliptical periareolar, **(C)** perioareolar with inferior extension, **(D)** perioareolar with lateral extension.

a circular incision around the edge of the areola with or without lateral extension is employed for skin-sparing mastectomy (Fig. 2-2). In the case of a large breast or mild or moderate breast ptosis, the volume of the skin envelope must be reduced, and this can be achieved by increasing the size of a central elliptical incision or by using a reduction pattern incision according to the plastic surgeon's preference (see Fig. 2-2).

Nipple-sparing mastectomy, a type of skin-sparing mastectomy that preserves not only the breast skin but also the NAC, may also be employed in patients undergoing immediate breast reconstruction (Fig. 2-3). For best results, in nipple-sparing mastectomy, a periareolar incision not exceeding 30% of the circumference of the areola can be used. Incisions that encircle the areola should be avoided, as incisions exceeding 30% of the areolar circumference increase the risk of nipple necrosis.[1] Other incisions associated with a low risk of nipple necrosis include the inframammary fold incision and the radial incisions (see Fig. 2-3). The crescent incision is often utilized in women with breast ptosis, as it allows the surgeon good exposure and lifts the NAC to a more cosmetically appropriate position (see Fig. 2-3). At the time of nipple-sparing mastectomy, the mastectomy incision or a separate axillary incision can be accessed to perform nodal staging with either sentinel lymph node surgery or axillary lymph node dissection.

FIGURE 2-3 A–D: Nipple-sparing mastectomy incisions. The four most common nipple-sparing mastectomy incisions are shown. Note that it is important to avoid exceeding 30% of the circumference around the nipple areola complex to prevent necrosis.

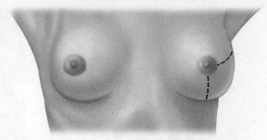

A. Radial

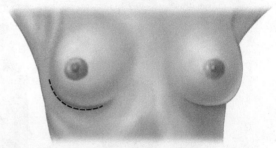

B. Inframammary

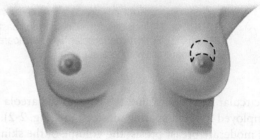

C. Crescent

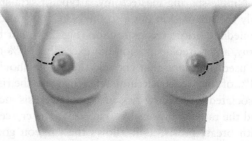

D. Periareolar

2. BOUNDARIES OF MASTECTOMY

Recommendation: Although the options for incisions and the amount of skin excised for simple total mastectomy, skin-sparing mastectomy, and nipple-sparing mastectomy vary, the anatomical boundaries guiding mastectomy remain uniform in order to remove the entire breast parenchyma.

Type of Data: Retrospective case series.

Strength of Recommendation: The consensus of the group supports this guideline based on historic evidence.

Rationale

The boundaries of the breast include the second rib superiorly, the upper border of the rectus sheath inferiorly, the lateral border of the sternum medially, and the latissimus dorsi muscle laterally.[2] The superior lateral boundary of any mastectomy should include the tail of the breast, which extends into the axilla a variable distance beyond the lateral margin of the pectoralis major muscle. Care should be taken to remove any glandular breast tissue that extends into the axilla. The breast should be dissected off the underlying pectoralis major muscle. Removal of the pectoral fascia with the breast is commonly but not uniformly advised. The fascia overlying the serratus anterior muscle and the rectus sheath should be preserved. Sutures should be placed to provide specimen orientation. Most mastectomies remove more than 95% of the breast; some breast tissue invariably remains. Thus, new primary cancers can, although rarely do, occur even after mastectomy. Therefore, meticulous resection and thorough removal of the breast tissue is essential to achieving optimal outcomes.

3. MASTECTOMY FLAP ELEVATION

Recommendation: Mastectomy flaps should be elevated in a manner that facilitates the removal of essentially all breast tissue to reduce the risk of recurrence and that preserves the overlying subcutaneous tissue and its vascular plexus to minimize the risk of flap necrosis.

Type of Data: Retrospective case series.

Strength of Recommendation: The consensus of the group supports this guideline based on historic evidence.

Rationale

Mastectomy flap thickness varies greatly among patients; the subcutaneous layer in thin patients may be only 2 to 3 mm thick. Persistent glandular tissue and residual disease have been reported to be more prevalent in patients with mastectomy flaps thicker than 5 mm.[3] Anatomic studies have confirmed the interdigitation of the subcutaneous fat and the underlying glandular portion of the breast. Because the border between the subcutaneous tissue and the breast may be poorly defined in patients with excessive adipose tissue in the breast, care must be taken to not extend mastectomy flaps into the deeper glandular plane and thus leave breast tissue in the mastectomy flap.[4] Thin mastectomy flaps dissected at the level of the dermis are predisposed to necrosis, whereas thick mastectomy flaps may include residual breast tissue that increases the risk of recurrence. Meticulous flap elevation is especially important in cases of skin-sparing or nipple-sparing mastectomy, in which the smaller incision may limit visualization of the upper and lateral borders of dissection depending on which incision is used. All margins at the site of known malignancy should be examined grossly and pathologic analysis of frozen sections performed as indicated to ensure that clear surgical margins are obtained. For patients in whom mammography has revealed diffuse microcalcifications, mammography of the mastectomy specimen with serial sections may be considered; if microcalcifications near a superficial margin are observed, additional skin or subcutaneous tissues can be excised at that site to obtain an adequate final margin.[5] In cases in which the tumor is close to the dermis, a negative margin of skin directly overlying the tumor must be achieved, or the skin must be excised.

Technical Considerations for Flap Elevation

Mastectomy flaps were historically developed using sharp dissection with a scalpel or scissors. Sharp dissection as the primary method of flap elevation for most surgeons was eventually replaced by electrocautery, which resulted in significantly less blood loss (Fig. 2-4).[6] Now, low-energy dissection devices provide an alternative to both sharp dissection and electrocautery for flap elevation. These devices generate temperatures that seal vascular and lymphatic structures, and they divide tissue with less collateral tissue injury and lower seroma volumes compared with sharp dissection or electrocautery.[7,8] To date, however, no specific device has been associated with better oncologic outcomes.

One optional adjunct to flap elevation with sharp dissection is tumescent solution injection, which has been reported to reduce operating room time without the blood loss or thermal injury associated with sharp dissection or electrocautery alone.[9] The tumescent solution is composed of normal saline, lidocaine, and epinephrine. After skin incision, a 20-gauge spinal needle is used to inject the solution into the space between the subcutaneous and glandular tissue to develop a bloodless plane (see Fig. 2-4). The blades of the scissors are opened approximately 1 to 1.5 cm and the scissors are pushed through the developed plane tissue to elevate the flap.[10] Although many breast surgeons have adopted this technique, some groups have reported that tumescent solution injection results in higher rates of flap necrosis than electrocautery does, possibly owing to the vasoconstriction it causes.[10–12] Surgeons should select the technique that they are confident will enable them to completely remove the breast with the fewest associated complications.

4. EXCISION OF THE PECTORALIS MAJOR MUSCLE

Recommendation: Although neoadjuvant systemic therapy should minimize the amount of direct muscle invasion encountered during mastectomy, localized excision of the pectoralis major muscle is sometimes necessary to achieve clear margins.

Type of Data: Older prospective trials and more recent case series.

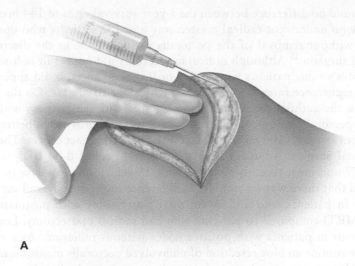

A

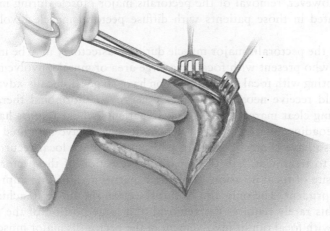

B

FIGURE 2-4 Flap elevation done sharply after injection of tumes-cent solution. Part **A** shows injection of tumescent solution with spinal needle and part **B** shows flap elevation with scissors.

Strength of Recommendation: The consensus of the group supports this guideline based on historic evidence.

Rationale

Resection of the pectoral muscle, an element of the classic Halstead radical mastectomy described in 1894,[13] was routinely performed during mastectomy for more than 70 years. However, the clinical benefit of such radical surgery was questioned once effective adjuvant radiotherapy and systemic therapies came into use. In 1978,

Baker et al found no difference between the 5-year survival rates of 144 breast cancer patients who underwent radical mastectomy and 188 patients who underwent mastectomy without removal of the pectoralis major muscle at the discretion of the operating surgeon.[11] Although radical mastectomy did not result in lower local recurrence rates among patients with stage I or II breast cancer, it did appear to result in lower recurrence rates among patients with stage III disease. On the basis of these findings, the authors concluded that compared with mastectomy without removal of the pectoralis major muscle, radical mastectomy provided a better chance of local control but not survival in patients with stage III breast cancer. The results of the National Surgical Adjuvant Breast and Bowel Project B-04 trial, first published in 1977 and most recently updated with 25-year follow-up data in 2002,[12] demonstrated that there was no significant difference in rates of overall survival or local control in patients who underwent total mastectomy with postmastectomy radiation (PMRT) compared to patients who had radical mastectomy. Local control was inferior in patients with positive nodes without radiation. As a result of this study, the routine en bloc resection of uninvolved pectoralis major muscles was abandoned. However, removal of the pectoralis major muscle during mastectomy may be indicated in those patients with diffuse pectoral muscle involvement at diagnosis.

Removal of the pectoralis major muscle during mastectomy may be indicated in some patients who present with focal or a large area of muscle involvement. Most patients presenting with focal muscle invasion have stage III, locally advanced cancers and should receive neoadjuvant chemotherapy or hormonal therapy to facilitate obtaining clear margins at surgery. In patients whose tumors have limited response to neoadjuvant therapy, muscle excision may have a limited treatment role; it may also have clinical benefit in patients who have local recurrences that are refractory to treatment.[14] In these patients, resection of the pectoralis major muscle at the site of focal invasion to obtain negative margins for improved local control seems prudent. The only aim of this resection should be to achieve a clear margin, and this rarely requires the removal of a large portion of the muscle. In most patients with focal tumor involvement of the pectoralis major muscle, a combination of resection of the area of involved pectoralis muscle plus PMRT are recommended.

Muscle invasion or T4 disease is considered a definite indication for PMRT in patients undergoing mastectomy. Several authors have demonstrated that in the absence of PMRT, close or positive margins and invasion of the pectoralis major muscle or its fascia increase the risk of local recurrence. For example, researchers in the Danish Breast Cancer Cooperative Group 82B and C trials studied a group of more than 1,500 high-risk patients who received no radiation and found that fascial invasion was an independent predictor of locoregional recurrence.[14] Similarly, a group from The University of Texas MD Anderson Cancer Center reported that in high-risk patients who did not receive PMRT, positive margins and fascial invasion were significant predictors of locoregional recurrence.[15] A systematic review confirmed that muscle or fascial invasion increased the relative risk for local recurrence (relative risk, 1.7) in patients who did not receive PMRT.[16] Although excision of focal muscular involvement followed by PMRT is often used to achieve clear margins, strong data supporting the benefit of muscle excision in this setting are lacking.

5. PREVENTION OF SEROMA/DRAIN PLACEMENT

Recommendation: Drains must be optimally placed to prevent seroma formation and reduce seroma-related morbidity after total mastectomy in order to avoid delays to adjuvant treatment.

Type of Data: Small prospective and multiple retrospective trials.

Strength of Recommendation: The group strongly recommends drain placement to limit seroma formation which could delay adjuvant treatment.

Rationale

Drains are placed at the completion of total mastectomy to evacuate fluid from the surgical site and prevent seroma formation. Seromas form from the inflammatory reaction to the surgical trauma. Electrocautery, which is widely used for mastectomy flap elevation, has been shown to exacerbate the inflammatory processes that lead to seroma formation.[17,18] With the exception of a body mass index greater than 30 kg/m^2, which is associated with prolonged seroma drainage,[19] no patient-, procedure-, or tumor-related factors have been found to affect seroma extent or duration. In patients at high risk of persistent seroma following total mastectomy, closure of the dead space with sutures and/or tissue sealants may be considered; however, this approach offers limited benefit in patients undergoing uncomplicated simple total mastectomy that does not include extensive axillary node dissection.

Persistent seroma can lead to mild or severe infections and/or delays in adjuvant therapy, thus potentially affecting oncologic outcomes.[20,21] The most widespread approach to reducing seroma-related morbidity after mastectomy is the use of closed-suction drainage. Small prospective trials have shown no difference in benefit between the use of multiple drains and a single drain[21–23] or between the use of low-pressure and high-pressure suction.[24] At least one closed suction drain should be placed at the time of wound closure; this drain should extend across the pectoralis major muscle towards the axillary space. Data from one randomized controlled trial supports placing a chlorhexidine disc at the drain site and using antiseptic bulb irrigation to reduce drain colonization.[25]

Various strategies have been employed to limit seroma formation without drain placement. For example, prospective trials have shown that fibrin sealant reduces the duration and quantity of wound drainage in patients undergoing total mastectomy and concomitant axillary node dissection.[26,27] Fixation of the flap with sutures may also result in earlier drain removal, although this approach is not widely used.[28,29] In most settings, removing the drain only after an output of <30 mL/day has achieved results in optimal outcomes.[30] Early drain removal without consideration of drainage volume is not recommended because it has been associated with a higher rate of postoperative complications.[28]

REFERENCES

1. Kuerer HM, ed. *Kuerer's Breast Surgical Oncology*. New York, NY: McGraw-Hill; 2010.
2. Garwood ER, Moore D, Ewing C, et al. Total skin-sparing mastectomy: complications and local recurrence rates in 2 cohorts of patients. *Ann Surg* 2009;249:26–32.
3. Harris JR, Lippman ME, Osborne CK, et al. *Diseases of the Breast*. Philadelphia, PA: Lippincott Williams & Wilkins; 2011.
4. Torresan RZ, dos Santos CC, Okamura H, et al. Evaluation of residual glandular tissue after skin-sparing mastectomies. *Ann Surg Oncol* 2005;12:1037–1044.
5. Nickell WB, Skelton J. Breast fat and fallacies: more than 100 years of anatomical fantasy. *J Hum Lact* 2005;21:126–130.
6. Newman LA, Kuerer HM, Hunt KK, et al. Presentation, treatment, and outcome of local recurrence afterskin-sparing mastectomy and immediate breast reconstruction. *Ann Surg Oncol* 1998;5:620–626.
7. Yilmaz KB, Dogan L, Nalbant H, et al. Comparing scalpel, electrocautery and ultrasonic dissector effects: the impact on wound complications and pro-inflammatory cytokine levels in wound fluid from mastectomy patients. *J Breast Cancer* 2011;14(1):58–63.
8. Cortadellas T, Córdoba O, Espinosa-Bravo M, et al. Electrothermal bipolar vessel sealing system in axillary dissection: a prospective randomized clinical study. *Int J Surg* 2011;9(8):636–640.
9. Miller E, Paull DE, Morrissey K, et al. Scalpel versus electrocautery in modified radical mastectomy. *Am Surg* 1988;54(5):284–286.
10. Abbott AM, Miller BT, Tuttle TM. Outcomes after tumescence technique versus electrocautery mastectomy. *Ann Surg Oncol* 2012;19:2607–2611.
11. Chun YS, Verma K, Rosen H, et al. Use of tumescent mastectomy technique as a risk factor for native breast skin flap necrosis following immediate breast reconstruction. *Am J Surg* 2011;201:160–165.
12. Seth AK, Hirsch EM, Kim JYS, et al. Additive risk of tumescent technique in patients undergoing mastectomy with immediate reconstruction. *Ann Surg Oncol* 2011;18(11):3041–3046.
13. Shoher A, Hekier R, Lucci A Jr. Mastectomy performed with scissors following tumescent solution injection. *J Surg Oncol* 2003;83:191–193.
14. Halstead W. The results of operations for the cure of cancer of the breast performed at the Johns Hopkins Hospital from June 1889 to January 1894. *Ann Surg* 1894;20:497–555.
15. Baker RR. A comparison of modified radical mastectomy to radical mastectomy in the treatment of operable breast cancer. *Ann Surg* 1978;189:553–557.
16. Fisher B, Jeong JH, Anderson S, et al. Twenty-five-year follow-up of a randomized trial comparing radical mastectomy, total mastectomy, and total mastectomy followed by irradiation. *N Engl J Med* 2002;347(8):567–575.
17. Nielsen HM, Overgaard M, Grau C, et al. Loco-regional recurrence after mastectomy in high-risk breast cancer—risk and prognosis. An analysis of patients from the DBCG 82 b&c randomization trials. *Radiother Oncol* 2006;79:147–155.
18. Katz A, Strom EA, Buchholz TA, et al. The influence of pathologic tumor characteristics on locoregional recurrence rates following mastectomy. *Int J Rad Oncol Biol Phys* 2001;50:735–742.
19. Rowell NP. Are mastectomy resection margins of clinical relevance? A systematic review. *Breast* 2010;19:14–22.
20. Hashemi E, Kaviani A, Najafi M, et al. Seroma formation after surgery for breast cancer. *World J Surg Oncol* 2004;2:44.
21. Porter KA, O'Connor S, Rimm E, et al. Electrocautery as a factor in seroma formation following mastectomy. *Am J Surg* 1998;176:8–11.
22. Kuroi K, Shimozuma K, Taguchi T, et al. Evidence-based risk factors for seroma formation in breast surgery. *Jpn J Clin Oncol* 2006;36(4)197–206.
23. Terrell GS, Singer JA. Axillary versus combined axillary and pectoral drainage after modified radical mastectomy. *Surg Gynecol Obstet* 1992;175:437–440.
24. Petrek JA, Peters MM, Cirrincione C, et al. A prospective randomized trial of single versus multiple drains in the axilla after lymphadenectomy. *Surg Gynecol Obstet* 1992;175:405–409.
25. Saratzis A, Soumian S, Willetts R, et al. Use of multiple drains after mastectomy is associated with more patient discomfort and longer postoperative stay. *Clin Breast Cancer* 2009;9:243–246.
26. Bonnema J, van Geel AN, Ligtenstein DA, et al. A prospective randomized trial of high versus low vacuum drainage after axillary dissection for breast cancer. *Am J Surg* 1997;173:76–79.
27. Degnim AC, Scow JS, Hoskin TL, et al. Randomized controlled trial to reduce bacterial colonization of surgical drains after breast and axillary operations. *Ann Surg* 2013;258(2):240–247.

28. Kuroi K, Shimozuma K, Taguchi T, et al. Effect of mechanical closure of dead space on seroma formation after breast surgery. *Breast Cancer* 2006;13(3):260–265.
29. Sakkary MA. The value of mastectomy flap fixation in reducing fluid drainage and seroma formation in breast cancer patients. *World J Surg Oncol* 2012;10:8.
30. Barton A, Blitz M, Callahan D, et al. Early removal of postmastectomy drains is not beneficial: results from a halted randomized controlled trial. *Am J Surg* 2006;191(5):652–656.

Nipple-Sparing Mastectomy: Key Question

In women with breast cancer or at high risk for breast cancer, what are the technical components of a nipple-sparing mastectomy for it to be performed in an oncologic fashion comparable to skin-sparing mastectomy?

INTRODUCTION

Many women still undergo mastectomy for breast cancer despite advances in local therapy. The significant psychological impact associated with mastectomy has driven the search to identify surgical approaches that optimize cosmetic outcomes while offering appropriate oncologic outcomes. The preservation of the nipple–areola complex (NAC) following breast cancer surgery increases a woman's perception of wholeness, and this has led to a resurgence of interest in nipple-sparing mastectomy (NSM). However, guidelines for selecting patients and performing NSM are lacking. We performed a systematic literature review to identify the optimal approaches to the main technical components of NSM that would enable surgeons to perform the procedure in an oncologic fashion comparable to that of skin-sparing mastectomy (SSM) in women who have breast cancer or who are at an increased risk for breast cancer.

METHODOLOGY

We performed a PubMed search with the assistance of professional medical librarians. All articles from 1978 to 2013 restricted to the English language using the Medical Subject Headings (MeSH) "genes, BRCA1," "genes, BRCA2," "hereditary breast," "ovarian cancer syndrome," "carcinoma, ductal, breast," "carcinoma, intraductal, noninfiltrating," "neoplasms, ductal, lobular, and medullary," "carcinoma in situ," "breast neoplasms/pathology," "breast neoplasms/surgery," "intraoperative complications," "postoperative complications," "necrosis," "treatment outcome," "neoplasm recurrence, local," "prognosis," "risk reduction behavior," and keywords brca1, brca2, hereditary breast, ovarian cancer syndrome, carcinoma ductal breast, breast neoplasms and (pathology OR surgery), breast and (neoplasm OR cancer OR carcinoma OR in situ OR invasive OR infiltrating), oncologic principles, oncologic technique, nipple coring, skin flap, incision, flap elevation, flap thickness, retroareolar tissue removal, retroareolar intraoperative assessment, nipple areola complex, nipple-areola complex, NAC, nipple areola complex sparing mastectomy, nipple-areola complex sparing mastectomy, NSM, total skin sparing mastectomy, intraoperative complications, postoperative complications, necrosis, treatment outcome, cosmesis, neoplasm recurrence locoregional, neoplasm recurrence locoregional, neoplasm recurrence local OR, prognosis, and risk reduction behavior were searched with a total of 370 abstracts identified.

Our search identified 370 abstracts; of these, 17 were duplicates, leaving 354 abstracts for review. Two reviewers identified 67 abstracts that focused on the oncologic technical considerations of NSM, including complications and oncologic outcomes. Each of the 67 articles summarized by these abstracts was then screened by two of six reviewers assigned randomly. Articles that lacked oncologic technical considerations or outcomes, had study populations of less than 30 patients, or had patient populations reported in another study already included in the review were excluded. An article's inclusion or exclusion was based on reviewer agreement. If the two reviewers did not agree on whether to include or exclude an article, a third reviewer was brought in to review the article, which was then included or excluded based on the third reviewer's decision. Forty-five articles were included in the final literature review. Our review included no randomized clinical trials; most studies reported outcomes from single institutions, and the vast majority were prospective or retrospective cohorts.

FINDINGS

Historical Prevalence of Nipple–Areola Complex Involvement in Mastectomy Specimens

The prevalence of tumor involvement in the NAC is one concern that affects the oncologic safety of NSM. Retrospective pathologic analyses of consecutive mastectomy specimens have found that 9% to 29% of patients undergoing mastectomy for breast cancer have NAC involvement.[1-6] This wide range likely reflects these studies' differing criteria for mastectomy. Factors associated with tumor in the NAC included a central location of the tumor, a tumor size greater than 5 cm, and a tumor-to-nipple distance of less than 2 cm. However, women who are considered appropriate candidates for NSM have been found to have a much lower rate of NAC involvement. Most series of women undergoing planned NSM have shown that fewer than 10% require excision of the NAC owing to positive findings on pathologic analysis (Table 2-1).

Patient Selection

The success of any surgical procedure relies in part on appropriate patient selection. Specific patient selection guidelines for NSM have not been established, but numerous studies have investigated patient selection for NSM in both the therapeutic and risk-reducing settings. Most series have limited the consideration for NSM to patients presenting with either ductal carcinoma in situ or stage I or II invasive cancer. Absolute contraindications for NSM include nipple changes, such as nipple discharge, nipple inversion, or ulceration of the NAC. Patients with inflammatory breast cancer, retroareolar tumors, Paget disease, and frozen section analysis–based confirmation of NAC involvement should not have NSM. Relative contraindications for NSM include tumor size (most commonly greater than 2.5 to 3.5 cm)[7-15] and nipple-to-tumor distance (often less than 2.0 to 2.5 cm).[8,10,11,13,15-17]

There is a general consensus that preoperative imaging should be used to rule out radiographically evident NAC involvement, with some advocating a possible role for preoperative magnetic resonance imaging.[8,18] There is less consensus regarding the roles of factors such as nodal metastases, smoking history, prior radiation, neoadjuvant therapy, and obesity in determining whether NSM can be performed. In patients with characteristics such as smoking history, prior radiation, or obesity, the risk of

TABLE 2-1 Studies Investigating the Prevalence of Tumor Extension to the Nipple–Areola Complex among Women Undergoing Nipple-Sparing Mastectomy for Cancer

Author	Year	No. of NSM Breasts with Cancer	Inclusion/Exclusion Criteria	No. of Breasts with NAC Involvement Identified Intraoperatively (Method)	Total No. of Breasts with NAC Involvement (%)
Crowe et al[7]	2004	85	Stage 0–II disease	8 (tissue cores)	9 (11%)
Margulies et al[21]	2005	50	Any patient without preoperative evidence of NAC involvement	3	4 (8%)
Psaila et al[11]	2006	139	T1 (74%) or T2 (19%) disease; recurrence after lumpectomy or RT (7%); tumor diameter <3.5 cm; tumor-to-cancer distance >2 cm	0	1 (1%)
Regolo et al[12]	2008	70	No clinically evident involvement of the NAC; tumor diameter <4 cm; tumor-to-cancer distance >1 cm as measured using US	2 (frozen section)	4 (6%)
Voltura et al[26]	2008	34	Stage 0–IIB disease	1	2 (6%)
Paepke et al[23]	2009	94	T1 (41%) or T2 (30%) disease	4 (frozen section)	13 (14%)
Radovanovic et al[30]	2010	214	Stage 0–IIIB disease with (17%) or without neoadjuvant chemotherapy	4 (frozen section)	4 (2%)
Boneti et al[18]	2011	156	Negative preoperative imaging; exclusion of patients with T3 or T4 disease, smoking history, or RT	4 (touch prep)	4 (3%)
de Alcantara et al[8]	2011	157	Stage 0–IIIA disease, DCIS (47%) or invasive breast cancer (52%)	4 (frozen section)	11 (7%)
Warren et al[28]	2012	412	Stage 0–IV disease		20 (5%)
Rulli et al[13]	2013	74	T0–T2 disease, DCIS (32%) or invasive breast cancer (64%), including node-negative disease (80%)	11	14 (19%)
Stolier et al[15]	2013	94	Invasive breast cancer (27%) or DCIS (14%); tumor-to-cancer distance >2 cm	9 (frozen section)	3 (3%)

DCIS, ductal carcinoma in situ; NAC, nipple–areola complex; NSM, nipple-sparing mastectomy; RT, radiation therapy; US, ultrasound.

NAC loss due to necrosis may be higher. It is still considered controversial regarding the oncologic safety of NSM in patients who have locally advanced tumors with lymph node metastasis or who have had neoadjuvant chemotherapy. NSM for patients who present with these factors should be considered on a case-by-case basis.

NSM for patients carrying BRCA mutations also continues to be controversial, as the few series that have included patients with BRCA mutations who underwent prophylactic NSM offer only short-term data so far.[14,17,19,20] However, the long-term cancer incidence rate of patients with BRCA mutations who undergo prophylactic NSM is anticipated to be low.

Intraoperative Management of the Nipple–Areola Complex

NSM preserves the skin of the NAC with the mastectomy flap. However, the extent to which the glandular and/or ductal tissue underlying and within the NAC should be excised requires clarification. Most authors who have described their technique for NSM report completely removing all ductal tissue from the nipple, leaving only the epidermis and dermis of the NAC. Nipple eversion during this aspect of the procedure may facilitate the complete removal of the ductal tissue within the nipple (the nipple "core"). To avoid thermal injury to the preserved skin of the NAC, surgeons should perform delicate, sharp dissection with a scalpel or scissors, rather than electrocautery.[7,12,14,15,17,21–25]

A few authors advocate preserving the nipple core and a few millimeters of glandular tissue beneath the NAC.[26–27] Voltura et al,[26] citing anatomical studies demonstrating that terminal ductal–lobular units are present in only 9% of nipple specimens, argue that complete removal of the nipple core is unwarranted. Petit et al[27] report preserving a 5-mm layer of glandular tissue beneath the NAC and treating this preserved tissue with radiation intraoperatively.

Based on the aforementioned evidence, all glandular and ductal tissue should be completely removed from the NAC during NSM for patients who will not receive radiation to the preserved NAC. The mastectomy flap must be meticulously elevated up to the edge of the NAC to preserve the blood supply to the NAC.

NSM Incision Placement

Correct incision placement is key to reducing surgical complications following NSM. Numerous incisions for NSM have been described, and familiarity with each, as well as working closely with the reconstructive surgeon to plan incision placement, will help to ensure that NSM yields optimal surgical and cosmetic outcomes. The most commonly used incisions are periareolar, radial, and inframammary incisions. Although no randomized studies of incision placement have been conducted, some general conclusions about incision placement for NSM can be derived from the findings of cohort studies. For example, periareolar incisions involving greater than 30% of the NAC are associated with a higher rate of NAC-related complications.[28] Overall, radial incisions are associated with the lowest rate of NAC compromise; studies comparing incision types have shown that the complication rate associated with radial incisions is significantly lower than those of periareolar and inframammary incisions.[20,29] In experienced hands, inframammary incisions yield both a low complication rate and provide good exposure, particularly in women with smaller breasts.[21,29] Medial incisions, which can compromise the second intercostal perforator, should generally be avoided.[7,15]

Incision through an existing surgical scar may result in complication rates as low as 4%,[18] but in general, this approach offers the least flexibility and is less relevant than other approaches given that most breast cancers are diagnosed on the basis of core biopsy rather than surgical excision findings. Those making the incisions should keep in mind the patient's unique breast size and shape. For example, a small report of 33 women undergoing concurrent NSM, mastopexy, and tissue expander placement demonstrated that nipple preservation is feasible in women with ptosis.[19] Good communication with the reconstruction team will yield the best cosmetic results with different breast shapes and sizes.

Reconstruction Types

Because NSM preserves the entire skin envelope overlying the breast, NSM is always performed in conjunction with breast reconstruction. The breast reconstruction approaches used with SSM are also options for NSM. These approaches include reconstruction using staged tissue expanders and an implant, reconstruction with one-stage implant placement, and reconstruction using autologous tissue. Consultation with a plastic surgeon experienced with NSM reconstruction will help determine the best reconstruction option for each patient.

Surgical Complications

Low surgical complication rates are a critical component of performing NSM in an oncologic fashion. Studies that have reported the surgical complications associated with NSM are shown in Table 2-2. The rate of nipple loss secondary to partial or complete NAC necrosis ranges from 0.7% to 7.3%.

Recurrence Rate

Achieving low rates of locoregional and distant recurrence is the key to performing NSM in an oncologic fashion similar to that of SSM. Studies with follow-up durations ranging from 10 to 139 months have shown that rates of local recurrence in the NAC or breast and rates of regional and distant recurrence following NSM are low (Table 2-3).

CONCLUSION

Technically successful NSM is a multistep process which begins outside the operating room with careful patient selection, planning of incision, and reconstruction. In the operating room, meticulous surgical technique for flap elevation and excision of ductal tissue under NAC are key to good outcomes. NSM has become more widespread in the past decade and represents a significant technical advance over traditional skin-sparing approaches. Although NSM is technically more demanding than traditional skin-sparing approaches, its cosmetic outcomes are clearly superior and result in high patient satisfaction. Although the prevalence of nipple involvement in consecutive mastectomy specimens is a source of valid concern, the likelihood

TABLE 2-2 Studies Investigating Surgical Complication Rates following Nipple-Sparing Mastectomy

Author	Year	No. of Patients	No. of Patients at the Beginning (%) with Partial NAC Necrosis	No. of Patients at the End with Complete NAC Necrosis	Nipple Loss	Skin Flap Necrosis or Epidermolysis	Infection	Loss of Implant	Comments
Crowe et al[7]	2004	149	2 (1)		1 (0.7)				
Margulies et al[21]	2005	50	5 (10)		2 (4)	1 (2)	1 (2)		
Komorowski et al[31]	2006	38	2 (5)	3 (8)		1 (3)			
Psaila et al[11]	2006	139		1 (0.7)		20 (14)			18% of patients experienced NAC pigmentation; 8% experienced desensitized NAC.
Regolo et al[12]	2008	102	2 (2)						
Petit et al[27]	2009	1001	55 (5)	35 (4)	50 (5)		25 (3)	43 (4)	All patients underwent subcutaneous mastectomy and received RT; 800 received ELIOT, and 201 received postoperative RT.

ELIOT, radiosurgical treatment combining subcutaneous mastectomy with intraoperative radiotherapy; NAC, nipple–areola complex; RT, radiation therapy.

TABLE 2-3 Studies Investigating Local and Distant Recurrences among Women Undergoing Nipple-Sparing Mastectomy for Breast Cancer

Author	Year	No. of Patients	No. of Patients Undergoing NSM for Prophylaxis	No. of Patients Undergoing NSM for Breast Cancer	Follow-Up Time, Months (Mean)	No. of Patients with Local Recurrence NAC (%)	No. of Patients with Local Recurrence Breast (%)	No. of Patients with Regional Recurrence (%)	No. of Patients with Distant Recurrence (%)
Crowe et al[7]	2004	149	40	109	41	0	0	2 (1)	2 (1)
Regolo et al[12]	2008	102	18	84	16	0	0	0	0
Gerber et al[16]	2009	60	0	60	101				14 (23)
Paepke et al[23]	2009	96	15	81	34	0	0	1 (1)	2 (2)
Petit et al[27]	2009	1,001	0	1,001	20	0	0	14 (1)	36 (4)
de Alcantara et al[8]	2011	353	196	157	10	0	0	0	1 (0.3)
Warren et al[28]	2012	657	412	245	28	0	7 (1)	4 (0.6)	8 (1)
Al-Mufarrej et al[19]	2013	64	64	0	139	0	0	0	0
Burdge et al[25]	2013	39	0	39	18	0	4 (10)	0	0
Rulli et al[13]	2013	60	0	60	50	2 (2)	0	3 (5)	0
Sakurai et al[24]	2013	788	0	788	87	29		65 (8)	0

NAC, nipple–areola complex; NSM, nipple-sparing mastectomy.

of finding tumor in the NAC in women undergoing planned NSM is low, likely owing to careful patient selection. Long-term follow-up data for NSM are lacking, although cohort studies with limited follow-up consistently suggest that the NSM is oncologically safe in both the therapeutic and prophylactic settings. NSM appears to be a safe alternative to SSM, especially for patients with early-stage disease, and familiarity with the approach will likely be an increasingly important requirement for breast surgeons.

REFERENCES

1. Gulben K, Yildirim E, Berberoglu U. Prediction of occult nipple-areola complex involvement in breast cancer patients. *Neoplasma* 2008;56:72–75.
2. Laronga C, Kemp B, Johnston D, et al. The incidence of occult nipple-areola complex involvement in breast cancer patients receiving a skin-sparing mastectomy. *Ann Surg Oncol* 1999;6: 609–613.
3. Wang J, Xiao X, Wang J, et al. Predictors of nipple–areolar complex involvement by breast carcinoma: histopathologic analysis of 787 consecutive therapeutic mastectomy specimens. *Ann Surg Oncol* 2012;19:1174–1180.
4. Li W, Wang S, Guo X, et al. Nipple involvement in breast cancer: retrospective analysis of 2323 consecutive mastectomy specimens. *Int J Surg Pathol* 2011;19:328–334.
5. Brachtel EF, Rusby JE, Michaelson JS, et al. Occult nipple involvement in breast cancer: clinicopathologic findings in 316 consecutive mastectomy specimens. *J Clin Oncol* 2009;27:4948–4954.
6. Mallon P, Feron J-G, Couturaud B, et al. The role of nipple-sparing mastectomy in breast cancer: a comprehensive review of the literature. *Plast Reconstr Surg* 2013;131:969–984.
7. Crowe JP Jr, Kim JA, Yetman R, et al. Nipple-sparing mastectomy: technique and results of 54 procedures. *Arch Surg* 2004;139:148–150.
8. de Alcantara Filho P, Capko D, Barry JM, et al. Nipple-sparing mastectomy for breast cancer and risk-reducing surgery: the Memorial Sloan-Kettering Cancer Center experience. *Ann Surg Oncol* 2011;18:3117–3122.
9. Kroll SS, Schusterman MA, Tadjalli HE, et al. Risk of recurrence after treatment of early breast cancer with skin-sparing mastectomy. *Ann Surg Oncol* 1997;4:193–197.
10. Maxwell GP, Storm-Dickerson T, Whitworth P, et al. Advances in nipple-sparing mastectomy: oncological safety and incision selection. *Aesthet Surg J* 2011;31:310–319.
11. Psaila A, Pozzi M, Barone Adesi L, et al. Nipple sparing mastectomy with immediate breast reconstruction: a short term analysis of our experience. *J Exp Clin Cancer Res* 2006;25:309–312.
12. Regolo L, Ballardini B, Gallarotti E, et al. Nipple sparing mastectomy: an innovative skin incision for an alternative approach. *Breast* 2008;17:8–11.
13. Rulli A, Caracappa D, Barberini F, et al. Oncologic reliability of nipple-sparing mastectomy for selected patients with breast cancer. *In Vivo* 2013;27:387–394.
14. Sacchini V, Pinotti JA, Barros AC, et al. Nipple-sparing mastectomy for breast cancer and risk reduction: oncologic or technical problem? *J Am Coll Surg* 2006;203:704–714.
15. Stolier AJ, Levine EA. Reducing the risk of nipple necrosis: technical observations in 340 nipple-sparing mastectomies. *Breast J* 2013;19:173–179.
16. Gerber B, Krause A, Dieterich M, et al. The oncological safety of skin sparing mastectomy with conservation of the nipple-areola complex and autologous reconstruction: an extended follow-up study. *Ann Surg* 2009;249:461–468.
17. Wagner JL, Fearmonti R, Hunt KK, et al. Prospective evaluation of the nipple–areola complex sparing mastectomy for risk reduction and for early-stage breast cancer. *Ann Surg Oncol* 2012;19:1137–1144.
18. Boneti C, Yuen J, Santiago C, et al. Oncologic safety of nipple skin-sparing or total skin-sparing mastectomies with immediate reconstruction. *J Am Coll Surg* 2011;212:686–693; discussion 693–695.
19. Al-Mufarrej FM, Woods JE, Jacobson SR. Simultaneous mastopexy in patients undergoing prophylactic nipple-sparing mastectomies and immediate reconstruction. *J Plast Reconstr Aesthet Surg* 2013;66:747–755.
20. Algaithy ZK, Petit JY, Lohsiriwat V, et al. Nipple sparing mastectomy: can we predict the factors predisposing to necrosis? *Eur J Surg Oncol* 2012;38:125–129.

21. Margulies AG, Hochberg J, Kepple J, et al. Total skin-sparing mastectomy without preservation of the nipple-areola complex. *Am J Surg* 2005;190:907–926.

22. Kim HJ, Park EH, Lim WS, et al. Nipple areola skin-sparing mastectomy with immediate transverse rectus abdominis musculocutaneous flap reconstruction is an oncologically safe procedure: a single center study. *Ann Surg* 2010;251:493–498.

23. Paepke S, Schmid R, Fleckner S, et al. Subcutaneous mastectomy with conservation of the nipple-areola skin: broadening the indications. *Ann Surg* 2009;250:288–292.

24. Sakurai T, Zhang N, Suzuma T, et al. Long-term follow-up of nipple-sparing mastectomy without radiotherapy: a single center study at a Japanese institution. *Med Oncol* 2013;30:1–7.

25. Burdge EC, Yuen J, Hardee M, et al. Nipple skin-sparing mastectomy is feasible for advanced disease. *Ann Surg Oncol* 2013;20:3294–3302.

26. Voltura AM, Tsangaris TN, Rosson GD, et al. Nipple-sparing mastectomy: critical assessment of 51 procedures and implications for selection criteria. *Ann Surg Oncol* 2008;15:3396–3401.

27. Petit J, Veronesi U, Orecchia R, et al. Nipple-sparing mastectomy with nipple areola intraoperative radiotherapy: one thousand and one cases of a five years experience at the European institute of oncology of Milan (EIO). *Breast Cancer Res Treat* 2009;117:333–338.

28. Warren Peled A, Foster RD, Stover AC, et al. Outcomes after total skin-sparing mastectomy and immediate reconstruction in 657 breasts. *Ann Surg Oncol* 2012;19:3402–3409.

29. Garwood ER, Moore D, Ewing C, et al. Total skin-sparing mastectomy: complications and local recurrence rates in 2 cohorts of patients. *Ann Surg* 2009;249:26–32.

30. Radovanovic Z, Radovanovic D, Golubovic A, et al: Early complications after nipple-sparing mastectomy and immediate breast reconstruction with silicone prosthesis: results of 214 procedures. *Scand J Surg* 2010;99(3):115–118.

31. Komorowski AL, Zanini V, Regolo L, et al: Necrotic complications after nipple-and areola-sparing mastectomy. *World J Surg* 2006;30(8):1410–1413.

CHAPTER 3

Axillary Lymphadenectomy

CRITICAL ELEMENTS

- Identification of Anatomical Structures for Level I and II Axillary Dissection
- Removal of Level III Nodes
- Removal of Rotter Nodes
- Removal of a Sufficient Number of Lymph Nodes for Axillary Staging
- Identification and Preservation of the Long Thoracic, Thoracodorsal, and Medial Pectoral Nerves
- Identification and Preservation of the Second and Third Intercostobrachial Nerves
- Drain Placement

1A. IDENTIFICATION OF ANATOMICAL STRUCTURES FOR LEVEL I AND II AXILLARY DISSECTION

Recommendation: Identification of the axillary vein and latissimus dorsi, pectoralis major, pectoralis minor, serratus anterior, and subscapularis muscles is essential for the resection of sufficient level I and II axillary nodes for breast cancer staging and adjuvant treatment planning.

Type of Data: Retrospective case series.

Strength of Recommendation: The consensus of the group supports this guideline based on historic evidence.

Rationale

Breast cancer typically spreads to the axillary lymph nodes first, and axillary dissection is important for both local control and treatment planning. The anatomic borders of the axilla must be identified to adequately resect level I and II axillary lymph nodes (see Fig. 3-1). The axilla is a triangular space that is delineated by the axillary vein

49

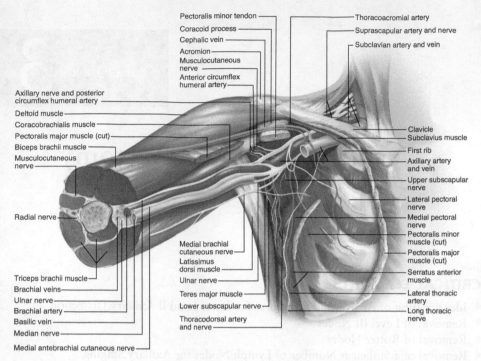

Pectoralis minor tendon
Coracoid process
Cephalic vein
Acromion
Musculocutaneous nerve
Anterior circumflex humeral artery

Thoracoacromial artery
Suprascapular artery and nerve
Subclavian artery and vein

Axillary nerve and posterior circumflex humeral artery
Deltoid muscle
Coracobrachialis muscle
Pectoralis major muscle (cut)
Biceps brachii muscle
Musculocutaneous nerve

Clavicle
Subclavius muscle
First rib
Axillary artery and vein
Upper subscapular nerve
Lateral pectoral nerve
Medial pectoral nerve
Pectoralis minor muscle (cut)
Pectoralis major muscle (cut)
Serratus anterior muscle
Lateral thoracic artery
Long thoracic nerve

Radial nerve

Medial brachial cutaneous nerve
Latissimus dorsi muscle
Ulnar nerve
Teres major muscle
Lower subscapular nerve
Thoracodorsal artery and nerve

Triceps brachii muscle
Brachial veins
Ulnar nerve
Brachial artery
Basilic vein
Median nerve
Medial antebrachial cutaneous nerve

FIGURE 3-1 Anatomy of the axilla.

superiorly, the latissimus dorsi muscle laterally, the serratus anterior muscle medially, the subscapularis muscle posteriorly, and the pectoralis minor and major muscles anteriorly. Lymph nodes in the axilla are identified by their location in one of three anatomical levels. Level I contains the axillary lymph nodes between the latissimus dorsi and the lateral border of the pectoralis minor muscle; level II contains the axillary lymph nodes between the lateral and medial borders of the pectoralis minor muscle; and level III encompasses the lymph nodes between the medial border of the pectoralis minor muscle and Halsted's ligament. Level III axillary nodes can be exposed by resecting or dividing the pectoralis minor muscle. Axillary lymph nodes are located primarily in level I (60% to 70% of nodes), followed by level II (20% to 30%) and level III (10% to 20%).[1–3] Axillary metastases are most often identified in level I nodes followed by level II nodes. Single-node metastasis occurs in level I nodes almost exclusively.[1,2] Metastases that occur in level II or III nodes in the absence of level I metastasis ("skip" metastases) are rare and typically occur in level II nodes.[2,4]

1B. REMOVAL OF LEVEL III NODES

Recommendation: The removal of level III axillary nodes is not typically indicated for patients with stage I or II breast cancer but should be considered to facilitate local disease control in patients with locally advanced breast cancer or N2 disease and patients in whom the nodes are identified by palpation intraoperatively.

Type of Data: Randomized controlled trials.

Strength of Recommendation: There is strong evidence to support this recommendation.

Rationale

Level III nodes account for less than 20% of axillary lymph nodes and are the least likely to have metastases.[1] Skip metastases in level III nodes occur in less than 1% of patients.[4] Two randomized controlled trials enrolling primarily patients with stage I or II disease revealed no differences in breast cancer staging or disease-free or overall survival rates between patients who underwent level I and II axillary dissection and those who underwent level I, II, and III axillary dissection after 10 years of follow-up. However, the patients who underwent level I, II, and III dissection had significantly longer operative times and more blood loss than patients who underwent level I and II dissection.[5,6] In patients with T3 breast cancer, who have a 32% risk of having positive nodes in all three levels, resection of level III nodes is reasonable if level I or II nodes are positive. Furthermore, in patients with more than four positive level I nodes, who have a >60% likelihood of level II and III metastases,[3] level III nodes can be resected to facilitate local control if clinically suspicious nodes are identified by digital palpation.[7]

1C. REMOVAL OF ROTTER NODES

Recommendation: The removal of Rotter nodes (i.e., the interpectoral nodes) is not typically recommended for patients with stage I or II breast cancer but should be considered to facilitate locoregional disease control in patients with locally advanced breast cancer or N2 disease and in patients for whom preoperative imaging studies reveal the nodes to be suspicious.

Type of Data: Case studies, retrospective reviews.

Strength of Recommendation: There is only retrospective data to support this recommendation. The consensus is that the risk of routine resection of asymptomatic Rotter nodes outweighs the small potential benefit.

Rationale

Rotter nodes were once routinely removed as part of radical mastectomy, which included the resection of the pectoralis major and minor muscles. Following the adoption of modified radical mastectomy, which included the dissection of level I and II lymph nodes but not the resection of the pectoralis major and minor muscles, several retrospective studies evaluated the clinical significance of Rotter nodes. These studies assessed the number of Rotter nodes that were positive for metastatic carcinoma, the tumor characteristics associated with positive Rotter nodes, and the frequency with which Rotter nodes were identified as the only positive nodes.[8-12] Positive Rotter nodes were more frequently identified in patients who had tumors in the upper outer quadrant of the breast, T3 disease, and/or positive axillary lymph nodes.[10] In case series, the incidence of isolated positive Rotter nodes was 0.3% among patients with stage I or II invasive breast cancer[8] but as high as 13% among patients with stage III disease, who comprised 50% of the cohort.[9]

2. REMOVAL OF A SUFFICIENT NUMBER OF LYMPH NODES FOR STAGING

Recommendation: A target minimum of 10 axillary lymph nodes should be removed to ensure a high level of confidence that the remaining lymph nodes are negative.

Type of Data: Several well-designed, nonrandomized controlled trials.

Strength of Recommendation: There is moderate evidence to support this recommendation.

Rationale
Before Chemotherapy
Axillary lymph node dissection (ALND) provides important prognostic information that can affect treatment decisions. The primary role of ALND is to provide a means of accurately staging breast cancer. ALND can also affect recurrence risk.

ALND primarily includes the resection of level I and II axillary lymph nodes. Fine-needle aspiration (FNA) can be performed to identify metastatic disease in level III nodes or Rotter nodes that positron emission tomography/computed tomography or infraclavicular ultrasonography reveal to be suspicious for disease involvement. Level III nodes or Rotter nodes that have biopsy-proven metastasis should be removed along with the level I and II nodes. Level I and II ALND should include tissue inferior to the axillary vein as well as tissue lateral to the latissimus dorsi muscle and medial to the pectoralis minor muscle.

Studies reviewing lymph node status and treatment outcomes in patients undergoing ALND have shown that a sample size of a minimum of 10 lymph nodes is needed to provide sufficient information to make sound treatment decisions in breast cancer patients.[13] Given the current practice of sentinel node biopsy for axillary staging in most breast cancer patients, an axillary dissection is now reserved as more of a therapeutic rather than diagnostic operation. The emphasis now is to use anatomical landmarks to guide therapeutic dissection of the axilla without concentration on number of nodes removed in order to provide sufficient local control for the axilla.

After Chemotherapy
The surgical techniques that guide axillary dissection are the same regardless of whether ALND is performed before or after chemotherapy. In both instances, the area of dissection is the same, and therapeutic dissection using anatomical landmarks is performed to clear the axillary nodes to provide local control of potential regional disease.

In contrast to patients undergoing surgery prior to any systemic treatment, some studies have shown that fewer lymph nodes are retrieved following neoadjuvant chemotherapy.[14] However, other investigations have found that axillary dissections performed before chemotherapy and axillary dissections performed after chemotherapy yield similar numbers of lymph nodes.[15,16] Therefore, adequate axillary node dissection after chemotherapy should include level I and II lymph nodes within the previously outlined boundaries rather than the absolute node count.

3A. IDENTIFICATION AND PRESERVATION OF THE LONG THORACIC, THORACODORSAL, AND MEDIAL PECTORAL NERVES

Recommendation: Complete axillary dissection should include the identification and preservation of the long thoracic, thoracodorsal, and medial pectoral nerves. The nodal tissue should be dissected from these nerves with minimal nerve manipulation and without skeletonization to ensure adequate oncologic resection with minimal nerve morbidity. The nodal contents between the long thoracic and thoracodorsal nerves should be dissected to achieve optimal axillary nodal clearance.

Type of Data: Retrospective case series.

Strength of Recommendation: Although the data is retrospective, there is strong consensus of the panel to follow this recommendation based on historical evidence and to limit patient morbidity.

Rationale

A major detraction from routine use of ALND is the increased morbidity and sequelae from nerve injury, which is a major complaint of breast cancer survivors. Nerve injury can cause muscle weakness or pain, limit movement, and result in anatomical abnormalities. Thus, the preservation of the main nerves in the axilla is necessary to help ensure optimal physical outcomes. The long thoracic nerve, which innervates the serratus anterior muscle, originates from the cervical nerve roots and travels within a fatty layer along the muscle surface. However, its exact anatomy varies among patients. Intentional or inadvertent transection of the nerve results in serratus muscle palsy that manifests as pain, weakness, limited shoulder elevation, and scapular winging.[17] Additional surgery and/or years of therapy may be necessary to recover function that is lost as a result of transecting the nerve.[18,19]

The thoracodorsal nerve, which innervates the latissimus dorsi muscle, arises primarily from the C7 and C8 cervical nerve roots and descends behind the axillary vein before joining with the thoracodorsal artery and vein to form the thoracodorsal neurovascular bundle. Although contemporary practice favors preserving the thoracodorsal nerve, this nerve can be resected if the nerve is encased by tumor. However, resecting the nerve is rarely necessary given the widespread use of systemic neoadjuvant chemotherapy. Transection of the thoracodorsal nerve results in weakness or atrophy of the latissimus dorsi muscle.

A complete ALND should include resection of the tissue between the long thoracic and thoracodorsal nerves. Retrospective studies have reported that nodal tissue anterior to the subscapularis muscle in this area is present in 56% to 67% of patients and that 10% of these nodes are positive.[20,21]

The medial pectoral nerve, which innervates the lower parts of the pectoralis major and pectoralis minor muscles, arises from the medial cord of the brachial plexus and is located lateral to the lateral pectoral nerve.[22] Transection of this nerve causes weakness and atrophy of the pectoralis minor muscle and the lateral and inferior portions of the pectoralis major muscle and results in muscle fibrosis. The nerve can be divided in cases of dense tumor involvement.

3B. IDENTIFICATION AND PRESERVATION OF THE SECOND AND THIRD INTERCOSTOBRACHIAL NERVES

Recommendation: The axilla should be carefully dissected to identify and preserve the intercostobrachial nerves (ICBNs). In the level I axilla, these nerves exit the chest wall through the intercostal and serratus anterior muscles and cross the axilla parallel to the axillary vessels. The second ICBN, which provides sensation to the skin of the medial and posterior upper arm, is generally the largest and most superior of the ICBNs. Unless the nerve is encased by tumor, this nerve should be spared by dissecting it from the axillary fat. Once released, the nerve is positioned inferior to the axillary vein.

Type of Data: Small prospective trials and a larger retrospective dataset.

Strength of Recommendation: There is moderate evidence to support this recommendation.

Rationale

Four small prospective trials with follow-up durations ranging from 3 to 38 months have investigated the value of ICBN preservation by randomizing patients to ALND with ICBN preservation or ALND without ICBN preservation. These trials, each of which enrolled fewer than 130 patients, revealed no significant difference in the rates of survival or axillary disease recurrence between patients who did and patients who did not have ICBN preservation. However, whereas Freeman et al,[23] Abdullah et al,[24] and Torresan et al[25] found that patients with ICBN preservation had significantly fewer sensory deficits and symptoms than patients with no ICBN preservation, Salmon et al[26] found that ICBN preservation provided no functional advantage. Findings from a retrospective study with a larger patient cohort and longer follow-up suggest that ligating or damaging the ICBNs during axillary surgery exacerbates sensory changes in the arm that may persist for years.[27]

4. DRAIN PLACEMENT

Recommendation: Optimal drain placement following standard level I, II, and/or III ALND is essential to preventing seroma in order to avoid delays to adjuvant treatment.

Type of Data: Multiple randomized trials and two meta-analyses.

Strength of Recommendation: There is strong evidence to support this recommendation.

Rationale

One of the most common complications of ALND is seroma. Seromas or subcutaneous fluid collections are often painful for patients and can increase infectious complications. Persistent seroma can lead to mild or severe infections and/or delays in adjuvant therapy, thus potentially affecting oncologic outcomes. Two meta-analyses have systematically reviewed nine randomized controlled trials that compared the outcomes of patients who underwent ALND with drainage to those of patients who underwent ALND with no or short-term drainage.[28,29] The numbers of patients included in each of these trials ranged from 40 to 227; more than 950 patients total were included.[28,29] Compared with patients who had no or only short-term drainage, patients who had volume-controlled axillary drainage (in whom drain removal was performed only after fluid volumes decreased to <30 to <50 mL/day) were significantly less likely to develop clinically significant seroma. Patients with drains had significantly fewer seromas, fewer aspirations, and smaller aspiration volumes. Overall, these findings were consistent regardless of whether ALND was performed with segmental resection or mastectomy. Although multiple studies have compared the different techniques and instruments or devices used for ALND, as well as the use of different pharmacologic agents to potentially decrease drainage following ALND,[30] comparisons of these studies and their patient cohorts are hindered by potential differences in techniques, drain usage, drain removal criteria, and extent of disease and axillary dissection.

REFERENCES

1. Berg JW. The significance of axillary node levels in the study of breast carcinoma. *Cancer* 1955;8(4):776–778.
2. Veronesi U, Luini A, Galimberti V, et al. Extent of metastatic axillary involvement in 1446 cases of breast cancer. *Eur J Surg Oncol* 1990;16(2):127–133.
3. Veronesi U, Rilke F, Luini A, et al. Distribution of axillary node metastases by level of invasion. An analysis of 539 cases. *Cancer* 1987;59(4):682–687.
4. Boova RS, Bonanni R, Rosato FE. Patterns of axillary nodal involvement in breast cancer. Predictability of level one dissection. *Ann Surg* 1982;196(6):642–644.
5. Tominaga T, Takashima S, Danno M. Randomized clinical trial comparing level II and level III axillary node dissection in addition to mastectomy for breast cancer. *Br J Surg* 2004;91(1): 38–43.
6. Kodama H, Nio Y, Iguchi C, et al. Ten-year follow-up results of a randomised controlled study comparing level-I vs level-III axillary lymph node dissection for primary breast cancer. *Br J Cancer* 2006;95(7):811–816.
7. Danforth DN Jr, Findlay PA, McDonald HD, et al. Complete axillary lymph node dissection for stage I-II carcinoma of the breast. *J Clin Oncol* 1986;4(5):655–662.
8. Cody HS III, Egeli RA, Urban JA. Rotter's node metastases. Therapeutic and prognostic considerations in early breast carcinoma. *Ann Surg* 1984;199(3):266–270.
9. Chandawarkar RY, Shinde SR. Interpectoral nodes in carcinoma of the breast: requiem or resurrection. *J Surg Oncol* 1996;62(3):158–161.
10. Vrdoljak DV, Ramljak V, Muzina D, et al. Analysis of metastatic involvement of interpectoral (Rotter's) lymph nodes related to tumor location, size, grade and hormone receptor status in breast cancer. *Tumori* 2005;91(2):177–181.
11. Kay S. Evaluation of Rotter's lymph nodes in radical mastectomy specimens as a guide to prognosis. *Cancer* 1965;18(11):1441–1444.
12. Durkin K, Haagensen CD. An improved technique for the study of lymph nodes in surgical specimens. *Ann Surg* 1980;191(4):419–429.
13. Kiricuta CI, Tausch J. A mathematical model of axillary lymph node involvement based on 1446 complete axillary dissections in patients with breast carcinoma. *Cancer* 1992;69(10):2496–2501.

14. Neuman H, Carey LA, Ollila DW, et al. Axillary lymph node count is lower after neoadjuvant chemotherapy. *Am J Surg* 2006;191(6):827–829.
15. Straver ME, Rutgers EJ, Oldenburg HS, et al. Accurate axillary lymph node dissection is feasible after neoadjuvant chemotherapy. *Am J Surg* 2009;198(1):46–50.
16. Boughey JC, Donohue JH, Jakub JW, et al. Number of lymph nodes identified at axillary dissection. *Cancer* 2010;116(14):3322–3329.
17. Wiater JM, Flatow EL. Long thoracic nerve injury. *Clin Orthop Relat Res* 1999;(368):17–27.
18. Nath RK, Lyons AB, Bietz G. Microneurolysis and decompression of long thoracic nerve injury are effective in reversing scapular winging: long-term results in 50 cases. *BMC Musculoskelet Disord* 2007;8:25.
19. Nath RK, Melcher SE. Rapid recovery of serratus anterior muscle function after microneurolysis of long thoracic nerve injury. *J Brachial Plex Peripher Nerve Inj* 2007;2:4.
20. Rabie AS, Eldweny HI, Abdel Maksoud IG, et al. Value of internerve tissue dissection during axillary lymphadenectomy for early breast cancer. *J Egypt Natl Canc Inst* 2007;19(4):249–253.
21. Mostafa A, Mokbel K, Engledow A, et al. Is dissection of the internerve tissue during axillary lymphadenectomy for breast cancer necessary? *Eur J Surg Oncol* 2000;26(2):153–154.
22. Porzionato A, Macchi V, Stecco C, et al. Surgical anatomy of the pectoral nerves and the pectoral musculature. *Clin Anat* 2012;25(5):559–575.
23. Freeman SR, Washington SJ, Pritchard T, et al. Long term results of a randomised prospective study of preservation of the intercostobrachial nerve. *Eur J Surg Oncol* 2003;29(3):213–215.
24. Abdullah TI, Iddon J, Barr L, et al. Prospective randomized controlled trial of preservation of the intercostobrachial nerve during axillary node clearance for breast cancer. *Brit J Surg* 1998;85(10):1443–1445.
25. Torresan RZ, Cabello C, Conde DM, et al. Impact of the preservation of the intercostobrachial nerve in axillary lymphadenectomy due to breast cancer. *Breast J* 2003;9(5):389–392.
26. Salmon RJ, Ansquer Y, Asselain B. Preservation versus section of intercostal-brachial nerve (IBN) in axillary dissection for breast cancer—a prospective randomized trial. *Eur J Surg Oncol* 1998;24(3):158–161.
27. Baron RH, Fey JV, Borgen PI, et al. Eighteen sensations after breast cancer surgery: a 5-year comparison of sentinel lymph node biopsy and axillary lymph node dissection. *Ann Surg Oncol* 2007;14(5):1653–1661.
28. Droeser R, Frey D, Oertli D, et al. Volume-controlled vs no/short-term drainage after axillary lymph node dissection in breast cancer surgery: a meta-analysis. *Breast* 2009;18(2):109–114.
29. He XD, Guo ZH, Tian JH, et al. Whether drainage should be used after surgery for breast cancer? A systematic review of randomized controlled trials. *Med Oncol* 2011;28:S22–S30.
30. Van Bemmel A, Van de Velde C, Schmitz R, et al. Prevention of seroma formation after axillary dissection in breast cancer: a systematic review. *Eur J Surg Oncol* 2011;37(10):829–835.

Lymphadenectomy: Key Question

For women with breast cancer and a positive sentinel lymph node, do level I and II axillary dissection, sentinel lymph node biopsy followed by limited axillary dissection, and sentinel lymph node biopsy followed by radiation therapy all result in axillary recurrence rates of less than 5%?

INTRODUCTION

Sentinel lymph node (SLN) biopsy is the standard procedure for staging invasive breast cancer in patients who have a clinically negative axilla. Before 2011, most guidelines advised that patients found to have positive SLNs on SLN biopsy should undergo completion axillary lymph node dissection (cALND) following breast-conserving surgery. However, observational studies have revealed that selected patients have a low chance of axillary recurrence regardless of whether they undergo cALND. For example, Yi et al[1] identified nearly 27,000 patients from the Surveillance, Epidemiology, and End Results database who had invasive breast cancer and did not undergo cALND and found that their axillary recurrence rate was only 0.1% at a median follow-up time of 50 months. Similarly, Bilimoria et al[2] identified more than 97,000 patients with SLN-positive breast cancer from the United States National Cancer Data Base and found no significant difference in regional control or survival between patients who underwent cALND and those who had observation alone. These studies' findings clearly suggest that selected patients with SLN-positive breast cancer can forgo cALND.

In 1999, the American College of Surgeons Oncology Group initiated the Z0011 trial, which randomized breast cancer patients with a positive SLN to either cALND or observation following breast-conserving surgery.[3] The trial demonstrated that there was no difference in local control or overall survival in patients who had a cALND versus standard adjuvant treatment including radiation, therefore negating the need for routine use of cALND in patients with early stage disease undergoing breast cancer treatment. These results were soon embraced by the surgical oncology community and changed practice substantially. For example, the National Comprehensive Cancer Network (NCCN)[4] now advises that cALND can be omitted in patients who meet the Z0011 criteria: NCCN recommends SLN resection alone without cALND dissection in women ≥18 years of age with T1/T2 tumors, fewer than three positive SLNs, and who are undergoing breast-conserving surgery and whole-breast irradiation. The panel recommends level I or II axillary dissection (1) when patients have clinically positive nodes at the time of diagnosis that is confirmed by FNA or core biopsy or (2) when sentinel nodes are not identified. For patients who do not meet the inclusion criteria of Z0011 trial, the NCCN recommends cALND for axilla management.[4] The disadvantage of cALND is the increased morbidity compared to SLN biopsy. Radiation for local control of the axilla has been a known alternative for many years. For example, B-04 randomized women with known positive axillary nodes to radiation versus cALND and found no difference in overall survival or local control.[5] We conducted an extensive literature review to determine whether cALND, axillary radiotherapy, or observation offer similar regional control and survival in patients who do not meet the Z0011 criteria. Herein, we summarize the findings of reported studies, including a previously completed systematic review, investigating axilla management with radiation therapy (RT) or with observation alone.

METHODOLOGY

We searched the PubMed online database in October 2013 to identify studies that evaluated the need for additional axillary management in patients with SLN-positive breast cancer. We used PubMed's Advanced Search Builder to identify articles indexed using the Medical Subject Headings "lymph node excision" (OR "axillary node dissection" OR "axillary node dissections") AND "sentinel lymph node biopsy" (OR "sentinel node biopsy" OR "limited axillary dissection") AND "radiotherapy" (OR "radiation therapy") AND "neoplasm recurrence, local" (OR "recurrence") AND "breast" (OR breast neoplasms) AND "neoplasms." Reviews were excluded from the search. We identified 284 articles for review; within this search we identified a previously completed systematic review which served as the basis of this literature review.[6] In addition to the previously published systematic review, we included randomized controlled trials that would provide level 1 evidence to address this topic.

FINDINGS

Observation or Completion Axillary Lymph Node Dissection

The findings of studies of patients with SLN-positive breast cancer who underwent cALND or had observation are summarized in Table 3-1. In the International Breast Cancer Study Group Trial 23-01, a multicenter randomized, noninferiority, phase III trial, breast cancer patients with micrometastasis (<2 mm) in the SLNs only were randomized to observation alone (467 patients) or cALND (464 patients). At a median follow-up time of 5 years, only four (0.8%) patients in the observation group and one (0.2%) patient in the cALND group developed axillary recurrences; disease-free survival (DFS) and overall survival (OS) did not differ significantly between the groups.[7] The 23-01 trial's findings clearly suggest that cALND can be omitted in breast cancer patients who have SLN micrometastases. In contrast to the 23-01 trial, the Z0011 trial included patients with SLN macrometastases (>2 mm). Similar to the 23-01 trial, findings from the Z0011 trial suggest that cALND can be omitted in selected patients. At a median follow-up time of 6.3 years, four (0.9%) patients in the observation group and two (0.5%) patients in the cALND group had regional recurrence[8]; the groups' rates of DFS and OS did not differ significantly.[9] Consistent with these findings, many observational studies have reported that breast cancer patients with SLN macrometastases in whom cALND is omitted have a low axillary recurrence rate. Selection bias notwithstanding, these studies provide additional evidence that cALND can be omitted in selected patients with SLN-positive breast cancer who have favorable clinicopathologic features, including patients with T1 or T2 tumors who are clinically node-negative and have one or two positive sentinel lymph nodes.

TABLE 3-1 Patients with Sentinel Lymph Node–Positive Breast Cancer Followed with Observation Alone

Author, Year	Study Design	Study Period	Median Follow-Up Time, Years	Surgery for Primary Tumor	No. of Patients	No. of Patients with Regional Recurrence (%)	5-Year Disease-Free Survival Rate %	5-Year Overall Survival Rate %
Giuliano et al, 2011[3],*	Multicenter randomized study	1999–2004	6.3	BCS	425	4 (0.9)	83.9	92.5
Galimberti et al, 2013[21],†	Multicenter randomized study	2001–2010	5.0	BCS or mastectomy	467	4 (0.8)	87.8	97.5
Milgrom et al, 2012[22]	Single-center retrospective study	1997–2009	4.8	BCS or mastectomy	535	6 (1.1)	94.8% (mastectomy), 91% (BCS)‡	97.8% (mastectomy), 92.6% (BCS)‡
Yegiyants et al, 2010[23]	Single-center prospective cohort	1997–2004	6.6	BCS	47	2 (4.3)	Not reported	1 (2)**
Schrenk et al, 2005[24]	Multicenter retrospective study	1996–2003	4.0	BCS or mastectomy	20	0 (0)	Not reported	1 (5)**
Guenther et al, 2003[25]	Multicenter prospective study	1996–2001	2.6	Not reported	46	0 (0)	1 (2.2)**	0 (0)**
Fant et al, 2003[26]	Single-center retrospective study	1998–2000	2.5	Not reported	31	0 (0)	Not reported	Not reported

BCS, breast-conserving surgery.
*A total of 436 patients were included in determining the 5-year disease-free survival rate and the 5-year overall survival rate.
†All patients had micrometastatic disease.
‡Four-year disease-free survival rate/overall survival rate.
**Number of deaths (%).

This recommendation is based on strong evidence (level 1B) from randomized controlled trials supported by observational studies.

Axillary Radiation Therapy

Studies that evaluated the use of RT without cALND for control of axillary disease were completed before the SLN biopsy era and provide support for the omission of cALND in patients with SLN-positive breast cancer (Table 3-2). For example, in the National Surgical Adjuvant Breast and Bowel Project B-04 trial, 1079 breast cancer patients with clinically negative nodes were randomized to radical mastectomy, total mastectomy plus axillary RT, or total mastectomy with delayed ALND in the event of regional recurrence. An analysis of long-term follow-up data did not reveal a significant difference in OS among the three groups.[10] Similarly, Veronesi et al[11] conducted a randomized trial of 435 breast cancer patients with clinically negative nodes to observation or axillary RT following breast-conserving surgery and found no significant differences in recurrence or survival between the two groups at a median follow-up time of 63 months. In another study, Louis-Sylvestre et al[12] prospectively randomized 658 breast cancer patients who had primary tumors less than 3 cm in diameter and clinically negative lymph nodes to ALND or axillary RT following breast-conserving surgery. Although the OS rates of the two groups (73.8% and 75.5%) were virtually identical after 15 years of follow-up, the axillary recurrence rate of the RT group (3%) was significantly higher than that of the ALND group (1%; $P = .04$). In this study, 21% of patients in the ALND group had positive lymph nodes, and a similar proportion of patients in the axillary RT group had been assumed to have positive lymph nodes.

Studies in the SLN biopsy era have demonstrated that patients with positive SLNs who receive axillary RT can achieve a low rate of axillary recurrence (Table 3-3). For example, Sanuki et al[13] retrospectively analyzed 104 patients who had cT1-2cN0M0, SLN-positive breast cancer and received breast-conserving surgery and axillary RT and found no axillary recurrence at a median follow-up time of 4.6 years. In a prospective cohort study, Gadd et al[14] found that only 1 of 73 patients with cT1-2N0M0, SLN-positive breast cancer who underwent breast-conserving surgery and axillary RT had axillary recurrence at a median follow-up of 32 months.

The multicenter randomized prospective "After Mapping the Axilla: Radiotherapy or Surgery? (AMAROS)" trial was initiated in 2001 to directly compare the efficacy of axillary RT to that of cALND in patients with SLN-positive breast cancer.[15] Of the 4,806 patients in the trial, 744 in the cALND arm and 681 in the axillary RT arm had a positive SLN. At a median follow-up of 6.1 years, there was no significant difference in axillary recurrence; four (0.54%) patients in the cALND arm and seven (1.03%) patients in the axillary RT arm had axillary recurrence. The 5-year OS and DFS rates of the cALND arm (93.27% and 86.90%, respectively) and axillary RT arm (92.52% and 82.65%, respectively) did not differ significantly ($P = .34$ and .18, respectively). This study demonstrates that axillary radiation therapy is as effective as axillary node dissection in reducing axillary recurrence in node-positive patients.

These studies' findings indicate with strong evidence (level 1) that axillary RT and cALND achieve similar local control and OS in patients with SLN-positive breast

TABLE 3-2   Patients with Sentinel Lymph Node Biopsy–Positive Breast Cancer who Underwent Completion Axillary Lymph Node Dissection

Author, Year	Study Design	Study Period	Median Follow-Up Time, Years	Surgery for Primary Tumor	No. of Patients	No. of Patients with Regional Recurrence (%)	5-Year Disease-Free Survival Rate %	5-Year Overall Survival Rate %
AMAROS trial, 2013[15]	Multicenter randomized study	2001–2005	6.1	BCS or mastectomy	744	4 (0.54)	86.9	93.3
IBCSG 23-01[21]	Multicenter randomized study	2001–2010	Median, 5.0	BCS or mastectomy	464	1 (0.2)	69 (15)	19 (4)
ACOSOG Z0011[3]	Multicenter randomized study	1999–2004	Median, 6.3	BCS	388	2 (0.5)	5-year DFS rate, 82.2%	52 (13)
GIVOM trial[28]	Multicenter randomized study	1999–2004	Median, 4.6	BCS or mastectomy	94	0 (0)	Not reported	Not reported
Mansel et al[29]	Multicenter randomized study	1999–2003	Mean, 1.0	BCS or mastectomy	83	0 (0)	Not reported	Not reported
Veronesi et al[30]	Single-center randomized study	1998–1999	Mean, 7.9	BCS	92	0 (0)	Not reported	Not reported
Canavese et al[31]	Single-center randomized study	1998–2001	Median, 5.5	BCS or mastectomy	31	0 (0)	Not reported	Not reported

ACOSOG, American College of Surgeons Oncology Group; AMAROS, After Mapping of the Axilla: Radiotherapy or Surgery; BCS, breast-conserving surgery; cALND, completion axillary lymph node dissection; GIVOM, Gruppo Interdisciplinare Veneto di Oncologia Mammaria; IBCSG, International Breast Cancer Study Group.

TABLE 3-3   Patients with Sentinel Lymph Node–Positive Breast Cancer who Received Axillary Radiotherapy

Author, Year	Study Design	Study Period	Median Follow-Up Time, Years	Surgery for Primary Tumor	No. of Patients	No. of Patients with Regional Recurrence (%)	5-Year Disease-Free Survival Rate %	5-Year Overall Survival Rate %
AMAROS trial, 2013[15]	Multicenter randomized study	2001–2005	6.1	BCS or mastectomy	681	7 (1.03)	82.65%	92.52%
Gadd et al, 2005[14]	Single-center prospective cohort study	2001–2004	2.6	BCS	73	1 (1.4)	Not reported	Not reported
Sanuki et al, 2013[13]	Single-center retrospective study	1988–2011	4.6	BCS	104	0 (0)	Not reported	1 (1)[†]
Mansel et al, 2006[27]	Multicenter randomized study	1999–2003	1.0[*]	BCS or mastectomy	33	0 (0)	Not reported	Not reported

AMAROS, After Mapping of the Axilla: Radiotherapy or Surgery; BCS, breast-conserving surgery.
[*]Mean follow-up time.
[†]Number of deaths (%).

cancer. For patients who are not candidates to forgo additional axillary treatment after SLN biopsy, axillary RT and axillary dissection have similar success.

Completion Axillary Lymph Node Dissection Plus Axillary Radiation Therapy

In the pre-SLN biopsy era, the combination of axillary RT and cALND was widely investigated. For example, the Danish Breast Cancer Cooperative Group conducted a subgroup analysis of 1,152 patients with node-positive disease[16] and found that the addition of postmastectomy radiation therapy (PMRT), which included axillary RT to cALND, reduced the 15-year locoregional failure rate from 51% to 10% (P <.001) in patients with four or more positive nodes and from 27% to 4% (P <.001) in patients with one to three positive nodes. The addition of axillary RT also improved the 15-year survival rate both in patients with one to three positive nodes (57% versus 48%; P = .03) and in patients with four or more positive nodes (21% versus 12%; P = .03). In a randomized trial from British Columbia,[17] 318 patients with node-positive disease who underwent mastectomy and cALND were randomized to chemotherapy alone versus PMRT plus chemotherapy. At 20 years of follow-up, locoregional DFS (74% versus 90%, respectively; relative risk [RR] = 0.36, 95% confidence interval [CI] = 0.18 to 0.71; P = .002) and OS (47% versus 37%; RR = 0.73, 95% CI = 0.55 to 0.98; P = .03) rates of the patients who received PMRT were significantly higher than those of the patients who received no further therapy. An individual patient-based meta-analysis from Early Breast Cancer Trialists' Collaborative Group further demonstrated the efficacy of PMRT in attaining locoregional control regardless of nodal status.[18] Postmastectomy radiotherapy can produce a substantial absolute reduction in this risk of local recurrence, and although it has little effect on breast cancer mortality during the first few years, it can produce a moderate, but definite, reduction in longer term cancer mortality.[19]

The National Cancer Institute of Canada Clinical Trials Group MA.20 trial[19] was initiated in 2000 to specifically investigate the efficacy of axillary RT in preventing axillary recurrence. A total of 1,832 breast cancer patients who underwent breast-conserving surgery and cALND were randomized to whole breast irradiation (WBI) alone or WBI plus comprehensive regional nodal irradiation (RNI). At a median follow-up time of 62 months, four (0.4%) patients in the WBI plus RNI group and 21 (2.3%) patients in the WBI alone group had regional recurrence only. Compared with WBI alone, WBI plus RNI was associated with significantly improved locoregional DFS (hazard ratio [HR] = 0.59, P = .02; 5-year risk, 96.8% and 94.5%, respectively), distant DFS (HR = 0.64, P = .002; 5-year risk, 92.4% and 87.0%, respectively), DFS (HR = 0.68, P = .003; 5-year risk, 89.7% and 84.0%, respectively), and OS (HR = 0.76, P = .07; 5-year risk, 92.3% and 90.7%, respectively). WBI plus RNI was also associated with a higher risk of pneumonitis (P = .01) and lymphedema (P = .004) than WBI alone. However, this study has only been presented in abstract form and reports recurrence rates associated with cALND alone that are higher than those of other published studies.

To date, no randomized controlled trials have compared the regional control rates of patients with SLN-positive breast cancer who underwent cALND, received axillary RT, or had observation alone. The findings of existing studies seem to suggest that regional treatment beyond SLN biopsy is not necessary for some patients who have a very low risk of axillary recurrence; in particular, there is strong evidence that additional axillary treatment is not necessary in patients who meet the Z0011 trial criteria or who have SLN micrometastasis. In contrast, as the findings of the MA-20 trial suggest, aggressive treatment with cALND and/or RT to the nodal basin may result in improved survival for patients at a high risk for axillary recurrence.

In determining whether cALND or axillary RT is appropriate for a patient, the surgeon must weigh the risks of each intervention against the benefits, and the patient should be educated about the associated complications with each procedure. The current challenge is to reliably identify the population of patients who require no additional treatment to the axilla and those for whom RT and/or cALND will improve survival. Current data suggests that patients who have high-risk primary tumors (such as high-grade tumors with extensive lymphovascular invasion), have undergone mastectomy and have macrometastasis, or have received neoadjuvant chemotherapy should undergo cALND if they have positive sentinel lymph nodes. Further investigation of these groups is necessary to determine the extent of treatment needed.

CONCLUSION

For breast cancer patients with T1 or T2 tumors and one or two positive SLNs who meet the Z0011 trial criteria, observation alone following breast-conserving surgery is adequate. This recommendation for omitting cALND is supported by level 1B evidence from randomized controlled trials and large observational studies. Observation alone is also adequate for patients with micrometastases in one or two SLNs who undergo lumpectomy or mastectomy, a recommendation that is also supported by level 1B evidence from randomized controlled trials. Selected patients with positive SLNs who are at high risk for axillary recurrence can receive axillary RT instead of undergoing cALND.

The combination of axillary RT and cALND might be beneficial for regional control in patients with SLN-positive disease, but the risk–benefit balance of this combined approach should be considered carefully. This recommendation is supported by level 2B evidence from randomized controlled trials with important limitations. Although both the "After Mapping the Axilla: Radiotherapy or Surgery?" and MA-20 trials demonstrated that axillary RT and cALND have similar risks and benefits, neither study included a control arm composed of patients who received no additional treatment.

REFERENCES

1. Yi M, Giordano SH, Meric-Bernstam F, et al. Trends in and outcomes from sentinel lymph node biopsy (SLNB) alone vs. SLNB with axillary lymph node dissection for node-positive breast cancer patients: experience from the SEER database. *Ann Surg Oncol* 2010;17(3): 343–351.
2. Bilimoria KY, Bentrem DJ, Hansen NM, et al. Comparison of sentinel lymph node biopsy alone and completion axillary lymph node dissection for node-positive breast cancer. *J Clin Oncol* 2009;27(18):2946–2953.
3. Giuliano AE, Hunt KK, Ballman KV, et al. Axillary dissection vs no axillary dissection in women with invasive breast cancer and sentinel node metastasis: a randomized clinical trial. *JAMA* 2011;305(6):569–575.

4. Carlson RW, Anderson B, Bensinger W, et al. NCCN practice guidelines for breast cancer. *Oncology* 2000;14(11A):33–49.

5. Fisher B, Jeong J-H, Anderson S, et al. Twenty-five-year follow-up of a randomized trial comparing radical mastectomy, total mastectomy, and total mastectomy followed by irradiation. *N Engl J Med* 2002;347(8):567–575.

6. Rao R, Euhus D, Mayo HG, et al. Axillary node interventions in breast cancer: a systematic review. *JAMA* 2013;310(13):1385–1394.

7. Veronesi U, Orecchia R, Zurrida S, et al. Avoiding axillary dissection in breast cancer surgery: a randomized trial to assess the role of axillary radiotherapy. *Ann Oncol* 2005;16(3): 383–388.

8. Giuliano AE, McCall L, Beitsch P, et al. Locoregional recurrence after sentinel lymph node dissection with or without axillary dissection in patients with sentinel lymph node metastases: the American College of Surgeons Oncology Group Z0011 randomized trial. *Ann Surg* 2010;252(3):426–432; discussion 32–33.

9. Giuliano AE, Hunt KK, Ballman KV, et al. Axillary dissection vs no axillary dissection in women with invasive breast cancer and sentinel node metastasis: a randomized clinical trial. *JAMA* 2011;305(6):569–575.

10. Fisher B, Jeong JH, Anderson S, et al. Twenty-five-year follow-up of a randomized trial comparing radical mastectomy, total mastectomy, and total mastectomy followed by irradiation. *N Engl J Med* 2002;347(8):567–575.

11. Veronesi U, Orecchia R, Zurrida S, et al. Avoiding axillary dissection in breast cancer surgery: a randomized trial to assess the role of axillary radiotherapy. *Ann Oncol* 2005;16(3):383–388.

12. Louis-Sylvestre C, Clough K, Asselain B, et al. Axillary treatment in conservative management of operable breast cancer: dissection or radiotherapy? Results of a randomized study with 15 years of follow-up. *J Clin Oncol* 2004;22(1):97–101.

13. Sanuki N, Takeda A, Amemiya A, et al. Outcomes of clinically node-negative breast cancer without axillary dissection: can preserved axilla be safely treated with radiation after a positive sentinel node biopsy? *Clin Breast Cancer* 2013;13(1):69–76.

14. Gadd M HJ, Taghian A, Hughes K, et al. Prospective study of axillary radiation without axillary dissection for breast cancer patients with a positive sentinel node. *Breast Cancer Res Treat* 2005;94:S13.

15. Donker M, van Tienhoven G, Straver ME, et al. Radiotherapy or surgery of the axilla after a positive sentinel node in breast cancer (EORTC 10981-22023 AMAROS): a randomised, multicentre, open-label, phase 3 non-inferiority trial. *Lancet Oncol* 2014;15(12):1303–1310.

16. Overgaard M, Nielsen HM, Overgaard J. Is the benefit of postmastectomy irradiation limited to patients with four or more positive nodes, as recommended in international consensus reports? A subgroup analysis of the DBCG 82 b&c randomized trials. *Radiother Oncol* 2007;82(3): 247–253.

17. Ragaz J, Olivotto IA, Spinelli JJ, et al. Locoregional radiation therapy in patients with high-risk breast cancer receiving adjuvant chemotherapy: 20-year results of the British Columbia randomized trial. *J Natl Cancer Inst* 2005;97(2):116–126.

18. Clarke M, Collins R, Darby S, et al. Effects of radiotherapy and of differences in the extent of surgery for early breast cancer on local recurrence and 15-year survival: an overview of the randomised trials. *Lancet.* 2005;366(9503):2087–2106.

19. Clarke M, Collins R, Darby S, et al. Effects of radiotherapy and of differences in the extent of surgery for early breast cancer on local recurrence and 15-year survival: an overview of the randomised trials. *Lancet* 2005;366(9503):2087–2106.

20. Whelan T, Olivotto I, Ackerman I, et al. NCIC-CTG MA. 20: an intergroup trial of regional nodal irradiation in early breast cancer. *J Clin Oncol* 2011;29(18)(suppl 1):LBA1003.

21. Galimberti V, Cole BF, Zurrida S, et al. Axillary dissection versus no axillary dissection in patients with sentinel-node micrometastases (IBCSG 23-01): a phase 3 randomised controlled trial. *Lancet Oncol* 2013;14(4):297–305.

22. Milgrom S, Cody H, Tan L, et al. Characteristics and outcomes of sentinel node-positive breast cancer patients after total mastectomy without axillary-specific treatment. *Ann Surg Oncol* 2012;19(12):3762–3770.

23. Yegiyants S, Romero LM, Haigh PI, et al. Completion axillary lymph node dissection not required for regional control in patients with breast cancer who have micrometastases in a sentinel node. *Arch Surg* 2010;145(6):564–569.

24. Schrenk P, Konstantiniuk P, Wolfl S, et al. Prediction of non-sentinel lymph node status in breast cancer with a micrometastatic sentinel node. *Brit J Surg* 2005;92(6):707–713.

25. Guenther JM, Hansen NM, DiFronzo LA, et al. Axillary dissection is not required for all patients with breast cancer and positive sentinel nodes. *Arch Surg* 2003;138(1):52–56.
26. Fant JS, Grant MD, Knox SM, et al. Preliminary outcome analysis in patients with breast cancer and a positive sentinel lymph node who declined axillary dissection. *Ann Surg Oncol* 2003;10(2):126–130.
27. Mansel RE, Fallowfield L, Kissin M, et al. Randomized multicenter trial of sentinel node biopsy versus standard axillary treatment in operable breast cancer: the ALMANAC Trial. *J Natl Cancer Inst* 2006;98(9):599–609.
28. Zavagno G, De Salvo GL, Scalco G, et al. A randomized clinical trial on sentinel lymph node biopsy versus axillary lymph node dissection in breast cancer: results of the Sentinella/GIVOM trial. *Ann Surg* 2008;247(2):207–213.
29. Mansel RE, Fallowfield L, Kissin M, et al. Randomized multicenter trial of sentinel node biopsy versus standard axillary treatment in operable breast cancer: the ALMANAC Trial. *J Natl Cancer Inst* 2006;98(9):599–609.
30. Veronesi U, Paganelli G, Viale G, et al. A randomized comparison of sentinel-node biopsy with routine axillary dissection in breast cancer. *N Engl J Med* 2003;349(6):546–553.
31. Canavese G, Catturich A, Vecchio C, et al. Sentinel node biopsy compared with complete axillary dissection for staging early breast cancer with clinically negative lymph nodes: results of randomized trial. *Ann Oncol* 2009;20(6):1001–1007.

CHAPTER 4

Sentinel Lymphadenectomy

CRITICAL ELEMENTS

- Identification of All Sentinel Nodes
- Technique for Injecting Localizing Tracer or Dye
- Preincision Evaluation of Drainage Pattern
- Node Removal Technique to Limit Seroma Formation

1. IDENTIFICATION OF ALL SENTINEL NODES

Recommendation: All sentinel nodes must be identified, removed, and subjected to pathologic analysis to ensure that sentinel lymph node mapping and sentinel lymphadenectomy provide accurate information for breast cancer staging. Sentinel nodes are defined by the presence of a tracer (radioactive tracer and/or colored dye) that has been previously injected into the affected breast or by the presence of a dominant palpable lymph node identified by the operating surgeon.

Type of Data: Randomized multicenter prospective trials.

Strength of Recommendation: The group strongly endorses this recommendation based on strong evidence.

Rationale

The original definition of a sentinel lymph node was "the first draining lymph node on the direct pathway from the primary tumor site."[1] According to the sentinel node hypothesis, tumor cells migrate from a primary tumor focus to the first draining lymph node(s) before involving distal lymph nodes. Sentinel lymph nodes are variably located but are usually within the level I or II axilla near the lateral thoracic vein.[2,3] The median number of sentinel nodes removed during a sentinel lymphadenectomy is between two and three; in the two largest randomized clinical trials comparing sentinel

67

lymphadenectomy to axillary node dissection, the mean numbers of sentinel nodes removed per procedure were 2.8 in the National Surgical Adjuvant Breast and Bowel Project B32 trial[3] and 2.2 in the ALMANAC (Axillary Lymphatic Mapping Against Nodal Axillary Clearance) trial.[4] For cases in which only one sentinel lymph node is removed, the reported false negative rate of the procedure is greater than 10%, potentially leading to the assignment of lower than actual disease stages to some breast cancers.[5]

Identification Using a Radioactive Tracer

Most commonly technetium sulfur colloid is injected in the breast an hour prior to the planned sentinel node biopsy, but the tracer can be injected the day before if more convenient. After the patient is under general anesthesia, a handheld gamma detection probe is held over the axilla to identify the area of greatest radioactivity. A 3- to 6-cm incision is then made near the area of greatest radioactivity within the region at the base of the axillary hairline. The clavipectoral fascia is opened to the level I axilla, and the area around the lateral thoracic vein and second intercostobrachial nerve is evaluated using the gamma detection probe. The first sentinel node is the node with the highest absolute radioactivity count. The nodes are excised using clip, tie, or sealing device closure of the indwelling lymphatics and vessels, and blunt dissection of the surrounding fat is performed to prevent the removal of multiple nonsentinel nodes. After the first sentinel node is excised, its ex vivo highest or 10-second radioactive count is obtained and recorded, and the radioactivity of the axillary basin is reassessed. All nodes whose radioactive count is at least 10% that of the most radioactive node are considered sentinel nodes and are removed in a similar fashion, and ex vivo radioactive counts are recorded for each node. Confirmation of an elevated ex vivo count of the node ensures that it is indeed a hot node and not that the count was falsely elevated in vivo due to scatter from the primary injection in the breast.

Identification Using Vital Blue (or Colored) Dye

For sentinel node identification with a blue dye, isosulfan or methylene blue are most commonly used. The dye is injected in the breast and massaged; subsequently, the axilla is incised and opened as described for sentinel node identification with a radioactive tracer. Blunt dissection is performed to identify the dye-filled lymphatic tract. This tract is then followed proximally and distally until a blue-stained sentinel node is identified (Fig. 4-1). If more than one dye-filled lymphatic tract is identified, each is followed until a blue node is identified. Blue-stained sentinel nodes are removed in a fashion similar to that used to remove sentinel nodes identified using a radioactive tracer. Another colored tracer in current use is indocyanine green; in cases in which this tracer is used, all nodes with fluorescent tracer uptake must be identified.

Identification Using a Dual-Tracer Approach

The majority of sentinel lymphadenectomy procedures utilize a dual-tracer technique.[6] If both a radioactive tracer and blue dye have been injected, nodes that are

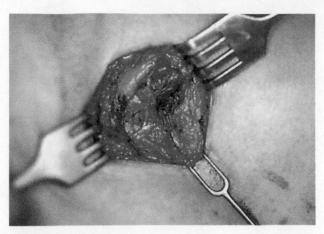

FIGURE 4-1 Sentinel node procedure demonstrating blue lymphatic leading to blue sentinel node. (Photo courtesy of Sarah Blair, MD, and Marek Dobke, MD.)

radioactive and/or stained blue are considered sentinel nodes. All blue-stained nodes should be assessed with a gamma detection probe for radioactivity, and all radioactive nodes that are removed should be assessed for the presence of blue dye. Some nodes may only be identified by one modality, as studies show that the procedure is the most accurate when dual tracer technique is utilized.[6]

Identification Using Palpation of the Axilla

As a component of sentinel lymphadenectomy, careful palpation of the level I and II axilla is essential to guiding the complete removal of all sentinel nodes. Nodes that feel abnormal on palpation should be categorized as sentinel nodes and removed regardless of whether they are radioactive or stained blue.[7]

2. TECHNIQUE FOR INJECTING LOCALIZING TRACER OR DYE

Recommendation: The site of localizing tracer or dye injection within the affected breast and/or subareolar plexus does not influence the identification of the axillary sentinel node(s).

Type of Data: Multiple single institutional series, small prospective randomized study, and systematic review.

Strength of Recommendation: Consensus of the group is that the evidence is strong.

Rationale

Over the past 15 years, several different techniques and combinations of techniques have been employed for the injection of radioactive tracer and/or dye for sentinel node identification. Pesek et al[5] published the most comprehensive and systematic

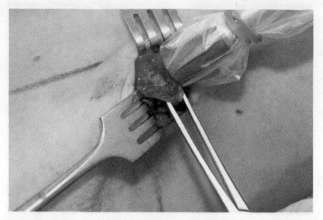

FIGURE 4-2 In cases of dual tracer, all blue nodes should be assessed for radioactivity and all radioactive nodes should be assessed for presence of blue dye. This illustrates checking for radioactivity in a blue node.

review of injection techniques for sentinel node identification. They concluded that of the seven different techniques and combinations of techniques they studied, including peritumoral (intraparenchymal) injection, sub- or (peri)areolar injection (Figs. 4-2 and 4-3), subdermal but nonintratumoral injection, intratumoral injection, peritumoral/subareolar injection, peritumoral/subdermal injection, and subareolar/subdermal injection, none had a significantly lower false negative rate than another; therefore, they could not justify recommending one technique over another.[5] A multicenter prospective randomized study found that, compared with peritumoral injection

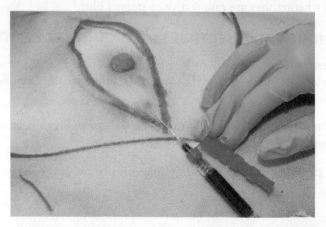

FIGURE 4-3 This demonstrates subdermal and perioareolar injection of blue dye in a patient undergoing mastectomy for clinically T2N0 breast cancer (Image courtesy of Sarah Blair MD and Marek Dobke MD)

of a radioactive tracer and blue dye, periareolar injection of a tracer and dye had a higher sentinel lymph node detection rate and higher within-node dye-tracer concordance.[7] One small study investigating radioactive tracer injection in both subareolar and peritumoral locations in individual patients (27 patients total) noted no difference in the number of axillary sentinel nodes identified using subareolar or peritumoral radioactive tracer injection; however, the study did find that peritumoral injection resulted in the localization of extra-axillary drainage sites (e.g., internal mammary [IM] nodes, paraclavicular nodes).[8,9] If extra-axillary sites are of interest, the radioactive tracer should be injected peritumorally. In developing quality metrics for sentinel node mapping (other than false negative rate, which requires a full axillary node dissection), Quan et al[6] did not include the tracer or dye injection site as one of the quality indicators because they found no data supporting one injection location over another. The findings of these studies demonstrate that no specific injection site ensures the lowest false negative rate and highest sentinel node identification rate. However, surgeons should monitor their performance of dye and radioactive tracer injection to ensure that the injection sites they use result in the identification of all sentinel nodes, an average number of removed sentinel nodes greater than 1.9, and a sentinel node positivity rate of 20% to 30%.[6]

Radioactive Tracer

Technetium-99m (99mTc)–labeled sulfur colloid is the radioactive tracer most commonly utilized for sentinel node identification; however, newer agents such as 99mTc-tilmanocept, whose use in sentinel lymphadenectomy has been approved by the U.S. Food and Drug Administration, are at least equally effective.[10] Usually, a nuclear medicine specialist injects the nuclear tracer the day of or the day before surgery, but it has also been injected by surgeons intraoperatively.[11,12] With either approach, the expected average number of sentinel nodes identified is two. The 99mTc-labeled sulfur colloid tracer, which can be filtered or unfiltered, is administered in volumes of 0.1 to 1.0 mL. The tracer can be injected at one site or multiple sites. In the National Surgical Adjuvant Breast and Bowel Project B-32 clinical trial, it was injected into multiple sites around the tumor and in the dermis above the tumor.[13] The tracer's radioactivity, which typically ranges from 0.25 mCi to 2.5 mCi at injection, depends on the time between the injection and operative intervention; higher doses are given when longer times between injection and surgery are expected.

Vital Blue (or Colored) Dye

Isosulfan blue dye is the most commonly used colored dye for sentinel node identification (Fig. 4-3). At the time of surgery, 1 to 5 mL of undiluted dye is injected into the site or sites of choice, and the breast is massaged for 2 to 5 minutes to travel through the lymphatic vessels. In 0.7% to 1.1% of cases, isosulfan blue dye has been associated with severe anaphylactic reactions requiring patient resuscitation.[13] Methylene blue dye, which has been used as a substitute for isosulfan blue dye, is less expensive and has a lower risk of allergic reaction but has been reported to have more frequent side effects such as skin necrosis, induration, and erythema (14). Methylene blue dye used for sentinel node identification is commonly diluted in normal saline at a 1:2 ratio.[14]

Documentation

All removed sentinel lymph nodes must be accurately labeled in the operating room. Detailed information must be given for each sentinel lymph node, including its description as a radioactive, blue-stained, or both radioactive and blue-stained ("hot and blue") node; a palpable hard node; or an unstained node found at the termination of a blue-stained lymphatic channel. The location of the node—axillary level I, II, or III or IM—should also be described. If a radioactive tracer was used for sentinel node identification, documentation for each removed node must include either a 10-second ex vivo radioactive count or the highest radioactive count recorded with the resected node placed on the tip of the gamma detector probe. Accurate documentation of the characteristics of the sentinel node(s) is an important indicator of the quality of sentinel lymphadenectomy (15).

3. PREINCISION EVALUATION OF DRAINAGE PATTERN

Recommendation: For sentinel node identification using a radioactive tracer, preincision skin localization of the area of highest radioactivity facilitates a minimally invasive approach to exposure in the axilla and the identification of any extra-axillary sites of nodal drainage (see Fig. 4-4). Lymphoscintigraphy is not required for sentinel node localization unless an extra-axillary site of drainage is suspected.

Type of Data: Retrospective review.

Strength of Recommendation: No strong data to recommend but low risk with potential benefit associated with adding this step.

Rationale

In cases involving nodal mapping using a radioactive colloid, surgeons should confirm an area of radioactivity concentration within the axilla and localize the area of highest radioactivity before making the incision for axillary sentinel node biopsy. These preincision steps are important regardless of whether preoperative lymphoscintigraphy is performed or whether the radioactive tracer is used with or without a colored dye. Routine lymphoscintigraphy to identify areas of high radioactivity is not recommended on the basis of a retrospective analysis of prospective data indicating that the procedure does not improve the success rate of sentinel node identification.[15–17] However, lymphoscintigraphy should be considered if (1) a surgeon or institution is in the early phases of learning sentinel lymphadenectomy or (2) there is concern that extra-axillary drainage is likely (for example, in a patient undergoing repeat sentinel node mapping for recurrent cancer) (20).

Identification of the Axillary "Hot Spot"

The majority of sentinel lymph nodes are encountered in the level I axilla within a 5-cm diameter circle centered midway between the pectoralis major and latissimus dorsi muscles at the inferior border of the axillary hairline (16). The surgeon should initiate cutaneous scanning prior to incision. Scanning should progress in either increasingly larger concentric circles or radially until an area of elevated radioactivity (the "hot spot") is identified. Marking the skin overlying the hot spot (Fig. 4-4) and confirming a diminution in the radioactive counts moving from the axillary hot spot medially towards the injection site in the breast helps identify the best location for the skin incision in the axilla, minimizing unnecessary blunt dissection of the axilla and disruption of nonsentinel nodes. In cases in which an axillary hot spot cannot be identified and lymphoscintigraphy has not been performed, lymphatic mapping with a radioactive tracer alone may not facilitate the successful removal of all sentinel nodes, and blue dye should be injected for intraoperative lymphatic mapping. The operative record should indicate whether an axillary hot spot was identified before incision.

Internal Mammary Node Removal

For patients in whom preoperative lymphoscintigraphy reveals a radioactive IM lymph node, surgeons may consider pursuing IM node removal, particularly if an axillary sentinel node is not identified or if pathologic analysis reveals the axillary sentinel node to be negative. Preincision scanning for the hot spot in such patients should be performed along the IM node chain, particularly in the second and third intercostal spaces along the lateral border of the sternum. If preoperative lympho-scintigraphy was not performed and no axillary hot spot is present, scanning along the parasternal border, particularly in the second and third intercostal spaces, is useful to determine whether an IM hot spot is present. Although the prognosis of patients with IM drainage and/or metastasis[18] is worse than that of patients without these conditions, no studies have shown that removing IM nodes conveys a survival advantage.[19] Furthermore, because isolated IM metastasis is rare, IM node removal is seldom performed.[20] Because adjuvant treatment decisions are more likely to be made from molecular panels and not necessarily low-volume regional metastasis, the

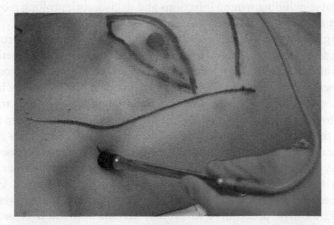

FIGURE 4-4 Demonstrates preincision localization of the area of highest count with the gamma probe in order to plan the axillary incision closest to the in-vivo sentinel nodes for resection. (Image courtesy of Sarah Blair, MD, and Marek Dobke, MD.).

rarity of IM node removal seldom affects adjuvant treatment decisions.[21] In addition, IM node removal is associated with an increased complication rate compared to sentinel node biopsy in the axilla.[19]

4. NODE REMOVAL TECHNIQUE TO LIMIT SEROMA FORMATION IN ORDER TO PREVENT DELAY TO ADJUVANT TREATMENT

Recommendation: Because no one method or device has been found to result in a lower incidence of seroma formation following sentinel lymphadenectomy, surgeons should use the approach that their experience indicates will have optimal outcomes.

Type of Data: Retrospective or small prospective studies, one systematic review.

Strength of Recommendation: No strong data for specific method to avoid seromas.

Rationale

The morbidity that may result from sentinel node biopsy is minimal compared with that which may result from conventional axillary lymph node dissection. The most frequently observed complication of sentinel lymph node biopsy is seroma, an accumulation of serous fluid under the skin. Persistent seroma can lead to mild or severe infections and/or delays in adjuvant therapy, thus potentially affecting oncologic outcomes.[22,23] In a randomized controlled trial by McCaul et al,[24] sentinel node biopsy had a significantly lower rate of seroma than conventional axillary lymph node dissection did. In their analysis of the outcomes following sentinel node surgery in the ACOSOG Z0011 trial, Lucci et al reported a seroma rate of only 6% after sentinel lymph node biopsy alone.[25] Although seroma is not a serious complication, it can lead to adverse events (including wound infections and dehiscence), prolong recovery time, increase treatment costs, and/or delay the initiation of adjuvant therapy.

Various surgical methods have been utilized in an effort to reduce seroma formation following sentinel node biopsy. However, whether one or another method results in better outcomes is unclear and no standard surgical technique for seroma prevention or treatment exists. One area of focus for reducing seroma following sentinel lymphadenectomy is lymph vessel sealing and axillary hemostasis, which traditionally have been performed using electrocautery, suture ligation, or vascular clip placement. Each of these techniques, whose use is based on surgeon preference, has its own potential complications. Suture ligation is time-consuming, and the knots used to secure the sutures may slip, causing the ligation to fail. Vascular clips may become dislodged. Electrocautery ligation may cause thermal damage to adjacent tissues. Given these techniques' potential complications, the use of electrothermal bipolar vessel sealing systems during axillary procedures to prevent seroma formation is becoming increasingly popular, although the method has not been found to significantly improve seroma rates. In a recent Italian study, 116 women were randomly assigned to conventional node dissection performed using a scalpel and monopolar cautery or to node dissection performed using an electrothermal bipolar vessel sealing system. The use of a bipolar vessel sealing system offered only marginal advantages over the conventional technique, and the groups had similar incidences of seroma.[26] Furthermore, no study has shown that the use or nonuse of additional devices (e.g., laser scalpels, argon diathermy electrodes, ultrasonic scalpels) during conventional node dissection using a scalpel and monopolar cautery significantly affects seroma incidence. Therefore, surgeons should use the technique with which they have had the most success in obtaining optimal surgical outcomes.

REFERENCES

1. Morton DL, Wen DR, Wong JH, et al. Technical details of intraoperative lymphatic mapping for early stage melanoma. *Arch Surg* 1992;127(4):392–399.
2. Clough KB, Nasr R, Nos C, et al. New anatomical classification of the axilla with implications for sentinel node biopsy. *Br J Surg* 2010;97(11):1659–1665.
3. Krag DN, Anderson SJ, Julian TB, et al. Sentinel-lymph-node resection compared with conventional axillary-lymph-node dissection in clinically node-negative patients with breast cancer: overall survival findings from the NSABP B-32 randomised phase 3 trial. *Lancet Oncol* 2010; 11(10):927–933.
4. Goyal A, Newcombe R, Mansel R. Clinical relevance of multiple sentinel nodes in patients with breast cancer. *Brit J Surg* 2005;92(4):438–442.
5. Pesek S, Ashikaga T, Krag LE, et al. The false-negative rate of sentinel node biopsy in patients with breast cancer: a meta-analysis. *World J Surg* 2012;36(9):2239–2251.
6. Quan ML, Wells BJ, McCready D, et al. Beyond the false negative rate: development of quality indicators for sentinel lymph node biopsy in breast cancer. *Ann Surg Oncol* 2010;17(2):579–591.
7. Cody HS III. Clinical aspects of sentinel node biopsy. *Breast Cancer Res* 2001;3:104–108.
8. Rodier J-F, Velten M, Wilt M, et al. Prospective multicentric randomized study comparing periareolar and peritumoral injection of radiotracer and blue dye for the detection of sentinel lymph node in breast sparing procedures: FRANSENODE trial. *J Clin Oncol* 2007;25(24):3664–3669.
9. Fearmonti RM, Gayed IW, Kim E, et al. Intra-individual comparison of lymphatic drainage patterns using subareolar and peritumoral isotope injection for breast cancer. *Ann Surg Oncol* 2010;17(1):220–227.
10. Wallace AM, Han LK, Povoski SP, et al. Comparative evaluation of [99mTc] tilmanocept for sentinel lymph node mapping in breast cancer patients: results of two phase 3 trials. *Ann Surg Oncol* 2013;20(8):2590–2599.
11. Johnson CB, Boneti C, Korourian S, et al. Intraoperative injection of subareolar or dermal radioisotope results in predictable identification of sentinel lymph nodes in breast cancer. *Ann Surg* 2011;254(4):612–618.
12. Stell VH, Flippo-Morton TS, Norton HJ, et al. Effect of intraoperative radiocolloid injection on sentinel lymph node biopsy in patients with breast cancer. *Ann Surg Oncol* 2009;16(8):2300–2304.
13. Krag DN, Anderson SJ, Julian TB, et al. Technical outcomes of sentinel-lymph-node resection and conventional axillary-lymph-node dissection in patients with clinically node-negative breast cancer: results from the NSABP B-32 randomised phase III trial. *Lancet Oncol* 2007;8(10):881–888.
14. Zakaria S, Hoskin TL, Degnim AC. Safety and technical success of methylene blue dye for lymphatic mapping in breast cancer. *Am J Surg* 2008;196(2):228–233.
15. Burak WE Jr, Waler MJ, Yee LD, et al. Routine preoperative lymphoscintigraphy is not necessary prior to sentinel node biopsy for breast cancer. *Am J Surg* 1999;177(6):445–449.
16. McMasters KM, Wong SL, Tuttle TM, et al. Preoperative lymphoscintigraphy for breast cancer does not improve the ability to identify axillary sentinel lymph nodes. *Ann Surg* 2000;231(5):724–731.
17. Goyal A, Newcombe RG, Mansel R. Role of routine preoperative lymphoscintigraphy in sentinel node biopsy for breast cancer. *Eur J Cancer* 2005;41(2):238–243.
18. Kong AL, Tereffe W, Hunt KK, et al. Impact of internal mammary lymph node drainage identified by preoperative lymphoscintigraphy on outcomes in patients with stage I to III breast cancer. *Cancer* 2012;118(24):6287–6296.
19. Lacour J, Bucalossi P, Caceres E, et al. Radical mastectomy versus radical mastectomy plus internal mammary dissection. Ten year results of an international cooperative trial in breast cancer. *Cancer* 1983;51(10):1941–1943.

20. Chagpar AB, Kehdy F, Scoggins CR, et al. Effect of lymphoscintigraphy drainage patterns on sentinel lymph node biopsy in patients with breast cancer. *Am J Surg* 2005;190(4):557–562.

21. Jain S, Gradishar WJ. The application of oncotype DX in early-stage lymph-node-positive disease. *Curr Oncol Rep* 2014;16(1):1–6.

22. Huang J, Barbera L, Brouwers M, et al. Does delay in starting treatment affect the outcomes of radiotherapy? A systematic review. *J Clin Oncol* 2003;21(3):555–563.

23. Downing A, Twelves C, Forman D, et al. Time to begin adjuvant chemotherapy and survival in breast cancer patients: a retrospective observational study using latent class analysis. *Breast J* 2014;20(1):29–36.

24. McCaul J, Aslaam A, Spooner RJ, et al. Etiology of seroma formation in patients undergoing surgery for breast cancer. *Breast* 2000;9(3):144–148.

25. Lucci A, McCall LM, Beitsch PD, et al. Surgical complications associated with sentinel lymph node dissection (SLND) plus axillary lymph node dissection compared with SLND alone in the American College of Surgeons Oncology Group Trial Z0011. *J Clin Oncol* 2007;25(24):3657–3663.

26. Nespoli L, Antolini L, Stucchi C, et al. Axillary lymphadenectomy for breast cancer. A randomized controlled trial comparing a bipolar vessel sealing system to the conventional technique. *Breast* 2012;21(6):739–745.

BREAST SURGERY AS AN ESSENTIAL COMPONENT OF MULTIDISCIPLINARY BREAST CANCER MANAGEMENT

The preceding chapters on breast surgery will be important and valuable for all surgeons treating breast cancer, including surgical trainees preparing for their boards. They establish a standardized surgical approach that all of us as breast surgeons should be following, regardless of our practice setting, frequency of seeing breast cancer patients, or level of training and experience. The management of breast cancer, including the surgical procedure itself, is among the most complex decision making in all of medicine and one of the most rapidly changing. Most patients will receive some combination or sequence of surgery, systemic therapy (hormone therapy, targeted therapy, or chemotherapy), and radiation therapy. Selecting these options is enhanced by the use of biomarkers that identify both metastatic risk and selection of treatments based on molecular and/or genetic markers. Then there is the individual's perception of "quality of life" issues that must also be taken into account. **The many advances being made enable us to better customize our multidisciplinary management to improve the quality and quantity of breast cancer patients <u>regardless of their presenting stage of disease</u>**.

This series of chapters on surgical management of breast cancer, along with the other chapters in this book, represent a brilliant strategy by the editors to define optimal standards of intraoperative surgery as an essential component of multidisciplinary cancer care. Without standards, patients may get the wrong operation, however well done technically (errors of commission), or they may get inadequate surgery (errors of commission) that diminish the primary goal of surgery to properly stage the patient's disease and to achieve complete local and regional cancer control. Either of these scenarios can result in recurrent disease that may result in debilitating symptoms and cause the patient to undergo reoperation. Or it may thwart the value of the systemic treatment (chemotherapy and/or hormone therapy), which in turn may cause a misinterpretation of recurrent disease as a failure of systemic treatment instead of an avoidable surgical failure. As a result, patients go through the devastating emotional consequences of a "cancer relapse" and the physical consequence of going to second-line systemic treatments (with lower success rates and oftentimes greater toxicity) that could have been avoided with a properly conducted operation in the correct setting. We and others have published about the value of surgical specialization, the importance of surgical standards, and how quality of surgical management can make a difference in all three goals of surgery: proper pathologic staging, local and regional cancer control, and even improved survival rates.[1–6]

The goal of making the final decision about surgical management of the breast cancer—in partnership with each patient—is to maximize the long-term results with regards to local disease control, symmetry of the breasts, cosmetic appearance, and emotional state. We are achieving this today in the clinical setting where women with breast cancer are evaluated by a multidisciplinary team of breast specialists and patient advocates/survivors in a dedicated breast center. These women come prepared with a more informed and empowered ability to participate in decision making with regard to their breast management. The teamwork and coordination between the breast imaging specialists, breast oncology surgeons, breast reconstruction surgeons, and breast radiation oncologists have also resulted in better staging and consistent patient recommendations. To ensure that all women have access to a range of surgical treatment options, we should continue to make refinements in breast surgery and a consistency of surgical outcomes, wherever the patient is being treated. In addition, we need to ensure that all women have access to educational material that is evidence-based, understandable, and balanced.

In conclusion, surgeons are constantly making recommendations to our cancer patients that balance both quantity and quality of life; nowhere is this more important than in breast cancer. Patients benefit from our surgical perspective as part of the treatment planning for early-stage (and some late-stage) breast cancer. To provide contemporary breast cancer care, surgeons need to think and function as BOTH a surgeon and an oncologist, including being part of a multidisciplinary team, being knowledgeable about counseling their patients about systemic therapy (preoperative or postoperative), knowing how to adopt molecular and genetic biomarkers into treatment planning, and participating in multidisciplinary planning so that their patients have a treatment plan with the best combination and sequence of their breast cancer management. After this planning, there is the importance of properly conducting the breast cancer surgery itself as described in the next chapters.

There are so many criteria for defining proper outcomes of breast cancer surgery (including cosmetic or "oncoplastic" outcomes), and the editors have properly focused on the essential purpose of surgery, which is "to delineate the highest oncologic safety to prevent tumor recurrences." In this context, these chapters, written by breast surgical experts, nicely describe the optimal standards of surgical care so that each patient can have results that have the least risk of morbidity and that achieve maximal locoregional disease control, optimal cosmetic results, and minimal risk for relapse.

Charles M. Balch, MD, FACS
Professor of Surgery
University of Texas Southwestern Medical Center
Dallas, Texas

REFERENCES

1. Balch CM, Durant JR, Bartolucci AA; Southeastern Cancer Study Group. The impact of surgical quality control in multi-institutional group trials involving adjuvant cancer treatments. *Ann Surg* 1983;198:164–167.
2. Skinner KA, Helsper JT, Deapen D, et al. Breast cancer: do specialists make a difference? *Ann Surg Oncol* 2003;10(6):606–615.
3. Kingsmore D, Hole D, Gillis C. Why does specialist treatment of breast cancer improve? The role of surgical management. *Br J Cancer* 2004;90:1920–1925.
4. Kingsmore DB, Ssemwogerere A, Hole DJ, et al. Increased mortality from breast cancer and inadequate axillary treatment. *Breast* 2003;12:36–41.
5. Lovrics P, Hodgson N, O'Brien MA, et al. Results of a surgeon-directed quality improvement project on breast cancer surgery outcomes in South-Central Ontario. *Ann Surg Oncol* 2014;21:2181–2187.
6. Yen TW, Laud PW, Sparapani RA, et al. Surgeon specialization and use of sentinel lymph node biopsy for breast cancer. *JAMA Surg* 2014;149(2):185–192.

Oncologic Elements of Operative Record—Breast

Clinical Staging				
Operative Intent	Primary excision	Re-excision	Prophylactic	
Procedure Summary				
Mastectomy				
Type	Total	Skin-sparing	Nipple-sparing	
Fascia removed	Yes	No		
Muscle excised	Yes	No		
Partial Mastectomy				
Method of localization	Needle	Radioactive seed	Ultrasonography	Palpation
Skin excision with specimen	Yes	No		
Depth of resection	___ cm to fascia	Fascia resected		
Margin status checked with pathologist	Yes	No		
Margin status if checked	Positive	Negative		
Specimen radiography	Yes	No		
Clip detected	Yes	No		
Sentinel Lymph Node Biopsy				
Tracer	Radioactive tracer	Blue dye	Dual tracer	
Nodes palpable	Yes	No		
Radioactive counts of node	___			
Background counts	___			
Intraoperative assessment	None	Frozen section	Imprint cytology	
Axillary Dissection				
Level of dissection	I and II	III		
Axillary vein identified and cleared	Yes	No		
Latissimus dorsi muscle identified and cleared	Yes	No		
Serratus anterior muscle identified and cleared	Yes	No		
Long thoracic nerve identified and preserved	Yes	No		
Thoracodorsal nerve identified and preserved	Yes	No		
Drain placed	Yes	No		

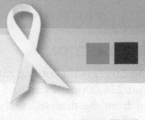

SECTION II

LUNG

INTRODUCTION

Lung cancer is the leading cause of cancer-related death in the United States. In 2013, about 226,000 new cases of lung cancer were diagnosed, and about 160,000 people died from the disease.[1] Only 15.9% of lung cancer patients are alive 5 years after their diagnosis.[2] Improvements in treatment approaches and a better understanding of early detection, prognostic markers, and targeted therapy have elicited much progress against the disease in the past 10 years. As we gain more knowledge to further refine diagnostic and treatment modalities, the care of lung cancer patients will only become more complex and nuanced.

About 85% of lung cancers are non–small cell lung cancer (NSCLC), and approximately 90% of NSCLCs are related to tobacco exposure. Despite recent advances in both screening and imaging, only approximately 30% of NSCLCs are diagnosed at an early stage, meaning that the majority of these cancers are diagnosed when they are no longer amenable to complete surgical resection. The paradigm of care for NSCLC patients lies in multidisciplinary evaluation, a process that integrates the expertise of specialists such as surgeons, medical oncologists, radiation oncologists, pulmonologists, radiologists, and pathologists to provide individualized therapy. Within this paradigm, surgical resection has long been the standard treatment for patients with resectable stage I to IIIA NSCLC. However, surgeons' practices for providing such treatment vary greatly. Large database analysis have revealed differences in morbidity, mortality, and long-term patient outcome when lung resections are performed by specialty-trained thoracic surgeons over cardiothoracic surgeons or general surgeons.[3] Setting standards to define systematic approaches to staging lung cancer and treating lung cancer patients is imperative to minimizing such wide variations in surgical practice. Doing so will improve the consistency and completeness of common thoracic oncologic surgeries and thereby improve patient outcomes.

Scope

Although surgery is often integrated with other modalities in lung cancer care, this section focuses on only the technical components and considerations governing the key operations that are important to ensuring that lung cancer patients receive high-quality multidisciplinary care. These key operations include procedures that are the cornerstones of clinical staging (e.g., mediastinal staging) and surgical treatment (e.g., lung resection).

The section also provides a broad set of collective recommendations guiding the surgical care of lung cancer patients. These recommendations take into account the fact that patients' care requirements depend on individual clinical scenarios and may vary to a high degree and that best practices are continuously evolving as new evidence accrues. Each key operation is discussed in terms of its oncologic principles, specific steps, and common but avoidable pitfalls, and both minimally invasive and open approaches to these operations are discussed. At the end of each chapter, a clinically relevant question regarding a topic of current debate and ongoing scientific research is explored.

In this section, we purposefully avoid duplicating clinical guidelines for lung cancer care, such as those established by the American College of Chest Physicians,[4] by not straying into the realm of clinical management algorithms. Although such guidelines can serve as a resource to guide the delivery of patient care, they do not explicitly address the technical aspects of the surgeries that impact outcomes. In fulfilment of this need, the following chapters describe the way in which insights taken from clinical science should be integrated into surgical approaches for lung cancer. In addition, because lung cancer surgery has many "craft" issues, stylistic tips to improve the ease or efficiency with which surgeons can perform a particular maneuver or step of an operation are also provided. Whenever possible, we describe the way in which the recommendations were derived and the level of evidence on which these recommendations were based. In this way, we distinguish sound consensus opinions regarding the minimum expected elements of a procedure from suggestions aimed at optimizing the outcomes of the procedure.

Purpose

The purpose of this section is to describe a minimal standard for the actions that should be taken in the surgical care of lung cancer patients, with the ultimate goal of improving the quality of care these patients receive. In this way, the aim of the following chapters is to "raise the floor" rather than define the absolute ceiling of what can be achieved; further improvement is always possible. This standard should serve as a guide for surgeons who are focused on delivering high-quality care to achieve the best outcomes for their patients. Underpinning this section is the belief that the vast majority of surgeons are committed to this goal and that the lack of a definition of what constitutes good quality care is a major impediment to achieving it.

The recommendations given in the following chapters are as data-driven and evidence-based as possible. However, many of the issues discussed in this section generally have not been addressed directly in previous studies. Thus, some recommendations must be extrapolated from indirect data. In addition, the consensus opinion of the selected experts tasked with writing the following chapters permeated the production of this section, which included identifying key questions, defining gaps in knowledge or performance, judging the applicability of indirect data, and debating the validity of opinions in the absence of data. The result of this process reflects not only the authors' efforts to provide recommendations that are as grounded in data as possible but also their use of whatever means necessary to establish a minimal standard for the surgical care of patients with lung cancer.

Quality of Care

Quality care has been defined as "the degree to which health services . . . increase the likelihood of desired health outcomes and are consistent with current professional knowledge."[5] This section focuses on those aspects of lung cancer surgery that, if performed with consistent accuracy and care, likely contribute to better outcomes. However, defining and implementing quality metrics, which generally requires validation that such measures are clearly linked to better outcomes and can be applied in a variety of settings, is beyond the scope of this chapter. In addition, implementing quality metrics is inherently linked to measurement; this chapter focuses only on what should be done and does not address the ways in which one might measure this.

Multidisciplinary Care

Although it is not a matter of surgical care, strictly speaking, working in a multidisciplinary fashion is so integral to modern cancer care that it merits emphasizing. Great surgical care done on an island will always have more limited impact. The knowledge required to effectively treat lung cancer patients is expanding rapidly and is far beyond what any one person can grasp. The care of lung cancer patients has come to involve many different treatment modalities, and providing optimal surgical care requires nuanced input from experts in multiple disciplines, including radiology and pathology.

The key to providing effective multidisciplinary care is the establishment of a regular forum in which experts from various fields discuss individual cases and collectively make treatment decisions. Simply obtaining input from another specialist when one believes it necessary is not enough. The forum enables surgeons to obtain other experts' input about knowledge gaps they otherwise would not have identified, let alone addressed. Optimal care is best ensured with multidisciplinary input.

Many European countries mandate that cancer cases be discussed in multidisciplinary forums. Similarly, the American College of Chest Physicians, after systematically reviewing the available literature, has recommended that patients with stage I to III lung cancer be evaluated by a multidisciplinary team.[6,7] However, quantifying the impact of this approach on patient outcomes has proven difficult, as outcomes are the result of multiple factors. Furthermore, recent studies have shown that the quality of multidisciplinary tumor board discussions can vary significantly.[8–11] A discussion of the implementation of a multidisciplinary tumor board is beyond the scope of this section; however, the setting in which surgical care is delivered (i.e., as part of a multidisciplinary team approach) and the quality of the team members' interactions are likely important factors contributing to lung cancer patients' quality of care and outcomes.

Staging Evaluation

Accurately identifying the clinical disease stage is a critical first step in caring for a patient with lung cancer. A detailed description of the way in which this is accomplished is the subject of clinical guidelines and beyond the scope of this section. Given the importance of accurate lung cancer staging, however, these guidelines are briefly reviewed here.

The first step in staging lung cancer is to make a clinical diagnosis and assess the certainty of this diagnosis. In the vast majority of patients with a lung mass, a diagnosis of lung cancer can be made quite reliably on the basis of radiographic findings and the patient's risk of developing lung cancer. If the probability of lung cancer is high (>80%), proceeding with stage evaluation is more efficient than obtaining a biopsy.

Stage evaluation begins with an assessment of the likelihood of distant metastases. This assessment begins with asking the patient about the organ-specific symptoms (e.g., headache, cognitive deficit, bone pain) and nonspecific symptoms (e.g., fatigue, anorexia) of distant metastases. Staging modalities include computed tomography (CT) and positron emission tomography (PET) imaging. Current NSCLC staging schema is shown in Figure I-1. Such a clinical evaluation is highly reliable (~95%) if negative in patients with a stage cI cancer by CT; however, there is a 30% false negative rate if the CT demonstrates mediastinal node enlargement suggesting more advanced stage disease (stage cIII). If the clinical evaluation is positive or if CT findings demonstrate mediastinal node enlargement (clinical stage III disease), additional

TNM Classification of Lung Cancer

TUMOR CHARACTERISTICS				
	Size	**Location**	**Invasion**	**Other**
T1	≤ 3 cm	• Not in main bronchus	• Surrounded by lung or pleura	
T1a	≤ 2 cm			
T1b	2cm - 3 cm			
T2	3cm - 7cm	• Involves main bronchus ≥ 2 cm from carina	Invades: • visceral pleura	• Atelectasis to hilum but not entire lung
T2a	3cm - 5cm			
T2b	5cm - 7cm			
T3	> 7cm	• Pancoast • < 2 cm from carina • Tumor in same lobe	Invades: • chest wall • diaphragm • phrenic nerve • mediastinal pleura • pericardium	• Atelectasis of entire lung
T4			Invades: • mediastinum • heart • great vessels • trachea • recurrent laryngeal nerve • esophagus • vertebral body • carina	• Separate tumor in ipsilateral lung

LYMPH NODES	
N1	• Ipsilateral nodes • Direct extension
N2	• Ipsilateral mediastinal nodes
N3	• Contralateral nodes • Scalene or supraclavicular nodes

METASTASIS	
M1a	• Tumor in contralateral lung • Pleural nodules • Malignant effusion
M1b	• Distant metastasis

FIGURE I-1 TNM classification of non–small cell lung cancer based on American Joint Committee on Cancer 7th edition revisions to the staging schema. Used with the permission of the American Joint Committee on Cancer (AJCC), Chicago, Illinois. The original source for this material is the AJCC Cancer Staging Manual, Seventh Edition (2010) published by Springer Science and Business Media LLC, www.springer.com.

imaging studies for distant metastases are recommended and typically include PET and brain magnetic resonance imaging.[12]

If distant metastases are not present, determining the status of the mediastinal nodes becomes crucial. In the setting of a clinical stage I lung cancer indicated by CT with or without PET, the chance of mediastinal node involvement is so low that invasive pretreatment node biopsy is not recommended.[12] If CT reveals tumor infiltration into the mediastinum (i.e., if one can no longer recognize or measure discrete enlarged mediastinal nodes), one can be certain of mediastinal involvement based on imaging alone and invasive confirmation of node involvement is not needed.[12] However, invasive biopsy is needed to confirm CT or PET findings of discrete node enlargement (cIII disease), as the modalities have false positive rates of 15% to 40% in this setting. Similarly, in patients with central tumors or evidence of N1 node involvement, CT and PET findings that are negative for disease in the mediastinum must be confirmed using invasive methods owing to false negative rates of 20% to 30%.[12]

Confirmation of mediastinal node status can be accomplished invasively by mediastinoscopy, esophageal ultrasonography, or endobronchial ultrasonography and needle aspiration. Although many studies have compared these procedures, the decision to use one or another in a particular patient often depends on nuances in the ease with which particular nodes can be accessed; the availability, skill, and experience of the operator and cytologist or pathologist; and logistical concerns. Perhaps most important of these factors is the thoroughness with which a procedure is performed. Defining the technical aspects of these procedures is the focus of this section.

A general principle of mediastinal assessment is that it should be done systematically. Guidelines from the European Society of Thoracic Surgeons and the American College of Chest Physicians[12,13] recommend exploration and biopsy of representative nodes in the five mediastinal node stations (2R, 2L, 4R, 4L, and 7). Studies have shown that N2 involvement is detected approximately twice as often with systematic sampling than with selective nodal sampling.[14–17] Similarly, clinical guidelines recommend that intraoperative nodal staging involve systematic sampling or either a complete or lobe-specific mediastinal node dissection for the same reasons.[18–20]

Current Staging and Synoptic of Staging System

The recurrent theme of this chapter on lung cancer will be the careful assessment of lymph node involvement. Although T status is of importance, in patients without metastatic disease, nodal involvement (both N1 and N2) is perhaps the greatest determinant of treatment failure and decreased long-term survival (Fig. I-2).[21]

In some instances, the presence of nodal disease in the mediastinum (N2) (Fig. I-3) precludes surgical resection. This is an area of active debate to determine the best therapy for these patients.[22] It is best practice to review clinical staging data in a prospective manner, with a dedicated thoracic team including surgeons, pulmonologists, and medical and radiation oncologists to determine the role, if any, of neoadjuvant therapy in patients with more advanced disease.[6] Furthermore, accurate pathologic staging is necessary to determine the role of adjuvant therapy. The need for a meticulous and methodical approach to staging cannot be overemphasized.

Effects of Nodal Stage on Lung Cancer Staging

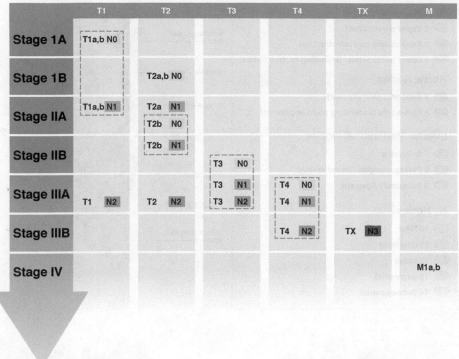

FIGURE I-2 Effect of nodal involvement on staging for non–small cell lung cancer. See Figure I-1 for designation of N0 to N3 descriptors.

Since the initial adoption of a staging system proposed by Dr. Clifton Mountain in the mid-1970s was created using a single institution database of patients, the Union Internationale Contre le Cancer and the American Joint Committee on Cancer have revised the staging system based on large international database of patients. The most recent changes were adopted in 2009, and this discussion focuses on this seventh version (see Fig. I-1).

Although the summary figure details the staging system, the authors wish to highlight some of the significant departures from the previous versions of the staging manual:

- T1 tumors are subclassified as T1a or T1b based on size.
- T2 tumors are subclassified as T2a or T2b based on size. T2a tumors also comprise other T2 descriptors as long as the tumor is ≤5 cm.
- Tumors >7 cm are considered T3.
- Multiple tumors in the same lobe are classified as T3.
- Additional tumors in another ipsilateral lobe are considered T4.

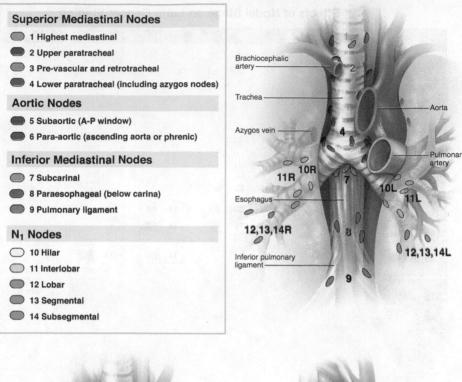

Superior Mediastinal Nodes

- 1 Highest mediastinal
- 2 Upper paratracheal
- 3 Pre-vascular and retrotracheal
- 4 Lower paratracheal (including azygos nodes)

Aortic Nodes

- 5 Subaortic (A-P window)
- 6 Para-aortic (ascending aorta or phrenic)

Inferior Mediastinal Nodes

- 7 Subcarinal
- 8 Paraesophageal (below carina)
- 9 Pulmonary ligament

N₁ Nodes

- 10 Hilar
- 11 Interlobar
- 12 Lobar
- 13 Segmental
- 14 Subsegmental

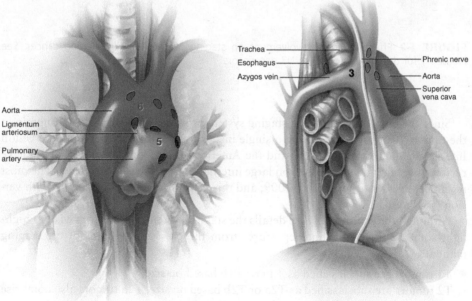

FIGURE I-3 Mountain–Dresler lymph node map. Adapted from Mountain CF, Dresler CM. Regional lymph node classification for lung cancer staging. *Chest* 1997;111:1718–1723, with permission.

Malignant effusions (pleural and pericardial), separate tumor nodules in the contralateral lung, and pleural nodules are considered M1a. More distant spread of disease is considered M1b.

N descriptors remain the same as in the prior edition.

REFERENCES

1. Siegel R, Naishadham D, Jemal A. Cancer statistics, 2012. *CA Cancer J Clin* 2012;62(1):10–29.
2. Howlader N, Noone A, Krapcho M, et al. *SEER Cancer Statistics Review, 1975–2009 (Vintage 2009 Populations)*. Bethesda, MD: National Cancer Institute; 2012.
3. Tieu B, Schipper P. Specialty matters in the treatment of lung cancer. *Semin Thorac Surg* 2012;24:99–105.
4. Detterbeck FC, Lewis S, Diekemper R, et al. Executive summary: diagnosis and management of lung cancer, 3rd ed: American College of Chest Physicians evidence-based clinical practice guidelines. *Chest* 2013;143(5)(suppl):7S–37S.
5. Mainz J. Defining and classifying clinical indicators for quality improvement. *Int J Qual Health Care* 2003;15(6):523–530.
6. Howington JA, Blum MG, Chang AC, et al. Treatment of stage I and II non-small cell lung cancer: diagnosis and management of lung cancer, 3rd ed: American College of Chest Physicians evidence-based clinical practice guidelines. *Chest* 2013;143:e278S–e313S.
7. Ramnath N, Dilling T, Harris L, et al. Treatment of stage III non-small cell lung cancer: diagnosis and management of lung cancer, 3rd ed: American College of Chest Physicians evidence-based clinical practice guidelines. *Chest* 2013;143(5)(suppl):e314S–e340S.
8. Lamb BW, Brown K, Nagpal K, et al. Quality of care management decisions by multidisciplinary cancer teams: a systematic review. *Ann Surg Oncol* 2011;18(8):2116–2125.
9. Lamb BW, Sevdalis N, Benn J, et al. Multidisciplinary cancer team meeting structure and treatment decisions: a prospective correlational study. *Ann Surg Oncol* 2013;20(3):715–722.
10. Lamb BW, Taylor C, Lamb JN, et al. Facilitators and barriers to teamworking and patient centeredness in multidisciplinary cancer teams: findings of a national study. *Ann Surg Oncol* 2013;20(5):1408–1416.
11. Lamb BW, Sevdalis N, Taylor C, et al. Multidisciplinary team working across different tumour types: analysis of a national survey. *Ann Oncol* 2012;23:1293–1300.
12. Silvestri GA, Gonzalez AV, Jantz M, et al. Methods of staging for non-small cell lung cancer: diagnosis and management of lung cancer, 3rd ed: American College of Chest Physicians evidence-based clinical practice guidelines. *Chest* 2013;143(5)(suppl):e211S–e250S.
13. De Leyn P, Lardinois D, Van Schil P, et al. ESTS guidelines for preoperative lymph node staging for non-small cell lung cancer. *Eur J Cardiothorac Surg* 2007;32(1):1–8.
14. Detterbeck F. Integration of mediastinal staging techniques for lung cancer. *Semin Thorac Cardiovasc Surg* 2007;19(3):217–224.
15. Gaer JAR, Goldstraw P. Intraoperative assessment of nodal staging at thoracotomy for carcinoma of the bronchus. *Eur J Cardiovasc Thorac Surg* 1990;4:207–210.
16. Wu Y, Huang ZF, Wang SY, et al. A randomized trial of systematic nodal dissection in resectable non-small cell lung cancer. *Lung Cancer* 2002;36(1):1–6.
17. Allen MS, Darling GE, Pechet TTV, et al. Morbidity and mortality of major pulmonary resections in patients with early-stage lung cancer: initial results of the randomized, prospective ACOSOG Z0030 trial. *Ann Thorac Surg* 2006;81(3):1013–1020.
18. Robinson L, Ruckdeschel J, Wagner HJ, et al. Treatment of non-small cell lung cancer–stage IIIA: ACCP evidence-based guidelines, 2nd ed. *Chest* 2007;132(3)(suppl):243S–265S.
19. Scott W, Howington J, Feigenberg S, et al. Treatment of non-small cell lung cancer–stage I & II: ACCP Evidence-based clinical practice guideline, 2nd ed. *Chest* 2007;132(3)(suppl):234S–242S.
20. Lardinois D, De Leyn P, Van Schil P, et al. ESTS guidelines for intraoperative lymph node staging in non-small cell lung cancer. *Eur J Cardiothorac Surg* 2006;30:787–792.
21. Detterbeck FC, Boffa DJ, Tanoue LT. The new lung cancer staging system. *Chest* 2009;136:260–271.
22. Veeramachaneni NK, Feins RH, Stephenson BJ, et al. Management of stage IIIa non-small cell lung cancer by thoracic surgeons in North America. *Ann Thorac Surg* 2012;94(3):922–926.

CHAPTER 5

Invasive Mediastinal Staging Overview

CRITICAL ELEMENTS

- Confirmation of Imaging Findings
- Mediastinal Staging for Central Tumors
- Mediastinal Staging Prior to Treatment
- Mediastinal Staging at the Time of Lung Resection

1. MEDIASTINAL STAGING FOR PATIENTS WITH SUSPECTED MEDIASTINAL NODAL INVOLVEMENT ON IMAGING

Recommendation: In general, for patients with known or suspected non–small cell lung cancer (NSCLC) who are potential surgical candidates, any positron emission tomography (PET) or computed tomography (CT) findings that suggest mediastinal nodal involvement should be confirmed with invasive mediastinal staging.

Type of Data: Retrospective.

Strength of Recommendation: Strong.

Rationale

Although PET and CT are critical components of the noninvasive clinical staging of NSCLC, both have surprisingly high false positive and false negative rates. Certain clinical presentations (e.g., granulomatous disease) can confound the interpretation of these imaging studies, which could result in inappropriate clinical stage assignment and improper care. Thus, guidelines for performing invasive staging of the mediastinum for NSCLC have been devised. More precise pretreatment staging should improve the care and survival of NSCLC patients.

Most guidelines for invasive mediastinal staging incorporate radiographic staging results, clinical T status, tumor location (central or peripheral), and available institutional technical expertise. Moreover, if PET or CT findings suggest the presence of disease in the hilum but not the mediastinum, invasive mediastinal staging is also recommended because of a substantial incidence of false negative radiographic mediastinal staging in such patients. If PET and CT results are discordant, invasive staging should be performed.

Invasive mediastinal staging techniques include cervical mediastinoscopy, endobronchial ultrasonography (EBUS), endoscopic ultrasonography (EUS), video-assisted thoracic surgery (VATS), and possibly transcervical extended mediastinal lymphadenectomy. The goal of these strategies is to accurately establish the pathologic disease stage to avoid unnecessary lung resection in patients with advanced disease and offer life-extending operations to patients whose clinical disease stage would otherwise be erroneously thought to be advanced because of false positive imaging results.

The negative predictive value of CT alone for mediastinal staging is 70% to 95% and that of PET alone is 80% to 99%. The combination of these two modalities has a negative predictive value of about 95%, indicating that in the absence of other indications, mediastinal staging is not necessary if both PET and CT reveal the mediastinal nodes to be normal.[1] CT or PET findings suggestive of abnormal mediastinal nodes in areas in which fungal or other granulomatous diseases are endemic creates challenges to accurate clinical decision making. Certainly, these findings may not represent tumor involvement of the nodes, and the imperative to document pathologic nodal status is even stronger in these instances.

2. MEDIASTINAL STAGING FOR CENTRAL TUMORS, CLINICAL N1 DISEASE, AND LARGER TUMORS IN THE ABSENCE OF MEDIASTINAL NODAL ABNORMALITIES ON COMPUTED TOMOGRAPHY AND POSITRON EMISSION TOMOGRAPHY

Recommendation: Patients with central tumors, regardless of T status or PET or CT findings, and patients with T2 or greater disease should undergo invasive mediastinal staging.

Type of Data: Retrospective.

Strength of Recommendation: Weak.

Rationale
For patients for whom PET and CT findings are negative for mediastinal and hilar (and systemic) disease, the use of invasive lymph node staging is predicated on the T status, the location of the primary lesion, and the characteristics of ipsilateral hilar nodes on clinical staging. Patients with clinical T1a/T1b peripheral lesions (stage IA disease) and no evidence for hilar or mediastinal adenopathy on PET and CT do not require additional mediastinal staging.[2] However, patients with T2 or greater primary

tumors, clinical evidence of hilar nodal involvement, or central tumors should undergo invasive mediastinal staging, even if their PET and CT findings are negative for disease in the mediastinum.[3]

There are some cogent arguments for offering invasive mediastinal staging to patients with negative PET and CT findings in the mediastinum who present with synchronous small lesions (T1a/T1b), regardless of whether these lesions are in the same lobe, in the same lung, or in opposite lungs. Also, patients for whom stereotactic body radiosurgery is planned should be subject to the same criteria as operative candidates. Local therapy with stereotactic radiosurgery may be of little value in the setting of nodal disease.

3. MEDIASTINAL STAGING PRIOR TO LUNG RESECTION

Recommendation: Proper mediastinal node staging requires a thorough understanding of the limitations of mediastinoscopy, EUS, EBUS, and VATS.

Type of Data: Retrospective.

Strength of Recommendation: Weak.

Rationale

The appropriate extent of mediastinal staging to some degree depends on the minimally invasive technique that is used, as this determines the accessibility of the nodes.[1] For traditional staging mediastinoscopy, sampled nodes should routinely include R4, L4, and 7 nodes. More stringent recommendations require that R2 and L2 specimens be obtained for all patients.

The different staging techniques afford variable access to the different lymph node stations. EBUS techniques have good lymph node yield when the nodes are enlarged and can access many level 10 and some level 11 nodes. EUS, on the other hand, offers access that is typically limited to level 7, 8, and 9 nodes. Thus, EUS can be used to diagnose the presence of mediastinal nodal involvement but is insufficient as a single staging modality to map the mediastinum. VATS typically permits access to only level 7 and ipsilateral nodes and so is useful for accessing nodes specifically targeted by PET or CT and for completing the staging of stations 5, 6, 8, and 9 when indicated. Cervical mediastinoscopy has been long held to be the gold standard of mediastinal lymph node staging and provides access to stations 2, 4, and 7 but not 5, 6, 8, or 9 nodal stations.

The first invasive modality performed for mediastinal staging should be bronchoscopic staging with EBUS, as it has a satisfactory lymph node yield, costs less, and has a lower complication risk than mediastinoscopy or VATS does.[4,5] If abnormal inferior mediastinal adenopathy is present, EUS may be performed initially or instead of EBUS[6] if institutional expertise is present. If it is not, mediastinoscopy should be performed first. The negative predictive value of mediastinoscopy is more than 90%, and the incidence of nodal involvement detected using the modality approaches 40%

overall. However, this latter value heavily depends on the indications for mediastinoscopy.[7] For example, in patients with clinical stage I disease, the incidence of nodal involvement detected by mediastinoscopy is only 3% and that detected by thoracotomy is only 5.6%.[2]

Newer staging modalities such as EBUS and EUS are dependent on ultrasound localization of lymph nodes. In EBUS-guided transbronchial needle aspiration, nodal biopsies are usually not attempted if the nodes cannot be visualized using ultrasonography, so these stations are often considered clinically negative. Nodes not visualized on ultrasonography are highly likely to be benign, and EBUS has a very low false negative rate for detecting nonbiopsied "normal" nodes.[8] In contrast, EUS has a false negative rate of 13% when the nodes are radiographically normal; however, this rate is higher—about 23%—in patients with other mediastinal nodal involvement. This indicates that mediastinoscopy or VATS should be used to complete mediastinal staging believed to be incomplete using EBUS alone or EBUS combined with EUS. (Please see Chapter 6 on the controversies of EBUS/EUS.) Comparative studies have demonstrated that mediastinoscopy offers a greater number of nodes sampled, a greater number of stations sampled, and more conclusive findings than EBUS or EUS.[9–11] Documentation of ipsilateral N2 disease alone is often insufficient to inform treatment recommendations; the status of the contralateral nodes must also be documented to enable surgeons to make specific recommendations regarding possible resection after induction therapy.

4. MEDIASTINAL STAGING AT THE TIME OF LUNG RESECTION

Recommendation: At the time of lung resection, on the right side, sampled/dissected nodes should include R10, R9, R8, 7, R4, and R2 nodes. On the left side, sampled/dissected nodes should include L10, L9, L8, 7, 6, 5, and L4 nodes and L2 nodes if accessible.

Type of Data: Retrospective.

Strength of Recommendation: Weak.

Rationale
The hilum and mediastinum should be thoroughly staged at the time of lung resection, even in patients who are undergoing nonanatomic parenchyma-sparing resections such as segmentectomy or wedge resection. There is no conclusive evidence that nodal dissection provides more complete staging information or results in better outcomes than nodal sampling does. On the right side, the sampled or dissected nodes should include the R9, R8, 7, R10, R4, and R2 nodes. On the left side, the sampled or dissected nodes should include the L9, L8, 7, 6, 5, and L4 nodes and the L2 nodes if accessible. Preservation of the recurrent laryngeal nerve takes precedence over complete nodal dissection in station 5.

TABLE 5-1 Literature Review

Author	Year	Study Design	No. of Patients	Main Question	Key Findings	Potential for Bias
Groth[1]	2008	Literature review	N/A	How accurate is radiographic mediastinal staging for NSLCL?	The accuracy of PET and/or CT is not as good as that of invasive mediastinal staging.	No
Schipper[8]	2008	Literature review	N/A	What is the comparative accuracy of minimally invasive to invasive techniques for mediastinal nodal staging in NSCLC?	No conclusive outcomes	No
Meyers[2]	2006	Retrospective review of single institution patient cohort	248	What is the incidence of occult mediastinal nodal involvement in patients with clinical stage I NSCLC?	The incidence of occult nodal metastases was 5.6%.	No
Licht[12]	2013	Retrospective review of national database	1513	What is the incidence of unsuspected mediastinal nodal disease in clinical stage I NSCLC?	The incidence of occult nodal metastases was 7.9%.	No
Crabtree[13]	2010	Retrospective single institution patient cohort	462	What is the incidence of unsuspected nodal disease in clinical stage IA NSCLC?	The incidence of occult nodal metastases was 3.5%.	No
Zhang[9]	2012	Prospective observational study of patients undergoing both EBUS and mediastinoscopy to stage NSCLC	36	What is the relative accuracy of mediastinoscopy compared to EBUS for assessing mediastinal nodes?	EBUS has a lower diagnostic yield and resulted in mediastinal understaging in patients with NSCLC.	Yes—EBUS operator skill not assessed

	Year	Study type	N	Question	Finding	
Smulders[10]	2005	Retrospective cohort study	156	What was the accuracy of mediastinoscopy in staging mediastinal nodes in patients with NSCLC?	Absence of mediastinal node involvement was correctly identified in 93.6%.	No
Annema[11]	2005	Prospective observational study	242	What is the impact of EBUS on the routine use of mediastinoscopy or thoracotomy for potentially resectable NSCLC?	EBUS eliminated 70% of surgical procedures.	No
Silvestri[4]	2013	Literature review and consensus process	N/A	What is the optimal algorithm for invasive mediastinal staging?	EBUS (and EUS) is the first choice for invasive mediastinal staging. If negative, these techniques should be followed by surgical biopsy.	No
ASGE[6]	2011	Literature review and practice guidelines statement	N/A	What is the utility of EUS in staging the mediastinum in patients with NSCLC?	EUS has utility for staging lower mediastinal and level 5 nodes.	No
ESTS[5]	2014	Unpublished				
Toloza[7]	2003	Systematic review and meta-analysis	N/A	What are performance characteristics of invasive mediastinal staging modalities?	TBNA sensitivity 0.76, NPV 0.71. EUS sensitivity 0.88, NPV 0.77. Mediastinoscopy sensitivity 0.81, NPV 0.91.	No

CT, computed tomography; EBUS, endobronchial ultrasonography; EUS, endoscopic ultrasonography; NPV, negative predictive value; NSCLC, non–small cell lung cancer; PET, positron emission tomography; TBNA, transbronchial needle aspiration.

REFERENCES

1. Groth SS, Whitson BA, Maddaus MA. Radiographic staging of mediastinal lymph nodes in non-small cell lung cancer patients. *Thorac Surg Clin* 2008;18(4):349–361.
2. Meyers BF, Haddad F, Siegel BA, et al. Cost-effectiveness of routine mediastinoscopy in computed tomography- and positron emission tomography-screened patients with stage I lung cancer. *J Thorac Cardiovasc Surg* 2006;131(4):822–829; discussion 822–829.
3. De Leyn P, Dooms C, Kuzdzal J, et al. Revised ESTS guidelines for preoperative mediastinal lymph node staging for non-small-cell lung cancer. *Eur J Cardio-Thorac Surg* 2014;45:787–798.
4. Silvestri GA, Gonzalez AV, Jantz MA, et al. Methods for staging non-small cell lung cancer: diagnosis and management of lung cancer, 3rd ed: American College of Chest Physicians evidence-based clinical practice guidelines. *Chest* 2013;143(5)(suppl):e211S–e250S.
5. DeLeyn P, Dooms C, Kuzdzal J et al. Revised ESTS guidelines for preoperative mediastinal lyph node staging for non-small cell lung cancer. *Eur J Cardiothorac Surg* 2012;45(5):787–798.
6. ASGE Standards of Practice Committee; Jue TL, Sharaf RN, Appalaneni V, et al. Role of EUS for the evaluation of mediastinal adenopathy. *Gastrointest Endosc* 2011;74(2):239–245.
7. Toloza EM, Harpole L, McCrory DC. Noninvasive staging of non-small cell lung cancer: a review of the current evidence. *Chest* 2003;123(1)(suppl):137S–146S.
8. Schipper P, Schoolfield M. Minimally invasive staging of N2 disease: endobronchial ultrasound/transesophageal endoscopic ultrasound, mediastinoscopy, and thoracoscopy. *Thorac Surg Clin* 2008;18(4):363–379.
9. Zhang R, Mietchen C, Krüger M, et al. Endobronchial ultrasound guided fine needle aspiration versus transcervical mediastinoscopy in nodal staging of non-small cell lung cancer: a prospective comparison study. *J Cardiothorac Surg* 2012;7:51.
10. Smulders SA, Smeenk FW, Janssen-Heijnen ML, et al. Surgical mediastinal staging in daily practice. *Lung Cancer* 2005;47(2):243–251.
11. Annema JT, Versteegh MI, Veseliç M, et al. Endoscopic ultrasound-guided fine-needle aspiration in the diagnosis and staging of lung cancer and its impact on surgical staging. *J Clin Oncol* 2005;23(33):8357–8361.
12. Licht PB, Jørgensen OD, Ladegaard L, et al. A national study of nodal upstaging after thoracoscopic versus open lobectomy for clinical stage I lung cancer. *Ann Thorac Surg* 2013;96(3):943–949; discussion 949–950.
13. Crabtree TD, Denlinger CE, Meyers BF, et al. Stereotactic body radiation therapy versus surgical resection for stage I non-small cell lung cancer. *J Thorac Cardiovasc Surg* 2010;140(2):377–386.

Endobronchial Ultrasonography/ Endoscopic Ultrasonography

CRITICAL ELEMENTS

- Identification of Lymph Nodes Suspicious for Cancer Metastasis
- Node Station Assessment Utilizing Endobronchial Ultrasonography/Endoscopic Ultrasonography

1. IDENTIFICATION OF LYMPH NODES SUSPICIOUS FOR CANCER METASTASIS

Recommendation: The standard endobronchial ultrasonography (EBUS) classification system of the sonographic features of lymph nodes is useful to determine whether lymph nodes are malignant or benign.

Type of Data: Retrospective.

Strength of Recommendation: Weak.

Rationale

Round lymph nodes whose short-axis diameter is larger than 1 cm, that have distinct margins and heterogeneous echogenicity, and that have coagulation necrosis sign but not central hilar structures are suspicious for malignancy and must be biopsied (Fig. 6-1).[1]

During EBUS-guided transbronchial needle aspiration (EBUS-TBNA) or endoscopic ultrasonography (EUS)–guided fine needle aspiration (EUS-FNA), all mediastinal and hilar lymph nodes should be assessed, characterized, and documented systematically. Lymph nodes should be identified according to the International Association for the Study of Lung Cancer lymph node map (Fig. I-3).[2] EBUS-TBNA and EUS-FNA should proceed from N3 nodes to N2 nodes and then to N1 nodes to prevent needle contamination and avoid accidental disease overstaging.

FIGURE 6-1 Sonographic characteristics, by EBUS or EUS, of mediastinal lymph nodes that favor benignancy or malignancy in lung cancer.

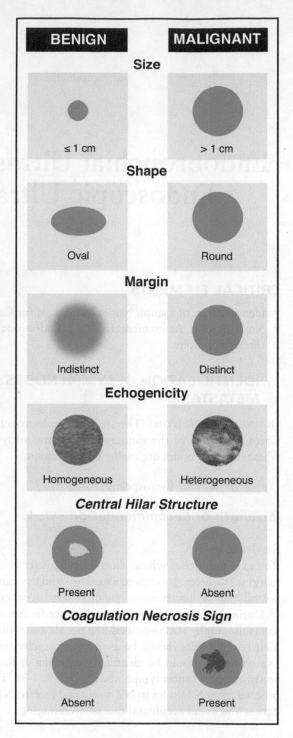

Morphology ultrasonography should be used to assess mediastinal lymph node stations 2R, 4R, 2L, 4L, and 7 during EBUS and stations 8 and 9 during EUS. When rapid on-site cytologic evaluation (ROSE) is available, a sample from one lymph node station should be confirmed as adequate for evaluation before the next station is sampled. When ROSE is not available, at least three passes of one lymph node station should be obtained unless a tissue block that is adequate for evaluation is grossly obtained during the first or second pass.[3]

2. NODE STATION ASSESSMENT UTILIZING ENDOBRONCHIAL ULTRASONOGRAPHY/ENDOSCOPIC ULTRASONOGRAPHY

Recommendation: Morphology ultrasonography should be used to assess mediastinal lymph node stations 2R, 4R, 2L, 4L, and 7 during EBUS and lymph node stations 8 and 9 during EUS.

Type of Data: Retrospective.

Strength of Recommendation: Weak.

Rationale

The recommendations for the extent of lymph node analysis are based on published guidelines.[4] Convex probe EBUS can access the upper paratracheal (stations 2R and 2L), lower paratracheal (stations 4R and 4L), subcarinal (station 7) and retrotracheal (station 3p) lymph nodes, as well as the hilar (station 10), interlobar (station 11), and lobar (station 12) nodes in the lower lobes. However, convex probe EBUS cannot access the prevascular (station 3a), subaortic (station 5), para-aortic (station 6), paraesophageal (station 8), pulmonary ligament (station 9), or lobar lymph nodes in the upper and middle lobes (Table 6-1).

EUS can access the pulmonary ligament (station 9), paraesophageal (station 8), subcarinal (station 7), retrotracheal (station 3p), and paratracheal (stations 2 and 4) lymph nodes. EUS usually cannot access the prevascular (station 3a), subaortic (station 5), para-aortic (station 6), or N1 lymph nodes. Some authors have reported that EUS can access stations 5 and 6, but the assessment of these nodes with EUS is

TABLE 6-1   Lymph Nodes Accessible by EBUS/EUS

EBUS	EUS
2	2
3p	3p
4	4
7	7
10	8
11	9
12*	

EBUS, endobronchial ultrasonography; EUS, endoscopic ultrasonography.
*Lower lobe lobar lymph nodes.

more difficult than that of other stations with EUS and requires significant expertise and experience to accomplish successfully.[5]

Technical Aspects

Although the instrumentation used for EUS and EBUS have some similarities, they also have distinct characteristics that limit the way in which each can be utilized. EBUS-TBNA is performed using a convex probe. A saline-filled balloon at the tip of the probe helps improve image quality. Samples are obtained using either a 21- or 22-gauge needle with real-time EBUS visualization. The needle has a number of safety features, including a mechanism that prevents the needle from protruding more than 40 mm and an internal sheath that prevents the needle from contaminating the working channel of the scope. In contrast, EUS-FNA is performed using a side-viewing videogastroscope with a dedicated curved linear array transducer attached to the tip of the probe. A number of different scopes from different companies are available for EUS-FNA, and all have minor differences in their overall diameter and size of the ultrasonography probe. A dedicated 22-gauge needle is usually used for EUS-FNA, but smaller (25-gauge) and larger (19-gauge) needles are also available. Similar to that performed using EBUS, tissue sampling using EUS is performed with the aid of real-time ultrasonography.

Both EBUS-TBNA and EUS-FNA can be performed on an outpatient basis utilizing either conscious sedation or general anesthesia. (When general anesthesia is used, the cough reflex is minimal, which may be an advantage during the procedure.) An endotracheal tube (size 8 minimum) or laryngeal mask airway is used to accommodate the scope. The size of the scope limits nasal insertion.

EBUS-TBNA should include an examination of the airway using regular flexible bronchoscopy. Ultrasonically visible vascular landmarks should be used to identify the specific lymph node stations according to the International Association for the Study of Lung Cancer lymph node map.[2] Doppler ultrasonography is used to identify surrounding vessels as well as the blood flow within lymph nodes. The needle is introduced into the lymph node with a sharp stab. The node is aspirated by removing the internal stylet and using a Vac-Lok syringe to apply negative pressure. (Because negative pressure can cause bloody samples of hypervascular lymph nodes, EBUS-TBNA of such nodes can be done without suction.) The needle is moved back and forth inside the lymph node to obtain samples. Finally, the needle is retracted into its sheath and removed from the bronchoscope.

The technique for EUS-FNA is similar to that for EBUS-TBNA. Anatomical landmarks such as the inferior vena cava, right and left atrium, azygos vein, main pulmonary artery, and aorta are identified. Any lymph nodes encountered are described and numbered according to the International Association for the Study of Lung Cancer lymph node map (see Fig. I-3 in the Introduction to Section II). Lymph nodes are then biopsied, usually with a 22-gauge needle, using real-time ultrasonography guidance. Finally, one cannot stress enough the importance of proper specimen handling during EBUS-TBNA and/or EUS-FNA. Institutional standards differ, and close collaboration between the surgeon and cytopathologist is essential. However, when ROSE is available, both EBUS-TBNA and EUS-FNA can be performed without the aid of a cytopathologist.

REFERENCES

1. Fujiwara T, Yasufuku K, Nakajima T, et al. The utility of sonographic features during endo-bronchial ultrasound-guided transbronchial needle aspiration for lymph node staging in patients with lung cancer: a standard endobronchial ultrasound image classification system. *Chest* 2010;138:641–647.
2. Rusch VW, Asamura H, Watanabe H, et al. The IASLC Lung Cancer Staging Project. A proposal for a new international lymph node map in the forthcoming seventh edition of the TNM classification for lung cancer. *J Thorac Oncol* 2009;4:568–577.
3. Lee HS, Lee GK, Lee HS, et al. Real-time endobronchial ultrasound-guided transbronchi al needle aspiration in mediastinal staging of non-small cell lung cancer: how many aspirations per target lymph node station? *Chest* 2008;134(2):368–374.
4. Howington JA, Blum MG, Chang AC, et al. Treatment of stage I and II non-small cell lung cancer: diagnosis and management of lung cancer, 3rd ed: American College of Chest Physicians Evidence-Based Clinical Practice Guidelines. *Chest* 2013;143(5)(suppl):e278S–e313S.
5. Liberman M, Durnceau A, Grunenwald E, et al. Initial experience with a new technique of endoscopic and ultrasonographic access for biopsy of para-aortic (station 6) mediastinal lymph nodes without traversing the aorta. *J Thorac Cardiovasc Surg* 2012;144(4):787–792; discussion 792–793.

Endobronchial Ultrasonography/ Endoscopic Ultrasonography: Key Question

When should negative endobronchial ultrasonography findings be confirmed by a more invasive procedure?

INTRODUCTION

Accurate staging is of paramount importance in the management of non–small cell lung cancer (NSCLC). The treatment of NSCLC, whether surgery, chemotherapy, radiotherapy, or a multimodality approach, depends on the stage of the disease. In NSCLC patients without metastatic disease, the status of the mediastinum is the most important determinant of candidacy for curative-intent treatment.

The first-line tests in the diagnosis and staging of NSCLC are imaging studies, including computed tomography (CT) and positron emission tomography (PET). Based on the most recent American College of Chest Physicians (ACCP) guidelines, the sensitivity and specificity of CT in identifying mediastinal lymph node metastasis are 55% and 81%, respectively, and those of PET are 77% and 86%, respectively.[1] These imaging studies have substantial false positive and false negative rates, and PET findings in particular must be confirmed with lymph node biopsy.

Traditionally, the gold standard for sampling lymph nodes in the mediastinum to confirm imaging studies' findings has been mediastinoscopy. Recently, however, endobronchial ultrasonography (EBUS)– or endoscopic ultrasonography (EUS)–guided needle aspiration techniques have also emerged as options for staging the mediastinum. In many institutions, EBUS-guided transbronchial needle aspiration (EBUS-TBNA) has replaced mediastinoscopy as the first-line means of sampling mediastinal lymph nodes, and mediastinoscopy is reserved to confirm the absence of N2 disease.[1,2]

As surgeons gain experience using EBUS-TBNA for lung cancer staging, the role of confirmatory mediastinoscopy and other invasive approaches to confirm EBUS-TNBA findings continues to diminish. Despite the impressive results obtained with EBUS-TBNA overall, confirmatory mediastinoscopy is still useful in certain situations. These situations are discussed in the following texts.

LITERATURE REVIEW

We conducted a Medline search of English language studies published from 2003 to 2013. We used the Medical Subject Heading term "endobronchial ultrasound"; the terms "negative predictive value," "false negative," "accuracy," and "sensitivity" were introduced to limit the number of studies identified. A total of 80 articles were found. Of the 80 abstracts we reviewed, 24 were excluded because the studies included patients who did not have lung cancer or examined EBUS in a role other than its use in invasive mediastinal staging. A careful review of the remaining 56 articles

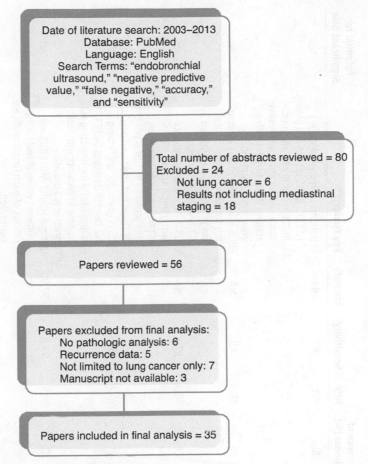

FIGURE 6-2 CONSORT diagram summarizing the literature search used for review of endobronchial ultrasound performance.

identified 35 articles that included data about the false negative rate, sensitivity, or negative predictive value of EBUS in the assessment of N2 disease in patients with NSCLC. This is summarized in Figure 6-2.

FINDINGS

Factors that affect the negative predictive value of EBUS

Multiple studies have demonstrated the utility of EBUS-TBNA as a staging modality in patients with NSCLC (Table 6-2).[3-30] The most important parameter defining the role of a staging modality in the preoperative staging of NSCLC is its ability to rule out mediastinal lymph node disease. In other words, a test for mediastinal disease must have a high sensitivity and high negative predictive value to prevent surgeons from performing a futile thoracotomy or thoracoscopic resection. However, both sensitivity and negative predictive value can be influenced by a number of factors.

TABLE 6-2 Studies Reporting Sensitivity and/or Negative Predictive Value of Real-Time Endobronchial Ultrasonography in the Mediastinal Staging of Confirmed or Highly Suspected Lung Cancer

Author, Year	Study Design	No. of Patients	Prevalence of N2 Disease (%)	NPV	Sensitivity	Accuracy	Key Findings	Potential for Significant Bias
Cornwell et al, 2013[3]	Retrospective	62	5	93	67	94	In patients with clinical stage I NSCLC, EBUS results in a lower incidence of nontherapeutic thoracotomy than noninvasive staging does, but this difference is not significant.	Yes
Herth et al, 2008[4]	Prospective observational	97	10	98.9	89	NA	EBUS is accurate in NSCLC staging for patients with clinical stage I NSCLC determined by CT and PET findings.	Yes
Herth et al, 2006[5]	Prospective observational	100	21	96.3	92.3	NA	EBUS is beneficial in patients with clinical stage I NSCLC. It prevents nontherapeutic thoracotomy in 1 of 6 patients. PET was not used routinely.	Yes
Hwangbo et al, 2009[6]	Prospective observational	126	26	96.7	90	97.4	EBUS is useful for confirming N2 disease detected by PET. It is also useful for detecting N2 disease in patients with radiographic N0 disease.	Yes
Lee et al, 2008[7]	Retrospective	102	30	96.9	93.8	97.9	Optimal results with EBUS are obtained when at least 3 aspirations of each lymph node are performed.	Yes
Yasufuku et al, 2011[8*]	Prospective controlled trial	153	35	91	81	93	EBUS is equivalent to mediastinoscopy in the mediastinal staging of NSCLC.	No

Study	Design						Comments	
Feller-Kopman et al, 2009*	Retrospective	131	35	89.7	85	NA	EBUS is an accurate and sensitive method for diagnosing and staging NSCLC.	Yes
Petersen et al, 2009[10]	Retrospective	157	43	90	85	NA	EBUS is accurate in staging the mediastinum in NSCLC patients. The routine confirmation of negative EBUS findings with mediastinoscopy has a minor role in NSCLC staging.	Yes
Sanz-Santos et al, 2012[11]	Retrospective	296	51	93.6	NA	NA	EBUS can be used to sample lymph node regions 4R, 4L, and 7 in more than 80% of patients. In such patients, EBUS has an NPV of >90% for mediastinal malignancy.	Yes
Nakajima et al, 2013[12]*	Retrospective	438	52	90	97	98	ROSE during EBUS results in a low incidence of nondiagnostic samples.	Yes
Jhun et al, 2012[13]	Retrospective	151	55	84.3	91.6	93.8	The diagnostic yield of EBUS is lower for left paratracheal lymph nodes. The diagnostic yield is not related to lymph node size.	Yes
Szlubowski et al, 2009[14]	Retrospective	226	57	89	83.5	92.9	EBUS is an effective and safe technique for mediastinal staging in NSCLC patients. In patients with negative EBUS results, surgical exploration of the mediastinum should be performed.	Yes

(continued)

TABLE 6-2 Studies Reporting Sensitivity and/or Negative Predictive Value of Real-Time Endobronchial Ultrasonography in the Mediastinal Staging of Confirmed or Highly Suspected Lung Cancer (continued)

Author, Year	Study Design	No. of Patients	Prevalence of N2 Disease (%)	NPV	Sensitivity	Accuracy	Key Findings	Potential for Significant Bias
Bauwens et al, 2008[15]	Retrospective	106	58	91	95	97	EBUS is a reasonable first step in the confirmation of N2 disease in NSCLC patients. Surgical mediastinal staging should be used to confirm negative EBUS findings.	Yes
Joesph et al, 2013[16]*	Retrospective	131	58	90	92	NA	ROSE does not affect clinical decisions made during staging EBUS.	Yes
Lee et al, 2012[17]	Retrospective	73	62	94	95	97	EBUS can be used to accurately assess the mediastinum in patients with NSCLC and radiographic N2 disease.	Yes
Cerfolio et al, 2010[18]	Retrospective	72	63	79	57	83	EBUS and EUS have high false negative rates, and negative results should be confirmed prior to thoracotomy.	Yes
Navani et al, 2012[19]	Retrospective	774	65	88	72	NA	EBUS samples are suitable for use in NSCLC subtyping and EGFR mutation analysis.	Yes
Kuo et al, 2011[20]	Retrospective	43	65	85.7	80.6	91	The diagnostic accuracy of EBUS is higher than that of PET in a tuberculosis-endemic population.	Yes
Hu et al, 2013[21]	Retrospective	231	67‡	92	88	87	Proficiency using EBUS requires 22 cases. Lymph node size is a predictor of success.	Yes
Yasufuku et al, 2005[22]*	Prospective observational	105	67	89.5	94.6	96.3	EBUS is an accurate staging procedure in patients with NSCLC.	Yes

Study	Type						Conclusions	
Rintoul et al, 2009[23]	Retrospective	109	71	60	91	92	EBUS can be used to accurately evaluate PET-positive hilar and mediastinal lymph nodes. Negative findings should be confirmed by surgical means.	Yes
Cetinkaya et al, 2011[24]	Retrospective	52	80	83	95	96	EBUS is safe and accurate in NSCLC staging.	Yes
Ernst et al, 2008[25]	Prospective cross-over	60	89	78	87	NA	The difference between EBUS and mediastinoscopy in determining the N status of patients with NSCLC is not statistically significant.	Yes
Gu et al, 2009[26]	Meta-analysis	1,299	NA	93	NA	NA	EBUS has a high NPV and is cost-effective in the mediastinal staging of NSCLC.	
Adams et al, 2009[27]	Meta-analysis	782	NA	NA	88	NA	EBUS has high sensitivity in the mediastinal staging of NSCLC.	
Abu-Hijleh et al, 2013[28]*	Retrospective	200	NA	75	87	91	EBUS is similar to surgical staging in patients with NSCLC. The NPV of EBUS is highest after the initial 25–50 cases. The accuracy of EBUS is independent of lymph node size or location and number of passes.	
Dong et al, 2013[29]*	Meta-analysis	1,066	NA	93	90	96	EBUS is accurate and safe in staging NSCLC.	
Whitson et al, 2013[30]*	Retrospective	120	NA	66†/85	83†/93	87†/95	The inclusion of nondiagnostic results yields a lower NPV, sensitivity, and accuracy.	

*ROSE was used.

†For the Whitson study, the first set of numbers includes nondiagnostic specimens. The values for when nondiagnostic studies are included are shown below in the same field.

‡Incidence of N1 and N2 disease.

CT, computed tomography; EBUS, endobronchial ultrasonography; EGFR, epidermal growth factor receptor; NA, not available; NPV, negative predictive value; NSCLC, non-small cell lung cancer; PET, positron emission tomography; ROSE, rapid on-site evaluation.

When examining the negative predictive values of EBUS reported in the literature, one must ask a number of questions to arrive at appropriate conclusions regarding the accuracy of staging.

What is the definition of false negative in the study?

There is no uniform definition of what constitutes a false negative EBUS result, and this has contributed to confusion regarding the applicability of the EBUS for mediastinal staging. For example, several reports have suggested that the false negative rate should include nondiagnostic results.[17,30] Although we agree that it is important to note the incidence of nondiagnostic results, we do not believe that such results should be included in the calculation of false negative rates. A nondiagnostic test is neither positive nor negative, and either a repeat EBUS or some other invasive staging modality should be performed to obtain diagnostic information.

The location of the malignant lymph nodes at the time of thoracotomy or thoracoscopic resection also presents an issue when defining a false negative EBUS result. One may ask, for example, whether a negative EBUS-directed biopsy of level 4L and 7 lymph nodes in a patient with a left upper lobe lesion constitutes a false negative result if metastases are found in level 5 or 6 lymph nodes at resection. Although such a finding signifies the inability of the test to prevent futile thoracotomy or thoracoscopic resection, it is not a false negative result per se, as level 5 and 6 lymph nodes cannot be evaluated using EBUS. This is not a failure of EBUS but rather a failure of the staging approach as a whole—CT, PET/CT, and EBUS may be insufficient for staging in this patient. Such situations are precisely why the most recent ACCP guidelines state that patients with tumors in the left upper lobe and an indication for invasive mediastinal staging should undergo evaluation with thoracoscopy, anterior mediastinotomy, or extended mediastinoscopy in the event that nodes outside the reach of standard cervical mediastinoscopy may be involved. We and others have used endoscopic transesophageal ultrasonography to assess these lymph nodes.[31,32]

Given the above considerations, we believe that a true false negative value includes an adequate sample of negative lymph nodes with abundant lymphocytes for nodal stations assessable to EBUS but not positive lymph nodes not assessable using EBUS (level 5, 6, 8, and 9 lymph nodes). The diagnostic yield (includes nondiagnostic samples) and the ability of EBUS to prevent futile resection (includes positive results in level 5, 6, 8, and 9 stations) are important results but are different than the false negative rate.

What is the pretest probability of the disease?

The impact of prevalence on negative predictive value is well known; the smaller the prevalence of mediastinal lymph node involvement, the better the negative predictive value. In our practice, there are two types of EBUS performed for mediastinal assessment of lung cancer patients; a staging EBUS and diagnostic or confirmatory EBUS. The technique is similar; however, the indications are different. In a staging EBUS, the patient has an intermediate suspicion of N2 or N3 involvement, a radiographically normal mediastinum (by CT and PET) and a central tumor or N1 lymph node enlargement, and no distant metastases (category C radiographic disease by ACCP guidelines).[1]

These patients receive a staging EBUS with systemic evaluation of all accessible mediastinal lymph nodes and biopsy of any lymph nodes with specific ultrasonographic criteria, such as lymph node size, shape, and echogenicity (see Fig. 6.2). The prevalence of mediastinal disease is low, and as specific reports have shown, the performance of EBUS in this setting yields a very high negative predictive value.[4,5] In patients with radiographically abnormal mediastinum (category B), especially if disease is bulky (category A), the prevalence of disease is higher, and the negative predictive value of EBUS tends to be lower.[23-25]

WHAT ADJUNCTS TO EBUS HAVE BEEN USED?

As mentioned earlier, most studies investigating EBUS for NSCLC staging focus on the modality's false negative rate and sensitivity. Ultimately, however, the important question is whether performing EBUS prevents futile resection in patients with N2 disease, and multiple recent studies have evaluated the addition of EUS-guided fine needle aspiration (EUS-FNA) to EBUS to increase the ability to prevent futile resection. Compared with EBUS alone, the combination of EBUS plus EUS-FNA has a greater sensitivity, negative predictive value, and diagnostic yield and heightened ability to reduce futile thoracotomy (Table 6-3).[33-40] Although the addition of EUS-FNA to EBUS enables access to additional lymph node stations, the assessment of level 5 and 6 lymph nodes using the combined technique remains difficult and is best done with thoracoscopy. (Anterior mediastinotomy and extended mediastinoscopy can also be used to assess these nodes but is not employed by the majority of surgeons owing to the ease with which thoracoscopy can be performed.)

Whether rapid on-site evaluation (ROSE) of the specimens has been used must also be considered. The usefulness of ROSE in conjunction with EBUS to improve accuracy is controversial, with studies reporting mixed results. Some reports note that the addition of ROSE to EBUS reduces the number of biopsies performed and potentially increases diagnostic yield; however, these findings have not been validated. One recent randomized trial demonstrated that although the addition of ROSE to EBUS elicited no improvement in the diagnostic yield of adequate specimens, patients who underwent EBUS with ROSE, possibly because fewer biopsies were attempted in these patients, had a lower complication rate than patients who underwent EBUS without ROSE.[41] Other studies have demonstrated the reduced utility of ROSE during EUS-FNA.[16]

SITUATIONS IN WHICH NEGATIVE EBUS FINDINGS SHOULD BE CONFIRMED WITH ADDITIONAL INVASIVE MEANS

Absence of lymphocytes

All patients with nondiagnostic EBUS results (i.e., an absence of lymphocytes) should undergo confirmatory mediastinoscopy (grade of recommendation: 1B). Some studies have reported a substantial incidence of malignancy in N2 nodes considered to be nondiagnostic specimens on EBUS.[19,30] Although nondiagnostic samples technically are not a false negative result, patients in whom EBUS yields nondiagnostic samples should be re-evaluated using another invasive test if no other samples yielded

TABLE 6-3 Studies Reporting Sensitivity and/or Negative Predictive Value of Real-Time Endobronchial Ultrasonography plus Endoscopic Ultrasonography in the Mediastinal Staging of Confirmed or Highly Suspected Lung Cancer

Author, Year	Study Design	No. of Patients	Prevalence of N2 Disease (%)	NPV	Sensitivity	Accuracy	Key Findings	Potential for Significant Bias
Szlubowski et al, 2010[33]	Prospective observational	120	22	88 for EBUS, 94 for EBUS-EUS	52 for EBUS, 76 for EBUS-EUS	89 for EBUS, 93 for EBUS-EUS	In the radiographically normal mediastinum, EBUS-EUS has a higher sensitivity and NPV than EBUS alone does. Confirmatory mediastinoscopy is not necessary if EBUS-EUS results are negative.	Yes
Wallace et al, 2008[34]	Prospective observational	138	30	97	93	NA	EBUS-EUS has higher sensitivity and NPV than EBUS alone does in NSCLC staging.	Yes
Hwangbo et al, 2010[35]	Retrospective	143	31	93 for EBUS, 96 for EBUS-EUS	84 for EBUS, 91 for EBUS-EUS	95 for EBUS, 97 for EUS	EBUS-EUS has a higher NPV, sensitivity, and accuracy than EBUS alone does, but this difference is not statistically significant.	Yes
Block et al, 2010[36]	Retrospective	42	36	87	84	NA	EBUS-EUS reduces the need for mediastinoscopy. Accuracy increases with user experience.	Yes
Annema et al, 2010[37]	Randomized controlled trial	123	49	85	85	NA	EBUS-EUS with confirmatory surgical staging in the event of negative results is more accurate than surgical staging alone. EBUS-EUS results in fewer nontherapeutic thoracotomies.	No
Herth et al, 2010[38]	Retrospective	139	52	92 for EBUS, 96 for EBUS-EUS	91 for EBUS, 96 for EBUS-EUS	91 for EBUS, 96 for EBUS-EUS	EBUS-EUS is more accurate than either EBUS or EUS alone.	Yes
Vilmann et al, 2005[40]	Prospective observational series	33	71	72 for EBUS, 100 for EBUS-EUS	85 for EBUS, 100 for EBUS-EUS	89 for EBUS, 100 for EBUS-EUS	EBUS-EUS is accurate and may replace surgical mediastinal staging methods.	Yes
Zielinski et al, 2013[39]	Retrospective observational	632	64	87.8	82.8	NA	Transcervical extended mediastinal lymphadenectomy has a higher sensitivity and NPV than EBUS-EUS.	Yes

EBUS, endobronchial ultrasonography; EBUS-EUS, combined endobronchial ultrasound-endoscopic ultrasound; EUS, endoscopic ultrasonography; NA, not available; NPV, negative predictive value; NSCLC, non–small cell lung cancer.

adequate information for staging purposes. For example, a patient with a right upper lobe tumor in whom EBUS yields a nondiagnostic level 7 sample but a positive 4R sample need not undergo additional tests to confirm the nondiagnostic result because the patient has N2 disease by definition; however, an additional procedure would be warranted if all the other samples were negative. The most likely next procedure would be mediastinoscopy.

Highly suspicious computed tomography or positron emission tomography findings

Patients with negative EBUS findings and highly suspicious CT or PET findings (category A or B radiographic disease by ACCP guidelines) should undergo additional invasive tests for mediastinal staging (grade of recommendation: 2B). The negative predictive value of EBUS in this setting is lower owing to the higher prevalence of disease, but this is also true of any other test, including mediastinoscopy. Multiple prospective comparative trials have reported that EBUS and mediastinoscopy have very similar results in this setting.[8,25] The addition of mediastinoscopy to EBUS has been reported to slightly improve the procedure's negative predictive value and sensitivity; however, this difference was statistically insignificant in most studies.[25] One study from the Mayo Clinic investigated the use of mediastinoscopy to confirm negative EBUS findings in patients with a high suspicion for N2 disease.[42] Of the more than 400 patients who underwent EBUS for lung cancer staging over a 2-year period, 29 with negative EBUS findings underwent confirmatory mediastinoscopy; of these 29 patients, eight (29%) were found to have N2 disease. Of the patients with negative EBUS and mediastinoscopy findings who proceeded to surgery, four were found to have N2 disease missed by both procedures. In all four of these patients, the disease was in lymph nodes that had been assessed by both EBUS and mediastinoscopy: two patients had disease in the level 4 lymph nodes, and two patients had disease in the level 7 lymph nodes.

Annema et al[37] showed that the combination of EBUS-EUS and mediastinoscopy has the highest sensitivity and negative predictive value in detecting disease involvement in the mediastinum. In this study, the disease prevalence was 44%. Surgical staging identified positive mediastinal lymph nodes that had not been detected by EBUS-EUS in an additional 9% of patients. The sensitivity and negative predictive value of EBUS-EUS alone were both 85%. The addition of surgical staging to endosonography increased the sensitivity to 94% and the negative predictive value to 93%.

Suspicious mediastinal lymph nodes not assessable using endobronchial ultrasonography

Patients in whom CT or PET reveals suspicious mediastinal lymph nodes that cannot be assessed with EBUS (level 5, 6, 8, and 9 lymph nodes) should undergo an additional procedure to sample those nodes (grade of recommendation: 1A). Disease within lymph node stations that cannot be assessed using EBUS is a common cause of false negative results.[6,8,10,11,14,25,37] Nevertheless, EBUS is a reasonable first-line study, as it can be used to document disease in the paratracheal lymph nodes and establish a diagnosis of N2 disease. However, in the event of negative EBUS findings, further testing should be undertaken. Options depend on the position of the lymph node.

For level 5 and 6 lymph nodes, thoracoscopy, anterior mediastinotomy, or extended mediastinoscopy have been used. Although they are rarely positive, level 8 and 9 lymph nodes can be sampled via EUS.

In addition, patients with a tumor in the left upper lobe in whom invasive mediastinal staging is indicated should undergo separate sampling of the level 5 and 6 lymph nodes if EBUS reveals other mediastinal node stations to be uninvolved (grade of recommendation: 2B). The relatively higher incidence of metastatic disease in the level 5 and 6 lymph nodes in patients with left upper lobe tumors, even in the absence of metastases in other mediastinal lymph nodes, presents a special situation in the staging of NSCLC. In these patients, staging EBUS can be performed; however, if EBUS findings are negative, additional assessment of the level 5 and 6 lymph nodes by thoracoscopy, anterior mediastinotomy, or extended mediastinoscopy is warranted.

CONCLUSIONS

Additional invasive staging should be considered if no lymphocytes were obtained in the EBUS specimen or if the pretest probability of cancer involvement was high. One should also take into consideration the ability of EBUS to assess the suspicious lymph node station. Some nodal stations are best assessed by other invasive means.

REFERENCES

1. Silvestri GA, Gonzalez AV, Jantz MA, et al. Methods for staging non-small cell lung cancer: diagnosis and management of lung cancer, 3rd ed: American College of Chest Physicians evidence-based clinical practice guidelines. *Chest* 2013;143(5)(suppl):e211S–e250S.
2. De Leyn P, Lardinois D, Van Schil PE, et al. ESTS guidelines for preoperative lymph node staging for non-small cell lung cancer. *Eur J Cardiothorac Surg* 2007;32(1):1–8.
3. Cornwell LD, Bakaeen FG, Lan CK, et al. Endobronchial ultrasonography-guided transbronchial needle aspiration biopsy for preoperative nodal staging of lung cancer in a veteran population. *JAMA Surg* 2013;148(11):1024–1029.
4. Herth FJ, Eberhardt R, Krasnik M, et al. Endobronchial ultrasound-guided transbronchial needle aspiration of lymph nodes in the radiologically and positron emission tomography-normal mediastinum in patients with lung cancer. *Chest* 2008;133(4):887–891.
5. Herth FJ, Ernst A, Eberhardt R, et al. Endobronchial ultrasound-guided transbronchial needle aspiration of lymph nodes in the radiologically normal mediastinum. *Eur Respir J* 2006;28(5):910–914.
6. Hwangbo B, Kim SK, Lee HS, et al. Application of endobronchial ultrasound-guided transbronchial needle aspiration following integrated PET/CT in mediastinal staging of potentially operable non-small cell lung cancer. *Chest* 2009;135(5):1280–1287.
7. Lee HS, Lee GK, Lee HS, et al. Real-time endobronchial ultrasound-guided transbronchial needle aspiration in mediastinal staging of non-small cell lung cancer: how many aspirations per target lymph node station? *Chest* 2008;134(2):368–374.
8. Yasufuku K, Pierre A, Darling G, et al. A prospective controlled trial of endobronchial ultrasound-guided transbronchial needle aspiration compared with mediastinoscopy for mediastinal lymph node staging of lung cancer. *J Thorac Cardiovasc Surg* 2011;142(6):1393–1400.
9. Feller-Kopman D, Yung RC, Burroughs F, et al. Cytology of endobronchial ultrasound-guided transbronchial needle aspiration: a retrospective study with histology correlation. *Cancer* 2009;117(6):482–490.
10. Ømark Petersen H, Eckardt J, Hakami A, et al. The value of mediastinal staging with endobronchial ultrasound-guided transbronchial needle aspiration in patients with lung cancer. *Eur J Cardiothorac Surg* 2009;36(3):465–468.
11. Sanz-Santos J, Andreo F, Castellà E, et al. Representativeness of nodal sampling with endobronchial ultrasonography in non-small-cell lung cancer staging. *Ultrasound Med Biol* 2012;38(1):62–68.

12. Nakajima T, Yasufuku K, Saegusa F, et al. Rapid on-site cytologic evaluation during endobronchial ultrasound-guided transbronchial needle aspiration for nodal staging in patients with lung cancer. *Ann Thorac Surg* 2013;95(5):1695–1699.
13. Jhun BW, Park HY, Jeon K, et al. Nodal stations and diagnostic performances of endobronchial ultrasound-guided transbronchial needle aspiration in patients with non-small cell lung cancer. *J Korean Med Sci* 2012;27(1):46–51.
14. Szlubowski A, Kuzdzał J, Kołodziej M, et al. Endobronchial ultrasound-guided needle aspiration in the non-small cell lung cancer staging. *Eur J Cardiothorac Surg* 2009;35(2):332–335.
15. Bauwens O, Dusart M, Pierard P, et al. Endobronchial ultrasound and value of PET for prediction of pathological results of mediastinal hot spots in lung cancer patients. *Lung Cancer* 2008;61(3):356–361.
16. Joseph M, Jones T, Lutterbie Y, et al. Rapid on-site pathologic evaluation does not increase the efficacy of endobronchial ultrasonographic biopsy for mediastinal staging. *Ann Thorac Surg* 2013;96(2):403–410.
17. Lee BE, Kletsman E, Rutledge JR, et al. Utility of endobronchial ultrasound-guided mediastinal lymph node biopsy in patients with non-small cell lung cancer. *J Thorac Cardiovasc Surg* 2012;143(3):585–590.
18. Cerfolio RJ, Bryant AS, Eloubeidi MA, et al. The true false negative rates of esophageal and endobronchial ultrasound in the staging of mediastinal lymph nodes in patients with non-small cell lung cancer. *Ann Thorac Surg* 2010;90(2):427–434.
19. Navani N, Brown JM, Nankivell M, et al. Suitability of endobronchial ultrasound-guided transbronchial needle aspiration specimens for subtyping and genotyping of non-small cell lung cancer: a multicenter study of 774 patients. *Am J Respir Crit Care Med* 2012;185(12):1316–1322.
20. Kuo C-H, Chen H-C, Chung F-T, et al. Diagnostic value of EBUS-TBNA for lung cancer with non-enlarged lymph nodes: a study in a tuberculosis-endemic country. *PLoS ONE* 2011;6(2):e16877.
21. Hu Y, Puri V, Crabtree TD, et al. Attaining proficiency with endobronchial ultrasound-guided transbronchial needle aspiration. *J Thorac Cardiovasc Surg* 2013;146(6):1387–1392.
22. Yasufuku K, Chiyo M, Koh E, et al. Endobronchial ultrasound guided transbronchial needle aspiration for staging of lung cancer. *Lung Cancer* 2005;50(3):347–354.
23. Rintoul RC, Tournoy KG, El Daly H, et al. EBUS-TBNA for the clarification of PET positive intrathoracic lymph nodes-an international multi-centre experience. *J Thorac Oncol* 2009;4(1):44–48.
24. Cetinkaya E, Seyhan EC, Ozgul A, et al. Efficacy of convex probe endobronchial ultrasound (CP-EBUS) assisted transbronchial needle aspiration for mediastinal staging in non-small cell lung cancer cases with mediastinal lymphadenopathy. *Ann Thorac Cardiovasc Surg* 2011;17(3):236–242.
25. Ernst A, Anantham D, Eberhardt R, et al. Diagnosis of mediastinal adenopathy—real-time endobronchial ultrasound guided needle aspiration versus mediastinoscopy. *J Thorac Oncol* 2008;3:577–582.
26. Gu P, Zhao Y, Jiang L, et al. Endobronchial ultrasound-guided transbronchial needle aspiration for staging of lung cancer: a systematic review and meta-analysis. *Eur J Cancer* 2009;45(8):1389–1396.
27. Adams K, Shah PL, Edmonds L, et al. Test performance of endobronchial ultrasound and transbronchial needle aspiration biopsy for mediastinal staging in patients with lung cancer: systematic review and meta-analysis. *Thorax* 2009;64:757–762.
28. Abu-Hijleh M, El-Sameed Y, Eldridge K, et al. Linear probe endobronchial ultrasound bronchoscopy with guided transbronchial needle aspiration (EBUS-TBNA) in the evaluation of mediastinal and hilar pathology: introducing the procedure to a teaching institution. *Lung* 2013;191(1):109–115.
29. Dong X, Qiu X, Liu Q, et al. Endobronchial ultrasound-guided transbronchial needle aspiration in the mediastinal staging of non-small cell lung cancer: a meta-analysis. *Ann Thorac Surg* 2013;96(4):1502–1507.
30. Whitson BA, Groth SS, Odell DD, et al. True negative predictive value of endobronchial ultrasound in lung cancer: are we being conservative enough? *Ann Thorac Surg* 2013;95(5):1689–1694.
31. Liberman M, Duranceau A, Grunenwald E, Martin J, Thiffault V, Khereba M, et al. New technique performed by using EUS access for biopsy of para-aortic (station 6) mediastinal lymph nodes without traversing the aorta. *Gastrointest Endosc* 2011;73(5):1048–1051.
32. Cerfolio RJ, Bryant AS, Eloubeidi MA. Accessing the aortopulmonary window (#5) and the para-aortic (#6) lymph nodes in patients with non-small cell lung cancer. *Ann Thorac Surg* 2007;84(3):940–945.
33. Szlubowski A, Zieliński M, Soja J, Annema JT, Şośnicki W, Jakubiak M, et al. A combined approach of endobronchial and endoscopic ultrasound-guided needle aspiration in the radiologically normal mediastinum in non-small-cell lung cancer staging–a prospective trial. *Eur J Cardiothorac Surg* 2010;37(5):1175–1179.

34. Wallace MB, Pascual JM, Raimondo M, Woodward TA, McComb BL, Crook JE, et al. Minimally invasive endoscopic staging of suspected lung cancer. *JAMA* 2008;299(5):540–546.

35. Hwangbo B, Lee GK, Lee HS, Lim KY, Lee SH, Kim HY, et al. Transbronchial and transesophageal fine-needle aspiration using an ultrasound bronchoscope in mediastinal staging of potentially operable lung cancer. *Chest* 2010;138(4):795–802.

36. Block MI. Transition from mediastinoscopy to endoscopic ultrasound for lung cancer staging. *Ann Thorac Surg* 2010;89:885–890.

37. Annema JT, van Meerbeeck JP, Rintoul RC, Dooms C, Deschepper E, Dekkers OM, et al. Mediastinoscopy vs endosonography for mediastinal nodal staging of lung cancer: a randomized trial. *JAMA* 2010;304(20):2245–2252.

38. Herth FJ, Krasnik M, Kahn N, Eberhardt R, Ernst A. Combined endoscopic-endobronchial ultrasound-guided fine-needle aspiration of mediastinal lymph nodes through a single bronchoscope in 150 patients with suspected lung cancer. *Chest* 2010;138(4):790–794.

39. Zielinski M, Szlubowski A, Kołodziej M, Orzechowski S, Laczynska E, Pankowski J, et al. Comparison of endobronchial ultrasound and/or endoesophageal ultrasound with transcervical extended mediastinal lymphadenectomy for staging and restaging of non-small-cell lung cancer. *J Thorac Oncol* 2013;8(5):630–636.

40. Vilmann P, Krasnik M, Larsen SS, Jacobsen GK, Clementsen P. Transesophageal endoscopic ultrasound-guided fine-needle aspiration (EUS-FNA) and endobronchial ultrasound-guided transbronchial needle aspiration (EBUS-TBNA) biopsy: a combined approach in the evaluation of mediastinal lesions. *Endoscopy* 2005;37(9):833–839.

41. Trisolini R, Cancellieri A, Tinelli C, et al. Rapid on-site evaluation of transbronchial aspirates in the diagnosis of hilar and mediastinal adenopathy: a randomized trial. *Chest* 2011;139:395–401.

42. Defranchi SA, Edell ES, Daniels CE, Prakash UB, Swanson KL, Utz JP, et al. Mediastinoscopy in patients with lung cancer and negative endobronchial ultrasound guided needle aspiration. *Ann Thorac Surg* 2010;90(6):1753–1757.

CHAPTER 7

Cervical Mediastinoscopy

CRITICAL ELEMENTS

- Nodal Station Assessment
- Patient Eligibility
- Preparing for Complications

1. NODAL STATION ASSESSMENT

Recommendation: Cervical mediastinoscopy can be used to evaluate lymph node stations 2R, 2L, 4R, 4L, and 7.

Type of Data: Retrospective.

Strength of Recommendation: Weak.

Rationale

Lung cancer patients with stage IIIA (ipsilateral) or stage IIIB (contralateral) mediastinal node involvement have poor long-term survival. The mediastinal nodes should be assessed before lung resection in patients who have accessible mediastinal lymph nodes that are greater than 1.5 cm in diameter and/or that positron emission tomography findings reveal to be positive. Patients without these characteristics but who nevertheless have a high likelihood of mediastinal nodal involvement should also undergo mediastinal lymph node assessment before lung resection. Such patients include those with tumors larger than 3 cm in diameter, central tumors (involving the inner third of the lung), and/or tumors of specific histologic types (i.e., large cell, neuroendocrine, and small cell tumors and adenocarcinomas) and/or those with multiple lung lesions. Patients who have tumors with a maximum standardized uptake value greater than 4 and/or positive N1 nodes on positron emission tomography (PET) should also undergo mediastinoscopy to assess the mediastinal nodes.

115

Mediastinal lymph nodes can be assessed using endobronchial ultrasonography or cervical mediastinoscopy. Cervical mediastinoscopy can be used to evaluate lymph node stations 2R, 2L, 4R, 4L, and 7. Endobronchial ultrasonography can evaluate these stations as well as station 10 and the hilar nodes in stations 11 and 12. The technique chosen depends on the surgeon's preference, institutional expertise, and the contraindications to cervical mediastinoscopy. A broad discussion of the available modalities is found in Chapter 5, Invasive Mediastinal Staging Overview.

2. PATIENT ELIGIBILITY

Recommendation: Caution and good surgical judgment should be exercised when offering cervical mediastinoscopy to patients with superior vena cava syndrome, abnormal anatomy, prior treatment to the operative field, and coagulopathy.

Type of Data: Retrospective.

Strength of Recommendation: Weak.

Rationale

Several authors have reported series of patients with superior vena cava (SVC) syndrome who underwent cervical mediastinoscopy. In these three series, 1 of 14 (7%) patients, 5 of 80 (6%) patients, and 2 of 39 (5%) patients, respectively, had significant bleeding requiring sternotomies. Airway obstruction due to hematoma was a life-threatening complication in one series. No patients in the three series died from undergoing mediastinoscopy. This complication is higher than reported in large series of patients without SVC syndrome undergoing this procedure.[1-3]

Anatomic characteristics that would exclude patients from mediastinoscopy include aortic arch aneurysm and innominate artery calcification, which increase the risk for stroke, and existing tracheostomy. Patients who have limited neck mobility, including those with ankylosing spondylitis, also would not be candidates for cervical mediastinoscopy.

Patients who have received remote neck and chest radiation, as well as those who have had recent adjuvant chemo- or radiotherapy, are candidates for mediastinoscopy. Mediastinoscopy can be repeated in patients who have received radiotherapy and in patients who present with a second malignancy. However, these patients may have inseparable adhesions that make performing repeat mediastinoscopy difficult. In addition, the lymph node sampling of a repeat mediastinoscopy is less sensitive than that of the primary mediastinoscopy.

Prior median sternotomy for cardiac surgery is not a contraindication to mediastinoscopy. Cardiac surgery typically does not violate the dissection plan used for mediastinoscopy, and mediastinoscopy outcomes in patients who have or have not had previous cardiac surgery are similar.

Nevertheless, surgeons should exercise good surgical judgment before offering mediastinoscopy and then intraoperatively in patients who have SVC syndrome or who have already undergone mediastinoscopy, have received neck radiation, or have undergone median sternotomy.

3. PREPARING FOR COMPLICATIONS

Recommendation: Proper preparation of both the patient and the operating room team and the use of video mediastinoscopy are essential to effectively managing emergency complications during cervical mediastinoscopy.

Type of Data: Retrospective.

Strength of Recommendation: Weak.

Rationale

Although rare, complications during cervical mediastinoscopy have been described. To ensure the successful and safe completion of the procedure, the entire operative team must be prepared to manage any complications, and the patient should be properly positioned and draped. These precautions will result in better outcomes with less morbidity.

The patient should be supine, with a roll placed transversely beneath the shoulders. The neck should be extended maximally and the head supported. The trachea should be easily palpable. Once the patient is under general anesthesia, an arterial line or pulse oximeter is placed in the right upper extremity to detect prolonged compression of the innominate artery. The availability of blood for potential transfusion should be confirmed. The draping should include the neck and chest in the unlikely event of life-threatening hemorrhage, airway injury, or pneumothorax requiring urgent intervention.

Plans for immediate emergent median sternotomy or thoracotomy in the event of hemorrhage or airway injury should be discussed during the preoperative time-out. All members of the nursing, circulating, and anesthesia teams must be aware of their roles in the event of an emergency situation.

To help ensure that all members of the operating room team are aware of what is happening surgically, video mediastinoscopy should be utilized so that all members of the surgery, anesthesia, and nursing teams can view the procedure simultaneously. However, video mediastinoscopy may not be feasible in all patients, as video mediastinoscopes, which are significantly larger than standard mediastinoscopes, may be too big to use in patients with limited space between the trachea and sternal notch and in patients with dense adhesions in this area. In these instances, a standard mediastinoscope must be used; therefore, both a video and standard mediastinoscope should be readily available. As only the surgeon is able to see the operative field with a standard mediastinoscope, proper communication is essential in the event of a complication.

Technical Aspects

Apart from issues of safety, studies have shown that video-assisted mediastinoscopy yields a higher number of lymph nodes than standard mediastinoscopy. However, owing to the larger size of the video instrument, video mediastinoscopy has been associated with slightly higher rates of recurrent nerve injury and pneumothorax. One recent report suggests that for patients with similar tumors, video mediastinoscopy not only yields a greater number of lymph nodes than standard mediastinoscopy but also far more frequently results in upstaging the disease. This results in fewer N2 false negatives undergoing surgery. The net effect is that patients who undergo video mediastinoscopy have better long-term survival than patients who undergo standard mediastinoscopy.

To successfully perform cervical mediastinoscopy, surgeons must know the anatomy of the innominate artery and vein, the aortic arch, the superior vena cava, the pulmonary artery, the azygous vein, the left recurrent nerve, the esophagus, and lymph node positions. Knowledge of this anatomy will result in an overall completion rate of 1%, including hemorrhage (0.3%), vocal cord dysfunction (0.5%), tracheal injury (0.01%), and pneumothorax (0.09%).[4] Other rare complications include incisional metastasis and chyle leak.

Prior to incision, the thyroid isthmus and either the innominate or carotid artery should be palpated to detect any vascular anomalies. Aberrant innominate artery and right common carotid artery originating from a common carotid trunk have been described. The incision (2 to 4 cm) should be made below the thyroid isthmus and above the sternal notch. The incision is carried down to the pretracheal fascia. Finger dissection between the anterior trachea and the pretracheal fascia is extended to the tracheal bifurcation and laterally along both sides of the trachea. Finger dissection should be used to lift the innominate artery off of the trachea, and the pretracheal plane should be opened digitally to access the paratracheal nodes. These nodes can often be palpated in both the left and right paratracheal spaces. The use of finger dissection may be responsible for the low incidence of recurrent nerve injury following mediastinoscopy. In a review of patients in whom vocal cord motion was monitored during mediastinoscopy, digital dissection of the anterior tracheal wall activated both recurrent nerves. Cautery in the left paratracheal plane activated the left recurrent nerve, but cautery in the subcarinal or right paratracheal space elicited little activity in the right recurrent nerve. The study's findings suggest that recurrent nerve injury is due to dissection and traction rather than cautery use.[5]

After the pretracheal plane has been opened, the mediastinoscope is inserted, and a suction dissector is used to open the subcarinal fascia.

After dissection has clearly revealed the lymph nodes in both the left and right paratracheal areas and in the subcarinal space, biopsy forceps can be used to sample these nodes. Several previous studies have reported that two to seven lymph nodes are sampled per procedure, but whether these studies were referencing individual nodes or pieces of nodes is unknown.[6–9] Interestingly, one study demonstrated that the volume of tissue sampled from a lymph node station was correlated with the presence of N2 disease. This study showed that biopsy of a greater number of lymph node stations did not increase the chances of detecting N2 disease. The author concluded that the larger volumes were taken from enlarged suspicious nodes.[10]

Catastrophic bleeding can be avoided by the use of aspiration, prior to biopsy, if there is any doubt as to the dissection of a lymph node. Lymph node stations 2R, 2L, 4R, 4L, and 7 should be subject to biopsy. The aortopulmonary window lymph nodes (stations 5 and 6) cannot be biopsied during standard mediastinoscopy.

Because mediastinoscopy is used to assess an area that has major vascular structures, hemostasis is necessary prior to closing the incision. The suction dissector can be used to control minor bleeding. In the event of major bleeding, the mediastinoscope should be left in place, and the area should be packed with gauze and hemostatic materials to control the bleeding. If these steps do not control the bleeding or if major vascular structures such as the pulmonary artery are injured, emergency median sternotomy or thoracotomy should be performed. In these cases, the preparatory measures discussed with the nursing and anesthesia teams prior to operation may be lifesaving. In Table 7-1, the reader will find a summary of significant publications on the utility, efficacy, and safety of cervical mediastinoscopy.

TABLE 7-1   Summary of Mediastinoscopy References

Author	Study Design	No. of Patients	Main Question	Key Findings	Potential for Bias
Turna et al, 2013[11]	Retrospective	433	Is there a survival difference between VID and MED?	VID had greater sensitivity, accuracy, and negative predictive value than MED. 5-year survival was 40% for VID vs. 66% for MED.	Yes
Zakkar et al, 2012[12]	Literature review and meta-analysis	6,123	Is VID better than conventional MED?	No randomized studies have compared VID and conventional MED.	
Kanzaki et al, 2011[13]	Retrospective	224	Which PET-negative patients have occult metastases at operation?	Patients with right upper lobe or right middle lobe adenocarcinoma >3 cm, and patients with SUV >4 had increased risk of occult metastases.	Yes
Cho et al, 2010[6]	Retrospective	521	How does the lymph node access, positive node detection rate, and complication rate of VID compare with those of conventional MED?	VID had a lower complication rate, detected more positive nodes, and accessed the same lymph node stations.	Yes
Yasufuku et al, 2011[7]	Prospective	153	Is EBUS or MED more sensitive in detecting positive lymph nodes?	The EBUS and MED had equal sensitivity and negative predictive values.	No
Anraku et al, 2010[8]	Retrospective	645	Does VID or conventional MED access more lymph node stations and detect more positive lymph nodes?	VID accessed more lymph node stations than MED.	Yes
Nelson et al, 2010[10]	Retrospective	567	Is biopsy sample volume related to the detection of metastatic disease?	Biopsy sample volume was a better predictor of metastatic disease than was the total number of stations sampled.	Yes
Al-Sarraf et al, 2008[14]	Retrospective	153	Which PET-negative patients have occult positive nodes at MED?	Patients with central tumors or right upper lobe tumors, N1 positive nodes, and nodes >1 cm on CT are more likely to have occult positive mediastinal nodes.	Yes

(continued)

TABLE 7-1 Summary of Mediastinoscopy References (continued)

Author	Study Design	No. of Patients	Main Question	Key Findings	Potential for Bias
Upadhyaya et al, 2008[15]	Case report	1			
Marra et al, 2008[16]	Prospective	104	Is repeat MED safe after induction chemotherapy?	Repeat MED after induction chemotherapy is possible in 98% of patients.	Yes
Roberts et al, 2007[5]	Prospective	15	What is the cause of laryngeal nerve injury during MED?	Blunt digital dissection, not cautery, causes recurrent nerve activation during MED.	No
Lee et al, 2007[17]	Retrospective	224	Which patients with negative PET findings have positive nodes at MED?	Central tumors, high SUV, adenocarcinoma, and large tumor size all predicted positive nodes at MED.	Yes
de Langen et al, 2006[18]	Meta-analysis	896 14 studies	What PET-negative mediastinal lymph node size should lead to MED?	5% PET-negative mediastinal lymph nodes 10–15 mm were positive with MED; 21% of PET-negative >1.5 were positive on MED.	No
Fibia et al, 2006[19]	Retrospective	142	What mediastinal lymph node size predicts positive mediastinal lymph nodes?	Adenocarcinoma and lymph nodes >1 cm increased the risk for positive mediastinal lymph nodes.	Yes
Lemaire et al, 2006[4]	Retrospective	2,145	What percentage of cancer patients have positive lymph nodes at MED, and what is the procedure's complication rate?	24% of cancer patients had positive lymph nodes at MED. The complication rate was 1.07%, and the mortality rate was 0.05%.	Yes
Stamatis et al, 2005[20]	Retrospective	279	Is repeat MED safe?	Repeat MED not possible in 2% and minor complications in 3%.	Yes
Dosios et al, 2005[3]	Retrospective	39	Is MED safe in patients with SVC syndrome?	MED had a diagnostic accuracy of 97%. There was no mortality but 8% had major complications, including hemorrhage and airway obstruction.	Yes

Study	Study type	n	Question	Results	Safe/Yes
Kumar et al, 2003[21]	Retrospective	28	Is MED safe in patients who have undergone cardiac surgery?	No complications were reported.	Yes
Venissac et al, 2013[9]	Retrospective	240	What does our experience with VID reveal?	On average, VID could be used to access 2.3 lymph node stations and biopsy 6 lymph nodes. Two patients had complications. Staging after thoracotomy remained unchanged in 93.6% of patients.	No
Le Pimpec Barthes et al, 2003[22]	Case report	1		The patient had chylothorax following MED.	
Qureshi et al, 2002[23]	Case report	1		Patient had right common carotid crossing trachea from left-sided common carotid trunk, precluding MED.	
Bataγiannis et al, 2002[24]	Case report	1		The patient had incisional metastasis following MED.	
Mineo et al, 1999[2]	Retrospective	80	Is MED safe in patients with SVC syndrome?	There was no mortality, but 6% of patients had significant bleeding.	Yes
Jahangiri et al, 1993[1]	Retrospective	14	Is MED safe in patients with SVC syndrome?	There was no mortality, but 7% of patients had bleeding requiring sternotomy.	Yes
Riquet et al, 1993[25]	Case report	1		The patient had chylous effusion after MED.	
Vallieres et al, 1987[26]	Retrospective	35	Which T1 patients (35) had positive N2 or N3 nodes?	23% had inoperable disease. 14% (5/35) had positive lymph node at MED. Large cell lung and adenocarcinoma had positive lymph nodes.	Yes

CT, computed tomography; EBUS, endobronchial ultrasonography; MED, mediastinoscopy; PET, positron emission tomography; SUV, standardized uptake value; SVC, superior vena cava; VID, video mediastinoscopy.

REFERENCES

1. Jahangiri M, Taggart DP, Goldstraw P. Role of mediastinoscopy in superior vena cava obstruction. *Cancer* 1993;71(10):3006–3008.
2. Mineo TC, Ambrogi V, Nofroni I, et al. Mediastinoscopy in superior vena cava obstruction: analysis of 80 consecutive patients. *Ann Thorac Surg* 1999;68(1):223–226.
3. Dosios T, Theakos N, Chatziantoniou C. Cervical mediastinoscopy and anterior mediastinotomy in superior vena cava obstruction. *Chest* 2005;128(3):1551–1556.
4. Lemaire A, Nikolic I, Petersen T, et al. Nine-year single center experience with cervical mediastinoscopy: complications and false negative rate. *Ann Thorac Surg* 2006;82(4):1185–1189.
5. Roberts JR, Wadsworth J. Recurrent laryngeal nerve monitoring during mediastinoscopy: predictors of injury. *Ann Thorac Surg* 2007;83(2):388–391.
6. Cho JH, Kim J, Kim K, et al. A comparative analysis of video-assisted mediastinoscopy and conventional mediastinoscopy. *Ann Thorac Surg* 2011;92(3):1007–1011.
7. Yasufuku K, Pierre A, Darling G, et al. A prospective controlled trial of endobronchial ultrasound-guided transbronchial needle aspiration compared with mediastinoscopy for mediastinal lymph node staging of lung cancer. *J Thorac Cardiovas Surg* 2011;142(6):1393–1400.
8. Anraku M, Miyata R, Compeau C, et al. Video-assisted mediastinoscopy compared with conventional mediastinoscopy: are we doing better? *Ann Thorac Surg* 2010; 89(5):1577–1587.
9. Venissac N, Alifano M. Mouroux J. Video-assisted mediastinoscopy: experience from 240 consecutive cases. *Ann Thorac Surg* 2003;71(1):208–212.
10. Nelson E, Pape C, Jørgensen OD, et al. Mediastinal staging for lung cancer: the influence of biopsy volume. *Eur J Cardiothorac Surg* 2010;37(1):26–29.
11. Turna A, Demirkaya A, Özkul S, et al. Video-assisted mediastinoscopic lymphadenectomy is associated with better survival than mediastinoscopy in patients with resected non-small cell lung cancer. *J Thorac Cardiovas Surg* 2013;146:774–780.
12. Zakkar M, Tan C, Hunt I. Is mediastinoscopy a safer and more effective procedure than conventional mediastinoscopy? *Interact Cardiovasc Thorac Surg* 2012;14(1):81–84.
13. Kanzaki R, Higashiyama M, Fujiwara A, et al. Occult mediastinal lymph node metastasis in NSCLC patients diagnosed as clinical N0-1 by preoperative integrated FDG-PET/CT and CT: risk factors, pattern, and histopathological study. *Lung Cancer* 2011;71(3):333–337.
14. Al-Sarraf N, Aziz R, Gately K, et al. Pattern and predictors of occult mediastinal lymph node involvement in non-small cell lung cancer patients with negative mediastinal uptake on positron emission tomography. *Eur J Cardiothorac Surg* 2008;33(1):104–109.
15. Upadhyaya PK, Bertelotti R, Laeeg A, et al. Beware of the aberrant innominate artery. *Ann Thorac Surg* 2008;85(2):653–654.
16. Marra A, Hillejan L, Fechner S, et al. Remediastinoscopy in restaging of lung cancer after induction therapy. *J Thorac Cardiovasc Surg* 2008;135(4):843–849.
17. Lee PC, Port JL, Korst JRJ, et al. Risk factors for occult mediastinal metastases in clinical stage I non-small cell lung cancer. *Ann Thorac Surg* 2007;84(1):177–181.
18. de Langen AJ, Raijmakers P, Riphagen I, et al. The size of mediastinal lymph nodes and its relation with metastatic involvement: a meta-analysis. *Eur J Cardiothorac Surg* 2006;29(1):26–29.
19. Fibia JJ, Molins L, Simon C, et al. The yield of mediastinoscopy with respect to lymph node size, cell type, and the location of the primary tumor. *J Thorac Oncol* 2006;1(5):430–433.
20. Stamatis G, Fechner S, Hillejan L, et al. Repeat mediastinoscopy as restaging procedure. *Pneumologie* 2005;59(12):862–866.
21. Kumar P, Yamada K, Ladas GP, et al. Mediastinoscopy and mediastinotomy after cardiac surgery: are safety and efficacy affected by prior sternotomy? *Ann Thorac Surg* 2003;76(3):872–876.
22. Le Pimpec Barthes F, D'Attellis N, Assouad J, et al. Chylous leak after cervical mediastinoscopy. *J Thorac Cardiovasc Surg* 2003;126(4):1199–1200.
23. Qureshi RA, Holgate AL, Harrington JM, et al. Unsuspected vascular anomaly at cervical mediastinoscopy. *Eur J Cardiothoracic Surg* 2002;21(5):927.
24. Baltayiannis N, Anagnostopoulos D, Bolanos N, et al. Incisional metastasis after cervical mediastinoscopy: a case report. *J BUON* 2002;7(3):287–290.
25. Riquet M, Darse-Derippe J, Saab M, et al. Chylomediastinum after mediastinoscopy: apropos of a case. *Rev Mal Respir* 1993;10(5):473–476.
26. Valliees E, Waters PF. Incidence of mediastinal node involvement in clinical T1 bronchogenic carcinomas. *Can J Surg* 1987;30(5):341–342.

Minimally Invasive and Open Approaches to Mediastinal Nodal Assessment

CRITICAL ELEMENT

- Lymph Node Dissection or Systematic Lymph Node Sampling in the Chest

Recommendation: The proper technique enables surgeons to access all lymph node stations using either a minimally invasive or an open approach.

Type of Data: Retrospective.

Strength of Recommendation: Weak.

Rationale

The staging and surgical treatment of lung cancer depends on the evaluation of both N1 and N2 nodal stations. Sampled or dissected nodes should include 9R, 8R, 7, 10R, 4R, and 2R nodes on the right side and 9L, 8L, 7, 6, and 5 nodes (and 4L and 2L nodes, if accessible) on the left side.[1] Specific strategies for accessing these nodal stations, as well as some technical maneuvers for avoiding complications during nodal assessment, are described below.[1–10]

Adequate lymph node dissection can be achieved using either a minimally invasive or open technique. Surgeons performing video-assisted thoracic surgery (VATS) may find it easier to approach a lymph node examination in an inferior-to-superior fashion. Details on lymph node dissection are outlined in Table 8-1.

Level 8 and 9 lymph nodes, which are adjacent to the inferior pulmonary vein, are exposed by releasing the inferior ligament and extending the dissection anteriorly and posteriorly to the hilum (Fig. 8-1A,B). The number and consistency of the nodal groups, especially those of stations 8 and 9, vary considerably. Nodes may be completely absent, discrete, or lumped in a fibrofatty tissue amenable to block dissection. To expose the 8R nodes, the surgeon opens the pleura between the esophagus and pericardium by extending the dissection from the inferior ligament to the esophageal hiatus (Fig. 8-2). The 8L and 9L stations are approached in a similar manner,

123

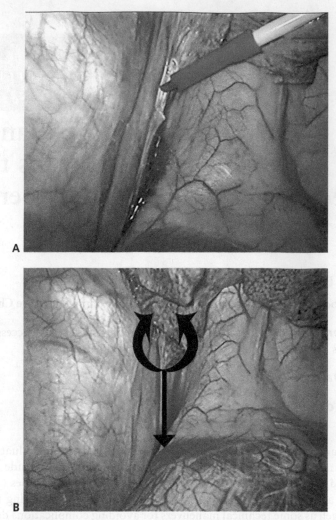

FIGURE 8-1   A,B: Thoracoscopic view of right-sided nodal dissection for stations 8 and 9. (Courtesy of Khalid Amer, FRCS [CTh].)

with care taken to avoid any hiatal hernias and preserve the vagus nerve in its medial location to the aorta.

Station 7 nodes are located between the right and left main bronchi. Nodes on the right are approached between the right main bronchus and the esophagus. The right lung is retracted anteriorly, and the pleural reflection at the back of the hilum is opened from the inferior ligament to the concavity of the azygos vein, medial to the vagus nerve (Fig. 8-3). In this step, all vagal bronchial branches could be divided with

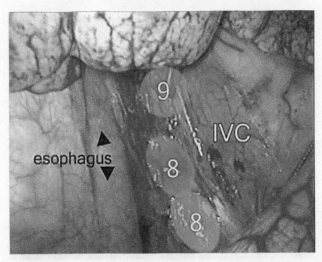

FIGURE 8-2 Exposure of station 8R by right thoracoscopy. IVC, inferior vena cava. (Courtesy of Khalid Amer, FRCS [CTh].)

impunity. (If diathermy is used, cutting these branches usually induces a cough reflex.) The bronchus intermedius and right main bronchus are identified and dissected proximally until the left main bronchus is identified. The subcarinal nodes are lifted off the pericardium (usually an avascular plane) and then dissected from their blood supply, with care taken to avoid injury to the membranous bronchus or esophagus (Fig. 8-4).

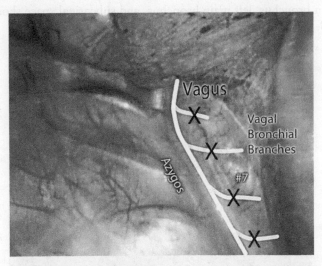

FIGURE 8-3 Right lung retracted forward to expose subcarinal nodes (level 7) via VATS approach. Small vagal branches towards lung can be divided without concern. (Courtesy of Khalid Amer, FRCS [CTh].)

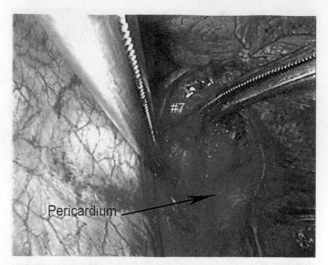

FIGURE 8-4 Mobilization of the subcarinal nodal packet via the right chest. The pericardium is the anterior border of the dissection plane. (Courtesy of Khalid Amer, FRCS [CTh].)

The nodes should be carefully labeled, as paraesophageal 8R and parabronchial 10R nodes could easily be mistaken for 7R nodes. In this location, injury to the thoracic duct is prevented by tucking the duct under the esophagus; lifting the esophagus off the vertebral bed may injure the thoracic duct. At the completion of this dissection, the right main bronchus, left main bronchus, and subcarinal space should be readily visible (Fig. 8-5).

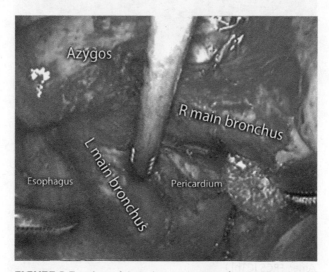

FIGURE 8-5 View of the subcarinal space after complete nodal dissection. (Courtesy of Khalid Amer, FRCS [CTh].)

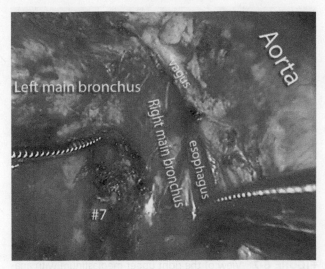

FIGURE 8-6 Subcarinal node dissection from the left chest. (Courtesy of Khalid Amer, FRCS [CTh].)

Accessing subcarinal station 7 nodes from the left is accomplished by following the lower lobe bronchus proximally, as it leads to the subcarinal space and right main bronchus (Fig. 8.6). One useful technique for bringing the carina forward from a deep level is to use a sturdy tape from an anterior port to retract the lower lobe bronchus. Dissection of the posterior aspect of the left hilum facilitates access to the nodes but places the recurrent laryngeal nerve at risk of injury. The location of the separation of the recurrent laryngeal nerve from the vagus nerve varies, and preserving the pleura between the vagus nerve and aorta may lessen the risk of injury to the laryngeal nerve.

Pre- and paratracheal station 2R and 4R nodes are located in a fibrofatty nodal block that can usually be dissected en bloc. These nodes are located in an anatomical triangle bound by the phrenic nerve, vagus nerve, and azygos vein (Fig. 8-7). The apex of the triangle is at the level of the brachiocephalic artery as it crosses the trachea towards the first rib. The lung is retracted downward to expose this triangle, and releasing the pleura between the azygos vein and main bronchus facilitates this exposure. Opening the pleura just lateral to the superior vena cava (SVC) instead of in the middle of the triangle also facilitates this dissection (Figs. 8-8 and 8-9). The right vagus nerve, as well as veins draining directly into the SVC, are present in the triangle, and small veins in this area should be actively sought out and controlled to prevent bleeding complications. In almost all cases, a single vein can be found draining directly into the posterior aspect of the SVC. If inadvertently cut, the vein may retract and bleed profusely, making it difficult to control. The left paratracheal nodes are perhaps the most challenging to expose because the aortic arch, ligamentum arteriosum, and recurrent nerve all hinder dissection. The most lateral of the 4L nodes lie on the tracheobronchial junction and are accessible from the back of the hilum. To expose these nodes, the main pulmonary artery is freed from the bronchus, and

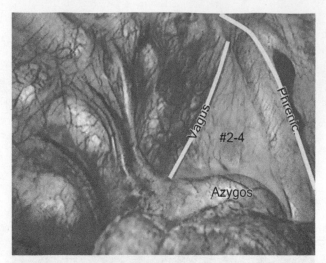

FIGURE 8-7 View of the right upper mediastinum with anatomical boundaries of paratracheal node dissection. (Courtesy of Khalid Amer, FRCS [CTh].)

a vessel loop is passed around the artery to facilitate its retraction. Gentle retraction of the carina in a downward direction and the artery in a cephalad direction exposes station 4L.

Similarly, station 5 and 6 nodes on the left exist in an anatomical triangle whose boundaries are the vagus nerve, phrenic nerve, and aortic arch. Dissection begins by retracting the lung posteriorly and downward. The fibrofatty nodal block is lifted off

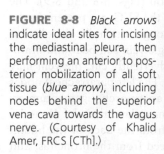

FIGURE 8-8 *Black arrows* indicate ideal sites for incising the mediastinal pleura, then performing an anterior to posterior mobilization of all soft tissue (*blue arrow*), including nodes behind the superior vena cava towards the vagus nerve. (Courtesy of Khalid Amer, FRCS [CTh].)

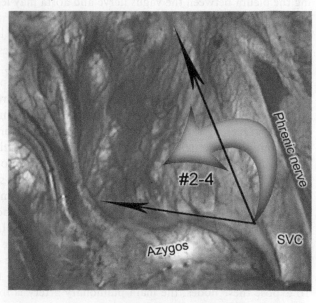

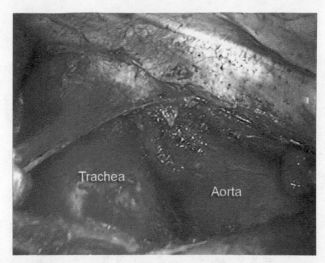

FIGURE 8-9 Right paratracheal node dissection basin after removal of all 2R and 4R nodal tissue. (Courtesy of Khalid Amer, FRCS [CTh].)

the main pulmonary artery into the aortopulmonary space, medial to the vagus nerve (Fig. 8-10). The phrenic nerve is identified on the most medial aspect of the triangle. The nodal block is dissected up to the origin of the left subclavian artery, and all nodes and fatty tissue superficial to the ligamentum are harvested. As long as the dissection is kept to the medial side of the vagus, the recurrent laryngeal nerve is free from potential injury.

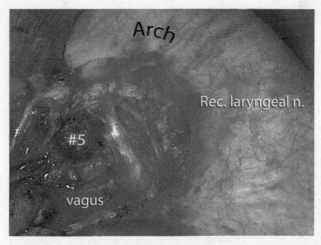

FIGURE 8-10 Exposure of level 5 (aortopulmonary window) nodes from behind the left hilum. (Courtesy of Khalid Amer, FRCS [CTh].)

TABLE 8-1 Structures Dissected/Divided

Level	Borders*	VATS Modifications	Comments
2	2R (includes nodes extending to the left lateral border of the trachea): Upper border: the apex of the right lung and pleural space and in the midline, the upper border of the manubrium Lower border: the intersection of caudal margin of the innominate vein with the trachea 2L: Upper border: the apex of the left lung and pleural space and in the midline, the upper border of the manubrium Lower border: the superior border of the aortic arch	Right dissection: • Incise the pleura to create a triangle adjacent to the SVC (posterior to the phrenic nerve), vertebral body (anterior to the vagus nerve), and azygos vein (superior border). • Retract the SVC and posterior mediastinum to open space. If performing VATS, a vagal sling and retraction sutures should be used. • Excise the 2/4 LN packet starting at the border of the SVC, dissecting posterior toward the trachea and aortic arch. • Additional 2R nodes may be found by retracting the brachiocephalic artery anteriorly. Additional 4R nodes may be found beneath the junction of the azygos vein and SVC. Left dissection: • This region is more difficult to approach from the left and generally requires exposure and dissection of the level 7 nodes. • Exposure can be improved by passing a silicone tape around the left main pulmonary artery and retracting the artery superiorly and away from the distal trachea, which is depressed inferiorly with a blunt soft retractor such as a peanut sponge.	Right dissection: Control (i.e., clip) veins draining directly into the SVC and large lymphatic channels. Avoid injury to the right recurrent nerve, which is generally 1–2 cm distal to the aortic arch beneath the brachiocephalic artery. Left dissection: Control (i.e., clip) large lymphatic channels and lymph node arteries. Avoid injury to the left recurrent nerve beneath the aortic arch.

4	4R (includes right paratracheal nodes and pretracheal nodes extending to the left lateral border of trachea):	
	Upper border: the intersection of the caudal margin of the innominate vein with the trachea	
	Lower border: the lower border of the azygos vein	
	4L (includes nodes to the left of the left lateral border of the trachea, medial to the ligamentum arteriosum):	
	Upper border: the upper margin of the aortic arch	
	Lower border: the upper rim of the left main pulmonary artery	
5	Includes subaortic lymph nodes lateral to the ligamentum arteriosum	• Incise the pleura to create a triangle adjacent to the phrenic nerve, vagus nerve, and left main pulmonary artery (superior border).	Nodes overlying the left superior vein belong to station 10L.
	Upper border: the lower border of the aortic arch	• Excise the 5/6 LN packet starting at the border of the superior vein, dissecting posterior to the pulmonary artery and anteromedial to the vagus nerve.	
	Lower border: the upper rim of the left main pulmonary artery	• Dissection of the level 6 packet proceeds to the aortic arch, and the fibrofatty packet is cleaned to the origin of the left subclavian artery. (Placing a tape around the phrenic nerve may protect it during this dissection.)	

(continued)

TABLE 8-1 Structures Dissected/Divided *(continued)*

Level	Borders*	VATS Modifications	Comments
6	Includes lymph nodes anterior and lateral to the ascending aorta and aortic arch Upper border: a line tangential to the upper border of the aortic arch Lower border: the lower border of the aortic arch		
7	Upper border: the carina of the trachea Lower border: on the left, the upper border of the lower lobe bronchus; on the right, the lower border of the bronchus intermedius	Right dissection: • Divide the posterior hilar pleura adjacent to the parenchyma from the inferior pulmonary vein to the azygos vein/superior right mainstem bronchus. • Divide the vagus nerve branches to the bronchus, sparing the main trunk. • Excise the nodal packet between the right and left mainstem bronchi and esophagus. Left dissection: • Divide the posterior hilar pleura adjacent to the parenchyma from the inferior pulmonary vein to the apex of the hilum anteromedial to the vagus nerve trunk.	Right dissection: Avoid injury to the membranous bronchus and esophagus. Do not include level 8 and 10R nodes. Left dissection: Control (i.e., clip) nodal artery branches from the aorta. Do not include level 4L nodes.

8	Includes nodes adjacent to the wall of the esophagus and to the right or left of the midline, excluding subcarinal nodes Upper border: on the left, the upper border of the lower lobe bronchus; on the right, the lower border of the bronchus intermedius Lower border: the diaphragm	• Divide the vagus nerve branches to the bronchus, sparing the main trunk; to spare the recurrent nerve, avoid dissecting between the vagus nerve and aorta. • Retract the lower lobe bronchus upward and anteriorly and simultaneously retract the esophagus posteriorly to expose the subcarinal nodes from the left. (This can be done using retraction tape if VATS is performed.) • Excise the nodal packet between the left and right mainstem bronchi and esophagus. • Divide the inferior pulmonary ligament. • Excise level 9 nodes within the ligament. • Reflect or dissect the pleura from the esophagus. • Excise level 8 nodes adjacent to the esophagus from the diaphragm to bronchus intermedius (right) or lower lobe bronchus (left).	Right dissection: Avoid injury to the vagus nerve, thoracic duct, azygos vein, and phrenic nerve. Left dissection: Avoid injury to the vagus nerve. Watch for hiatal hernia. Level 9 node quantity varies.
9	Includes nodes lying within the pulmonary ligament Upper border: the inferior pulmonary vein Lower border: the diaphragm		

*As defined by the International Association for the Study of Lung Cancer.

LN, lymph node; SVC, superior vena cava; VATS, video-assisted thoracic surgery.

From Rusch VW, Asamura H, Watanabe H, et al. The IASLC lung cancer staging project: a proposal for a new international lymph node map in the forthcoming seventh edition of the TNM classification for lung cancer. *J Thorac Oncol* 2009;4(5):568–577.

REFERENCES

1. De Leyn P, Dooms C, Kuzdzal J, et al. Revised ESTS guidelines for preoperative mediastinal lymph node staging for non-small-cell lung cancer. *Eur J Cardiothorac Surg* 2014;45(5):787–798.
2. Gossot D. *Atlas of Endoscopic Major Pulmonary Resections*. Paris: Springer-Verlag; 2010.
3. Naruke T, Tsuchiya R, Kondo H, et al. Lymph node sampling in lung cancer: how should it be done? *Eur J Cardiothorac Surg* 1999;16:17–24.
4. Toker A, Kaya S, Erus S, et al. Dissection of superior mediastinum in patients with left sided hilar lung cancer. 2009. http://www.ctsnet.org/sections/videosection/videos/vg2009_TokerA_DissectnSuperMediastnm. Accessed March 25, 2015.
5. Toker A, Tanju S, Ziyade S, et al. Alternative paratracheal lymph node dissection in left-sided hilar lung cancer patients: comparing the number of lymph nodes dissected to the number of lymph nodes dissected in right-sided mediastinal dissections. *Eur J Cardiothorac Surg* 2011;39(6):974–980.
6. Amer K. Thoracoscopic mediastinal lymph node dissection for lung cancer. *Semin Thorac Cardiovasc Surg* 2012;24(1):74–78.
7. D'Amico TA. Videothoracoscopic mediastinal lymphadenectomy. *Thorac Surg Clin* 2010;20(2):207–213.
8. Ziyade S, Pinarbasili NB, Ziyade N, et al. Determination of standard number, size and weight of mediastinal lymph nodes in postmortem examinations: reflection on lung cancer surgery. *J Cardiothorac Surg* 2013;8:94.
9. Darling GE, Allen MS, Decker PA, et al. Number of lymph nodes harvested from a mediastinal lymphadenectomy: results of the randomized, prospective American College of Surgeons Oncology Group Z0030 trial. *Chest* 2011;139(5):1124–1129.
10. Rami-Porta R. Leave no lymph nodes behind! *Eur J Cardiothorac Surg* 2013;44(1):e64–e65.

Minimally Invasive and Open Approaches to Mediastinal Nodal Assessment: Key Question

What is the difference between MLND and MLNS, and what circumstances dictate the use of one or the other during an anatomic pulmonary resection for non–small cell lung cancer?

INTRODUCTION

In lung cancer patients, the presence of lymph node metastases is a significant prognostic factor for survival and helps inform treatment decisions. Therefore, accurate lymph node assessment during surgical resection for clinical early-stage lung cancer is essential. Although imaging modalities such as computed tomography and positron emission tomography are helpful in the preoperative assessment of lymph nodes, their ability to detect mediastinal lymph node metastases is limited. Given the false negative rate of cervical mediastinoscopy, mediastinal lymph node evaluation should be performed during pulmonary resection regardless of whether mediastinoscopy or endobronchial ultrasonography has already been performed and omitted only in extenuating circumstances. Visual inspection alone of the lymph nodes at the time of lung resection is also inadequate. Thus, the gold standard for lymph node assessment is complete excision and microscopic analysis of the lymph nodes.

The assessment of mediastinal lymph nodes during surgery for early-stage lung cancer can involve either a mediastinal lymph node dissection (MLND) or a less extensive mediastinal lymph node sampling (MLNS). The value placed on either approach varies among surgeons, and no study has definitively shown one approach to be associated with better outcomes. Advocates for MLND assert that removing occult nodal metastases may decrease recurrence and improve survival; detractors note that more than two-thirds of patients with N2 disease will have recurrence with distant metastases, regardless of the strategy used, and cite the increased time and potential complications associated with MLND. The purpose of this review is to (1) appropriately define MLND and MLNS and (2) provide the best evidence identifying the situations in which MLND should be performed.

METHODOLOGY

A flow chart illustrating the literature review is given in Figure 8-11. We conducted a Medline search of studies published from 1995 to 2013 using the Medical Subject Heading terms "mediastinal lymph node dissection" and "lung cancer surgery." This search identified 1,052 articles. Filters were then applied to limit the search results to English language articles reporting clinical or comparative studies in humans for which abstracts were available. Of the 190 abstracts reviewed, 160 were excluded because they were case series or topic reviews, focused on metastatic disease to the

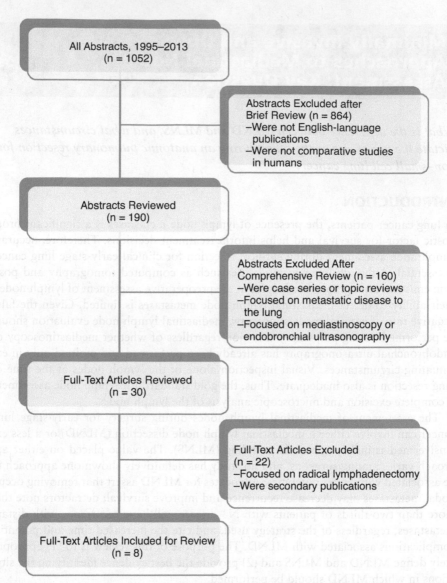

All Abstracts, 1995–2013
(n = 1052)

Abstracts Excluded after
Brief Review (n = 864)
–Were not English-language
  publications
–Were not comparative studies
  in humans

Abstracts Reviewed
(n = 190)

Abstracts Excluded After
Comprehensive Review (n = 160)
–Were case series or topic reviews
–Focused on metastatic disease to
  the lung
–Focused on mediastinoscopy or
  endobronchial ultrasonography

Full-Text Articles Reviewed
(n = 30)

Full-Text Articles Excluded
(n = 22)
–Focused on radical lymphadenectomy
–Were secondary publications

Full-Text Articles Included for Review
(n = 8)

FIGURE 8-11   Flow diagram for literature review process to address key question of MLND versus MLNS.

lung, or focused on mediastinoscopy or endobronchial ultrasonography. We carefully reviewed the remaining 30 articles and identified eight that evaluated MLND and systematic MLNS in similar populations (Table 8-2). The other 22 articles were excluded because they did not fulfill these criteria, focused on radical lymphadenectomy, or were secondary publications about series already included in the eight studies we identified.

TABLE 8-2 Summary of Studies Comparing Lymph Node Evaluation Strategies for Resectable Non–Small Cell Lung Cancer

Author	Year	Study Design	No. of Patients	Main Objective	Key Finding	Potential for Significant Bias
Darling et al[8]	2011	Randomized trial	1023	Determine whether MLND or MLNS is associated with better survival outcomes	MLND and MLNS were associated with equivalent survival outcomes in patients with intraoperative confirmation of N0 disease.	No
Doddoli et al[7]	2005	Retrospective cohort	465	Assess the therapeutic effect of the extent of lymph node dissection	More lymph nodes were sampled and survival was better with MLND.	Yes
Wu et al[10]	2002	Randomized trial	532	Determine whether MLND or MLNS is associated with better survival outcomes	MLND was associated with better survival than MLNS.	No
Keller et al[4]	2000	Retrospective cohort	373	Assess the impact of MLND and MLNS on patient survival	MLND was associated with better survival than MLNS.	Yes
Lardinois et al[6]	2005	Retrospective cohort	100	Compare clinical outcomes between patients undergoing MLND and those undergoing MLNS	MLND was associated with better disease-free survival than MLNS.	Yes
Watanabe et al[11]	2005	Retrospective cohort	411	Evaluate the feasibility of lymph node evaluation with VATS	VATS and thoracotomy had similar rates of lymph node evaluation and morbidity.	Yes
Boffa et al[13]	2012	Retrospective cohort	11,531	Compare the completeness of lymph node evaluation with VATS to that with thoracotomy	N1 upstaging was less frequent with VATS.	Yes
Merritt et al[12]	2013	Retrospective cohort	129	Compare the completeness of lymph node evaluation with VATS to that with thoracotomy	More nodes were dissected and upstaging was more frequent with thoracotomy.	Yes

MLND, mediastinal lymph node dissection; MLNS, mediastinal lymph node sampling; VATS, video-assisted thoracic surgery.

FINDINGS

Definitions of Mediastinal Lymph Node Sampling and Mediastinal Lymph Node Dissection

MLND has been described as an en bloc resection of all midline and ipsilateral mediastinal lymph node basins that leaves the trachea, phrenic nerves, aorta, and superior vena cava skeletonized.[1-3] This resection includes lymph node stations 2R/4R, 7, 8R, and 9R on the right and stations 5/6, 7, 8L, and 9L on the left. The major technical challenge in performing this resection is identifying the structural borders of each station. For stations 2R/4R, these borders are the superior vena cava anteriorly, the trachea and right upper lobe bronchus medially, and the esophagus posteriorly. For station 7, the structural borders are the pericardium anteriorly, the carina and right mainstem bronchus/bronchus intermedius superiorly, and the esophagus posteriorly. Stations 8R and 9R lymph nodes should be resected as they are visualized during the mobilization of the inferior pulmonary ligament. On the left, stations 5/6 are bordered by the phrenic nerve anteriorly, the vagus/recurrent laryngeal nerve posteriorly, and the pulmonary artery and left mainstem bronchus inferiorly. Station 7 is bordered by the pericardium anteriorly, the esophagus posteriorly, and the left mainstem bronchus superiorly. Stations 8L and 9L are resected in the same manner as stations 8R and 9R.

Systematic MLNS, which has been defined as an exploration of each nodal station with biopsy of at least one representative node from each station,[2,4] is considered the minimum standard for lymph node evaluation during the surgical resection of early-stage lung cancer. In contrast to systematic MLNS, selective MLNS is vaguely defined, although it has been described as "cherry picking," and involves the biopsy of only suspicious-looking lymph nodes. Selective MLNS has proven extremely limited in terms of providing adequate diagnostic and prognostic information and is no longer considered a reasonable option for the evaluation of the mediastinum in lung cancer patients.

Circumstances for Mediastinal Lymph Node Dissection or Mediastinal Lymph Node Sampling

In patients with non–small cell lung cancer (NSCLC), MLND or systematic MLNS should be performed at the time of anatomic lung resection to facilitate accurate pathologic staging.[3,5] However, the decision to perform MLND or systematic MLNS depends on a variety of factors. One such factor is the number of lymph nodes required to provide accurate pathologic staging. Studies have consistently shown that more lymph nodes are resected with MLND than with MLNS; on average, MLND yields 17 or 18 lymph nodes, whereas systematic MLNS usually yields approximately seven lymph nodes.[6-8] Therefore, MLND should be performed in situations in which a high lymph node yield is required to better stage the disease or to completely excise potential N2 disease.

MLND does not improve the long-term survival of patients with T1 or T2 tumors and N0 disease proven by systematic sampling at the time of anatomical lung resection.[8] However, suspicious lymph nodes encountered at the time of pulmonary resection should be immediately evaluated by frozen section analysis, as the discovery of metastatic spread to the lymph nodes may change intraoperative management. In the setting of an intraoperatively confirmed metastatic lymph node, MLND is recommended.

For patients with stage II (N1-positive) NSCLC, MLND is recommended and may improve survival.[3] Although few studies have specifically compared outcomes following MLND to those following MLNS, several subgroup analyses have demonstrated that MLND offers a survival advantage over MLNS in patients with stage II lung cancer.[4,6,9,10]

Surgical approach—thoracotomy, video-assisted thoracic surgery (VATS), or robot-assisted thoracic surgery—should not be a factor in deciding whether to perform MLND or systematic MLNS. However, whether an open approach or a minimally invasive approach offers a more thorough lymph node excision (by either MLND or MLNS) remains unclear. One study demonstrated that thoracotomy and minimally invasive approaches procure equal numbers of lymph nodes.[11] In contrast, another study found that the mean number of lymph nodes obtained with VATS (9.9 lymph nodes) was much lower than that obtained with open approaches (14.7 lymph nodes).[12] In addition, an analysis of the Society of Thoracic Surgeons General Thoracic Surgery Database demonstrated that compared with VATS, thoracotomy, owing to its higher rates of positive hilar lymph nodes, resulted in a higher rate of cancer upstaging in patients with clinical stage I lung cancer. This difference disappeared, however, among patients treated by surgeons who predominately used VATS.[13] Compared with systematic MLNS, MLND has been associated with small but clinically insignificant increases in operative time, blood loss volume, and chest tube drainage volume. In experienced centers, therefore, MLND adds minimal morbidity compared to systematic MLNS.

CONCLUSION

The key difference between MLND and systematic MLNS is that MLND removes more lymph nodes than MLNS does. For patients with suspected or documented stage II (N1 or T3) lung cancer, MLND should be performed to improve staging and long-term survival regardless of the surgical approach employed.

REFERENCES

1. Martini N. Mediastinal lymph node dissection for lung cancer. The Memorial experience. *Chest Surg Clin N Am* 1995;5(2):189–203.
2. Allen MS, Darling GE, Pechet TT, et al; ACOSOG Z0030 Study Group. Morbidity and mortality of major pulmonary resections in patients with early-stage lung cancer: initial results of the randomized, prospective ACOSOG Z0030 trial. *Ann Thorac Surg* 2006;81(3):1013–1019; discussion 1019–1020.
3. Lardinois D, De Leyn P, Van Schil P, et al. ESTS guidelines for intraoperative lymph node staging in non-small cell lung cancer. *Eur J Cardiothorac Surg* 2006;30(5):787–792.
4. Keller SM, Adak S, Wagner H, et al. Mediastinal lymph node dissection improves survival in patients with stages II and IIIa non-small cell lung cancer. Eastern Cooperative Oncology Group. *Ann Thorac Surg* 2000;70(2):358–365.
5. Howington JA, Blum MG, Chang AC, et al. Treatment of stage I and II non-small cell lung cancer: diagnosis and management of lung cancer, 3rd ed: American College of Chest Physicians evidence-based clinical practice guidelines. *Chest* 2013;143(5)(suppl):e278S–e313S.
6. Lardinois D, Suter H, Hakki H, et al. Morbidity, survival, and site of recurrence after mediastinal lymph-node dissection versus systematic sampling after complete resection for non-small cell lung cancer. *Ann Thorac Surg* 2005;80(1):268–274.
7. Doddoli C, Aragon A, Barlesi F, et al. Does the extent of lymph node dissection influence outcome in patients with stage I non-small-cell lung cancer? *Eur J Cardiothorac Surg* 2005;27(4):680–685.

8. Darling GE, Allen MS, Decker PA, et al. Randomized trial of mediastinal lymph node sampling versus complete lymphadenectomy during pulmonary resection in the patient with N0 or N1 (less than hilar) non-small cell carcinoma: results of the American College of Surgery Oncology Group Z0030 Trial. *J Thorac Cardiovasc Surg* 2011;141(3):662–670.
9. Izbicki JR, Passlick B, Pantel K, et al. Effectiveness of radical systematic mediastinal lymphadenectomy in patients with resectable non-small cell lung cancer: results of a prospective randomized trial. *Ann Surg* 1998;227(1):138–144.
10. Wu Y, Huang ZF, Wang SY, et al. A randomized trial of systematic nodal dissection in resectable non-small cell lung cancer. *Lung Cancer* 2002;36(1):1–6.
11. Watanabe A, Koyanagi T, Obama T, et al. Assessment of node dissection for clinical stage I primary lung cancer by VATS. *Eur J Cardiothorac Surg* 2005;27(5):745–752.
12. Merritt RE, Hoang CD, Shrager JB. Lymph node evaluation achieved by open lobectomy compared with thoracoscopic lobectomy for N0 lung cancer. *Ann Thorac Surg* 2013;96(4):1171–1177.
13. Boffa DJ, Kosinski AS, Paul S, et al. Lymph node evaluation by open or video-assisted approaches in 11,500 anatomic lung cancer resections. *Ann Thorac Surg* 2012;94(2):347–353.

CHAPTER 9

Lung Resection

CRITICAL ELEMENTS

- Surgical Approach
- Chest Exploration
- Flexible Bronchoscopy
- Lung Isolation
- Mediastinal Exploration for Gross Nodal Disease

1. SURGICAL APPROACH

Recommendation: Pulmonary resection can be approached safely through a thoracotomy or thoracoscopically depending on the extent of the disease and the surgeon's experience and preference.

Type of Data: Retrospective, Prospective.

Strength of Recommendation: Weak.

Rationale

Video-assisted thoracoscopic surgery (VATS) approaches, which are being used with increasing frequency, can be performed safely by experienced thoracic surgeons.[1-3] Compared with standard thoracotomy, VATS may cause less postoperative pain and morbidity while offering equivalent survival and recurrence rates.[4-6] VATS lobectomy has become a standard approach for early-stage lung cancer and is being used increasingly for more advanced disease. According to the American College of Chest Physicians Clinical Practice Guidelines, a minimally invasive approach is preferable to a thoracotomy for anatomic pulmonary resection for stage I non–small cell lung carcinomas in experienced centers.[7] In addition, VATS may enable patients to receive adjuvant chemotherapy earlier.[8] Relative contraindications to VATS include the

141

inability to completely resect the tumor with a lobectomy, the inability to tolerate one-lung ventilation, T3 or T4 tumors, and N2 or N3 disease.[9] The incisions used in thoracoscopic lobectomy include incisions for an inferior port for the camera and for one or two additional ports anteriorly or posteriorly in the sixth intercostal space for the retraction and passage of the stapler (Fig. 9-1). A 6- to 8-cm utility incision for removal of the specimen is made in the fourth intercostal space overlying the hilum. A specimen retrieval bag should be used to decrease the risk of tumor seeding at the incision.[10] Rib spreading should not be used.

Although thoracotomy or thoracoscopic approaches can be used to safely perform pulmonary resection, experienced surgeons must know which approach to use for each patient and when it is necessary to convert a thoracoscopic surgery to an open thoracotomy.

Regardless of VATS or open approach, the patient is positioned in the lateral decubitus position, and the operating table is flexed to help widen the intercostal spaces. All pressure points should be padded. The thoracotomy incision is positioned for optimal exposure of the hilum and should have the capacity to be

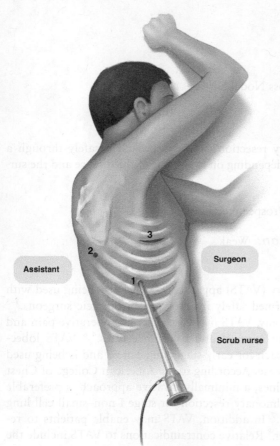

FIGURE 9-1 Example of positioning and incisions used for thoracoscopic (VATS) lobectomy.

rapidly extended if needed. An oblique skin incision is made 1 or 2 fingerbreadths below the scapular tip.

Although no controlled studies have compared standard posterolateral thoracotomy to muscle-sparing thoracotomy, muscle-sparing thoracotomy may cause less pain and result in better postoperative pulmonary function and shoulder function preservation.[11–13] The latissimus dorsi muscle is mobilized either posteriorly or anteriorly, and the serratus anterior muscle is mobilized anteriorly or spread along the direction of its fibers. The chest is entered through the fifth intercostal space, and a 1-cm segment of the inferior rib is resected to improve exposure. A standard posterolateral thoracotomy incision offers excellent exposure of the hilar structures. The latissimus dorsi muscle is divided, but the serratus anterior muscle can often be spared. If the serratus anterior muscle is divided, it should be divided close to the rib insertions to preserve innervation to the muscle. Surgeons should make an effort to avoid injuring the intercostal nerves, as such injury can cause chronic pain following thoracotomy. Several techniques to reduce the pain from intercostal nerve injury have been described, and these include using intracostal sutures placed through holes drilled in the inferior rib and harvesting a nondivided intercostal bundle prior to thoracotomy to minimize the compression of the intercostal nerves.[14,15]

2. CHEST EXPLORATION

Recommendation: The chest should be explored visually to evaluate for pleural dissemination of tumor. If such dissemination is confirmed by frozen section or cytologic analysis, the resection should be aborted.

Type of Data: Retrospective.

Strength of Recommendation: Weak.

Rationale

The chest should be thoroughly explored by palpating all lobes for additional nodules and examining the pleural surface. Suspicious lesions should be biopsied and subjected to frozen section analysis. Pleural effusion not identified preoperatively is infrequent and in one study occurred in only 45 of 1,279 (3.5%) patients undergoing lung resection. Of these 45 patients, 24 (53%) had positive pleural lavage cytology findings and 5-year survival rates of 6% to 8%, whereas the patients with negative cytology findings had outcomes similar to those of patients without an effusion.[16] In contrast, Naruke et al[17] found that 364 of 2,055 (17.7%) patients had previously unidentified pleural effusion at thoracotomy and that of these 364 patients, 74 (20.3%) had positive cytology findings. Pleural fluid or lavage cytology should be obtained and pleurodesis considered in patients found to have an unexpected pleural effusion. However, the use of pleural lavage cytology in the absence of pleural effusion remains controversial; in the American College of Surgeons Oncology Group Z0040 trial, only 29 of 1,047 (2.8%) lung cancer patients had a positive preresection intraoperative pleural lavage.[18]

3. FLEXIBLE BRONCHOSCOPY

Recommendation: If not performed preoperatively, flexible bronchoscopy should be performed following anesthesia induction for surgery to assess the segmental anatomy and determine whether endobronchial disease is present.

Type of Data: Retrospective.

Strength of Recommendation: Weak.

Rationale

Flexible bronchoscopy should be performed preoperatively or intraoperatively prior to pulmonary resection to assess the bronchial anatomy, suction any secretions, and determine whether, and if so, the extent to which endobronchial disease is present. In patients with central tumors, bronchoscopy findings may reveal that a more extensive resection, such as a bilobectomy, is necessary. In one study, flexible bronchoscopy in the preoperative work-up of 225 patients with solitary pulmonary nodules revealed unexpected endobronchial involvement in 10 (4.4%) patients.[19] In four of these patients, surgery was aborted owing to small cell lung cancer, pneumonia, or involvement of the right mainstem bronchus that caused inadequate pulmonary function precluding pneumonectomy. On the other hand, Goldberg et al[20] and Torrington et al[21] found that bronchoscopy did not provide additional benefits, although these series were smaller, including only 91 patients and 33 patients, respectively.

4. LUNG ISOLATION

Recommendation: Single-lung ventilation with a double-lumen endotracheal tube or bronchial blocker should be used to maintain lung isolation during pulmonary resection.

Type of Data: Retrospective, Prospective.

Strength of Recommendation: Weak.

Rationale

Lung isolation, which is performed after flexible bronchoscopy, has been possible since the introduction of the red rubber Robert–Shaw double-lumen endotracheal tube.[22] A left-sided double-lumen tube is generally used for lung isolation unless the left mainstem bronchus is distorted owing to the tumor or a descending aortic aneurysm or must be transected for left pneumonectomy or sleeve resection. A right-sided double-lumen tube has an opening for ventilation of the right upper lobe. Although an airway exchange catheter, which is especially useful in the difficult-to-intubate patient, can be used to place a double-lumen tube, care must be taken to avoid injuring the airway during the tube exchange.[23,24] Tube position should be confirmed by bronchoscopy, as one study found that auscultation alone for this purpose is unreliable, with one-third of patients requiring tube repositioning.[25] Because it can be displaced proximally during lateral positioning of the patient, the bronchial cuff should be located 5 mm below the carina and its position rechecked after the patient has been positioned. Compared with a bronchial blocker, double-lumen tubes can be placed more quickly and enable faster suctioning of the isolated lung, quicker lung collapse, and easier conversion between single- and double-lung ventilation. However, once single-lung ventilation is achieved, exposure is similar with either a bronchial blocker or a double-lumen endotracheal tube.[26,27] Bronchial blockers can also provide selective lobar isolation.

5. MEDIASTINAL EXPLORATION FOR GROSS NODAL DISEASE

Recommendation: Intraoperative evaluation of the mediastinum for gross nodal involvement should be performed prior to pulmonary resection for lung cancer.

Type of Data: Retrospective.

Strength of Recommendation: Weak.

Rationale

In lung cancer patients, mediastinal nodes that are positive on positron emission tomography or pathologically enlarged should be evaluated with minimally invasive techniques (i.e., endobronchial ultrasonography, mediastinoscopy, anterior mediastinotomy, or VATS) prior to lung resection. For patients who have involvement of the mediastinal nodes, resection should not be the primary treatment, as several studies,[28–34] as well as a meta-analysis[35] and an excellent evidence-based review,[36] have shown that the survival of patients with mediastinal nodal involvement who undergo surgical resection alone is inferior to that of those who undergo surgical resection following neoadjuvant therapy.

Given careful evaluation of the preoperative imaging, gross mediastinal disease should rarely be discovered at the time of a planned lung resection. Nevertheless, it is reasonable to examine the mediastinal nodal stations prior to resection to ensure that no gross (palpable or visible) nodal involvement is present. Such examination can be accomplished by opening the overlying mediastinal pleura as an initial step to node sampling or dissection. Gross disease can be palpable as enlarged, discrete nodes and/or as firm tissue that extends outside the nodal capsule and into the surrounding tissue. If such tissue is identified, it should be subjected to frozen section analysis. If frozen section analysis intraoperatively reveals gross N2 nodal disease, aborting the resection should be considered.

REFERENCES

1. Swanson SJ, Herndon JE II, D'Amico TA, et al. Video-assisted thoracic surgery lobectomy: report of CALGB 39802—a prospective, multi-institution feasibility study. *J Clin Oncol* 2007;25: 4993–4997.
2. McKenna RJ Jr, Houck W, Fuller CB. Video-assisted thoracic surgery lobectomy: experience with 1,100 cases. *Ann Thorac Surg* 2006;81:421–425; discussion 425–426.
3. Kim K, Kim HK, Park JS, et al. Video-assisted thoracic surgery lobectomy: single institutional experience with 704 cases. *Ann Thorac Surg* 2010;89:S2118–S2122.

4. Paul S, Altorki NK, Sheng S, et al. Thoracoscopic lobectomy is associated with lower morbidity than open lobectomy: a propensity-matched analysis from the STS database. *J Thorac Cardiovasc Surg* 2010;139:366–378.

5. Tomaszek SC, Cassivi SD, Shen KR, et al. Clinical outcomes of video-assisted thoracoscopic lobectomy. *Mayo Clin Proc* 2009;84:509–513.

6. Walker WS, Codispoti M, Soon SY, et al. Long-term outcomes following VATS lobectomy for non-small cell bronchogenic carcinoma. *Eur J Cardiothorac Surg* 2003;23:397–402.

7. Howington JA, Blum MG, Chang AC, et al. Treatment of stage I and II non-small cell lung cancer: diagnosis and management of lung cancer, 3rd ed: American College of Chest Physicians evidence-based clinical practice guidelines. *Chest* 2013;143:e278S–e313S.

8. Petersen RP, Pham D, Burfeind WR, et al. Thoracoscopic lobectomy facilitates the delivery of chemotherapy after resection for lung cancer. *Ann Thorac Surg* 2007;83:1245–1249; discussion 1250.

9. Hanna JM, Berry MF, D'Amico TA. Contraindications of video-assisted thoracoscopic surgical lobectomy and determinants of conversion to open. *J Thorac Dis* 2013;5:S182–S189.

10. Yim AP. Port-site recurrence following video-assisted thoracoscopic surgery. *Surg Endosc* 1995;9:1133–1135.

11. Hazelrigg SR, Landreneau RJ, Boley TM, et al. The effect of muscle-sparing versus standard posterolateral thoracotomy on pulmonary function, muscle strength, and postoperative pain. *J Thorac Cardiovasc Surg* 1991;101:394–401.

12. Lemmer JH Jr, Gomez MN, Symreng T, et al. Limited lateral thoracotomy. Improved postoperative pulmonary function. *Arch Surg* 1990;125:873–877.

13. Landreneau RJ, Pigula F, Luketich JD, et al. Acute and chronic morbidity differences between muscle-sparing and standard lateral thoracotomies. *J Thorac Cardiovasc Surg* 1996;112: 1346–1350.

14. Cerfolio RJ, Bryant AS, Maniscalco LM. A nondivided intercostal muscle flap further reduces pain of thoracotomy: a prospective randomized trial. *Ann Thorac Surg* 2008;85:1901–1906; discussion 1906–1907.

15. Cerfolio RJ, Price TN, Bryant AS, et al. Intracostal sutures decrease the pain of thoracotomy. *Ann Thorac Surg* 2003;76:407–411; discussion 411–412.

16. Ruffini E, Rena O, Bongiovanni M, et al. The significance of intraoperative pleural effusion during surgery for bronchogenic carcinoma. *Eur J Cardiothorac Surg* 2002;21:508–513.

17. Naruke T, Tsuchiya R, Kondo H, et al. Implications of staging in lung cancer. *Chest* 1997;112: 242S–248S.

18. Rusch VW, Hawes D, Decker PA, et al. Occult metastases in lymph nodes predict survival in resectable non-small-cell lung cancer: report of the ACOSOG Z0040 trial. *J Clin Oncol* 2011;29:4313–4319.

19. Schwarz C, Schonfeld N, Bittner RC, et al. Value of flexible bronchoscopy in the pre-operative work-up of solitary pulmonary nodules. *Eur Respir J* 2013;41:177–182.

20. Goldberg SK, Walkenstein MD, Steinbach A, et al. The role of staging bronchoscopy in the preoperative assessment of a solitary pulmonary nodule. *Chest* 1993;104:94–97.

21. Torrington KG, Kern JD. The utility of fiberoptic bronchoscopy in the evaluation of the solitary pulmonary nodule. *Chest* 1993;104:1021–1024.

22. Bjork VO, Carlens E. The prevention of spread during pulmonary resection by the use of a double lumen catheter. *J Thorac Surg* 1950;20:151.

23. Abdulatif M, Ismail E. Use of the Aintree intubation and airway exchange catheters through LMA-ProSeal for double-lumen tube placement in a morbidly obese patient with right main stem bronchus tumour. *Br J Anaesth* 2012;108:1038–1039.

24. Thomas V, Neustein SM. Tracheal laceration after the use of an airway exchange catheter for double-lumen tube placement. *J Cardiothorac Vasc Anesth* 2007;21:718–719.

25. Klein U, Karzai W, Bloos F, et al. Role of fiberoptic bronchoscopy in conjunction with the use of double-lumen tubes for thoracic anesthesia: a prospective study. *Anesthesiology* 1998;88: 346–350.

26. Campos JH. An update on bronchial blockers during lung separation techniques in adults. *Anesth Analg* 2003;97:1266–1274.

27. Campos JH, Kernstine KH. A comparison of a left-sided Broncho-Cath with the torque control blocker univent and the wire-guided blocker. *Anesth Analg* 2003;96:283–289.

28. Depierre A, Milleron B, Moro-Sibilot D, et al; French Thoracic Cooperative Group. Preoperative chemotherapy followed by surgery compared with primary surgery in resectable stage I (except T1N0), II, and IIIa non-small-cell lung cancer. *J Clin Oncol* 2002;20(1):247–253.

29. Nagai K, Tsuchiya R, Mori T, et al; Lung Cancer Surgical Study Group of the Japan Clinical Oncology Group. A randomized trial comparing induction chemotherapy followed by surgery with surgery alone for patients with stage IIIA N2 non-small cell lung cancer (JCOG 9209). *J Thorac Cardiovasc Surg* 2003;125(2):254–260.
30. Roth JA, Fossella F, Komaki R, et al. A randomized trial comparing perioperative chemotherapy and surgery with surgery alone in resectable stage IIIA non-small-cell lung cancer. *J Natl Cancer Inst* 1994;86(9):673–680.
31. Rosell R, Gómez-Codina J, Camps C, et al. A randomized trial comparing preoperative chemotherapy plus surgery with surgery alone in patients with non-small-cell lung cancer. *N Engl J Med* 1994;330(3):153–158.
32. Wagner H Jr, Lad T, Piantadosi S, et al. Randomized phase 2 evaluation of preoperative radiation therapy and preoperative chemotherapy with mitomycin, vinblastine, and cisplatin in patients with technically unresectable stage IIIA and IIIB non-small cell cancer of the lung LCSG 881. *Chest* 1994;106(6)(suppl):348S–354S.
33. Elias AD, Skarin AT, Leong T, et al. Neoadjuvant therapy for surgically staged IIIA N2 non-small cell lung cancer (NSCLC). *Lung Cancer* 1997;17(1):147–161.
34. Pass HI, Pogrebniak HW, Steinberg SM, et al. Randomized trial of neoadjuvant therapy for lung cancer: interim analysis. *Ann Thorac Surg* 1992;53(6):992–998.
35. Burdett SS, Stewart LA, Rydzewska L. Chemotherapy and surgery versus surgery alone in non-small cell lung cancer. *Cochrane Database Syst Rev* 2007;(3):CD006157.
36. Ramnath N, Dilling TJ, Harris LJ, et al. Treatment of stage III non-small cell lung cancer: diagnosis and management of lung cancer, 3rd ed: American College of Chest Physicians evidence-based clinical practice guidelines. *Chest* 2013;143(5)(suppl):e314S–e340S.

CHAPTER 10

Segmentectomy

CRITICAL ELEMENT

- Patient Selection for Segmentectomy

Recommendation: Segmentectomy should be an option in only select node-negative patients and is dependent on being able to achieve an adequate parenchymal margin.

Type of Data: Retrospective.

Strength of Recommendation: Weak.

Rationale

Sublobar resections are a treatment modality primarily used for early-stage non–small cell lung cancer (NSCLC) in patients with limited pulmonary reserve, where a larger anatomic resection would not be tolerated. Sublobar resections are also currently under prospective randomized evaluation in two independent trials as an alternative treatment strategy for healthy patients with small, peripheral, node-negative tumors. Lobectomy is currently the recommended treatment for stage I and II NSCLC according to the American College of Chest Physicians (ACCP) evidence-based guidelines for the diagnosis and management of lung cancer[1] and the National Comprehensive Cancer Network (NCCN) guidelines.[2] These recommendations are based primarily on results from the only randomized trial completed to date which compared lobectomy to sublobar resection for stage I NSCLC and noted a threefold increase in local recurrence and trend toward worse survival in those undergoing sublobar resection.[3]

A sublobar resection for NSCLC is defined as either an anatomic segmentectomy or a wide wedge resection. Segmentectomy is generally considered to be the oncologically superior of the two approaches, typically with wider margins and greater numbers of harvested lymph nodes than wedge resection.[4] Segmentectomy is therefore the preferred sublobar approach for primary resection of NSCLC when technically and medically

148

feasible. A systematic evaluation of the mediastinal lymph nodes is recommended for all sublobar resections performed for NSCLC.

Surgeons undertaking segmentectomy need to be familiar with segmental anatomy. There are 19 pulmonary segments, 10 on the right and 9 on the left, with the anterior basal and medial basal on the left considered a single segment. Although segmental resections have been described for nearly all bronchial segments, generally accepted segmental resections are outlined in Figure 10-1.[5,6] Suggested criteria for use of segmentectomy include small tumors (<3 cm), location in the peripheral one-third of the lung, and no endobronchial involvement. Such conditions allow for adequate surgical margins.[7,8] Careful review of the chest computed tomography (CT) is suggested preoperatively. This allows the surgeon to ascertain if the tumor is confined within the segmental boundary and appropriate for sublobar techniques.[5,6,9,10] It is also helpful for determining the adequacy of margins and identification of aberrant anatomy. Flexible bronchoscopy is indicated to ensure absence of endobronchial disease and delineating bronchial anatomy prior to division.[10] General anesthesia with single lung ventilation is beneficial to maintain a quiet operative field for open

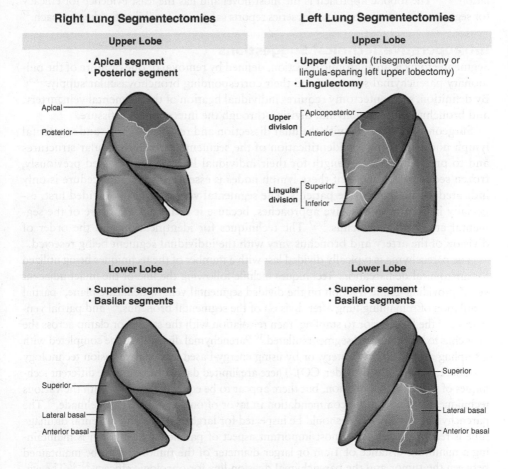

FIGURE 10-1   Pulmonary segments amenable to anatomic resection.

approaches and is mandatory to obtain the pneumothorax required for minimally invasive approaches. Lateral decubitus positioning with flexion is recommended. Thoracotomy, video-assisted thoracoscopic surgery (VATS), or robotic-assisted approaches are all acceptable for sublobar resections, and the approach should not alter the technical aspects of the procedure.[6] The optimal approach depends on the patient and tumor characteristics and the surgeon's expertise. The efficacy of minimally invasive techniques for wedge resection has been long accepted.[11] Numerous nonrandomized trials and single institution case series have demonstrated equivalent short- and long-term oncologic outcome for segmental resections by VATS and open techniques.[12-19] Although no prospective randomized trials comparing the different approaches have been completed, limited evidence suggests VATS may be better tolerated with reduced pain and length of stay and greater postoperative independence.[19-24] The greatest benefit from minimally invasive approaches appears to be in those patients with severe medical comorbidity. Data from the Society of Thoracic Surgery General Thoracic Surgery Database suggest significant reductions in perioperative morbidity and mortality with minimally invasive approaches to lung resections in high-risk population.[25,26] The robotic approach is the most novel and has the least evidence for efficacy for segmental resections, but a recent series reports safety and feasibility for the approach.[27]

Intraoperative Technical Suggestions

Segmentectomy is an anatomic resection, defined by removal of one or more of the pulmonary parenchymal segments and their corresponding bronchovascular supply.[2,3,6,7] By definition, segmentectomy requires individual ligation of the segmental vein, artery, and bronchus and parenchymal division through the intersegmental fissure.

Surgeons should begin with the hilar dissection and removal of hilar and segmental lymph nodes to allow for identification of the segmental bronchovascular structures and to provide adequate length for their individual ligation. As stressed previously, frozen section assessment of these lymph nodes is essential, as this procedure is only indicated for node-negative patients. The segmental vein is typically divided first, especially in minimally invasive approaches, because it facilitates exposure of the segmental artery and bronchus.[3,6,7] The techniques for identification and the order of division of the artery and bronchus vary with the individual segment being resected.

The parenchyma is typically divided last with a number of the techniques being utilized for anatomical demarcation. Techniques include following the line of the intact adjacent vein,[9] providing gentle traction on the divided segmental vein to delineate plane,[5] partial ventilation of remaining lung after division of the segmental bronchus,[5,9] and partial ventilation of the lung, prior to stapling, then reisolation with the stapler or clamp across the bronchus to leave resected segment inflated.[10] Parenchymal division can be completed with a stapling device, electrocautery, or by using energy-based coagulative fusion technology (LigaSure, Valley Labs, Boulder, CO). There are limited data comparing the different techniques of parenchymal division, but there appear to be equivalent results with the various techniques, and no clear recommendation in favor of one technique can be made.[28] The parenchymal division plane should be inspected for large air leaks and a pleural drainage tube is recommended. The most important aspect of parenchymal division is maintaining a minimum distance of 1 cm or larger diameter of the tumor should be maintained between the tumor and the parenchymal division line for oncologic efficacy.[25-27] The evidence for decreased local control with narrow resection margins is outlined in Table 10-1.

TABLE 10-1 Evidence for Decreased Local Control with Narrow Resection Margins

Author	Year	Type of Study (Prospective/Retrospective, Case Series/Cohort/Case Control/RCT/Modeling Study/Propensity Core Matches Analysis—e.g., Retrospective Case Series, Like Most of Our Literature, or Prospective RCT)	Number and Type of Resection	Definition of Close Margin	Local Recurrence Rate Close	Local Recurrence Rate Wide	Key Finding	Significant Potential for Bias (Yes/No)
El-Sherif[32]	2007	Retrospective case series	55 wedge 26 segment	<1 cm	14.6%	7.5%	Margins <1 cm are at high risk for locoregional recurrence.	Wedge more frequently associated with a close margin than segmentectomy
Schuchert[8]	2007	Retrospective case series	182 segment	M/T ratio ≤1	25%	6.2%	M/T ratio <1 is associated with higher rate of recurrence.	Recurrences not separated between locoregional and systemic
Sienel[33]	2007	Retrospective case series	49 segment	<1 cm	23%	0%	Local recurrence following segmentectomy is associated with resection margins <1 cm.	Not all patients with stage I disease
Sawabata[34]	2012	Retrospective case series	37 wedge	M/T ratio ≤1	38.5%	0%	All local recurrences occurred in cases of lung with M/T <1.	All tumors <2 cm
Mohiuddin[35]	201	Retrospective case series	367 wedge	<1.5 cm	HR 0.41 (ref margin 0.5 cm)		Risk of local recurrence can be decreased with margins ≥1.5 cm.	All tumors <2 cm

HR, heart rate; M/T, margin distance/tumor width ratio; RCT, randomized controlled trial.

Intraoperative touch prep of the specimen to assess the bronchial margin has been suggested[29] as a means of ensuring negative margins and improving oncologic efficacy. A slide is simply run over the specimen after it is removed from the patient but before the specimen is cut by the pathologist. A negative microscopic margin in combination with negative marginal cytology decreases the risk for local recurrence following sublobar resection.[30,31] This strategy was evaluated in the recent prospective trial by the American College of Surgeons Oncology Group (ACOSOG) Z40302, which examined the use of intraoperative brachytherapy following sublobar resection, and significant logistical hurdles were encountered, which appear to limit its widespread use of intraoperative touch preps.

REFERENCES

1. Howington JA, Blum MG, Chang AC, et al. Treatment of stage I and II non-small cell lung cancer: diagnosis and management of lung cancer, 3rd ed: American College of Chest Physicians evidence-based clinical practice guidelines. *Chest* 2013;143:e278S–e313S.
2. National Comprehensive Cancer Network. Clinical practice guidelines in oncology: non–small cell lung cancer. http://www.nccn.org/professionals/physician_gls/pdf/nscl.pdf. Accessed April 8, 2014.
3. Ginsberg RJ, Rubinstein LV; Lung Cancer Study Group. Randomized trial of lobectomy versus limited resection for T1 N0 non-small cell lung cancer. *Ann Thorac Surg* 1995;60:615–622; discussion 22–23.
4. Kent M, Landreneau R, Mandrekar S, et al. Segmentectomy versus wedge resection for non-small cell lung cancer in high-risk operable patients. *Ann Thorac Surg* 2013;96:1747–1755.
5. Gossot D. Totally thoracoscopic basilar segmentectomy. *Semin Thorac Cardiovasc Surg* 2011;23:67–72.
6. Pham D, Balderson S, D'Amico TA. Technique of thoracoscopic segmentectomy. *Oper Tech Thorac Cardiovasc Surg* 2008;13:188–203.
7. Sawabata N, Ohta M, Matsumura A, et al. Optimal distance of malignant negative margin in excision of non-small cell lung cancer: a multicenter prospective study. *Ann Thorac Surg* 2004;77:415–420.
8. Schuchert MJ, Pettiford BL, Keeley S, et al. Anatomic segmentectomy in the treatment of stage I non-small cell lung cancer. *Ann Thorac Surg* 2007;84:926–932; discussion 32–33.
9. Ceppa DP, Balderson S, D'Amico TA. Technique of thoracoscopic basilar segmentectomy. *Semin Thorac Cardiovasc Surg* 2011;23:64–66.
10. Schuchert MJ, Pettiford BL, Luketich JD, et al. Parenchymal-sparing resections: why, when, and how. *Thorac Surg Clin* 2008;18:93–105.
11. Lewis RJ. The role of video-assisted thoracic surgery for carcinoma of the lung: wedge resection to lobectomy by simultaneous individual stapling. *Ann Thorac Surg* 1993;56(3):762–768.
12. Roviaro GC, Rebuffat C, Varoli F, et al. Videoendoscopic thoracic surgery. *Int Surg* 1993;78:4–9.
13. Iwasaki A, Shirakusa T, Shiraishi T, et al. Results of video-assisted thoracic surgery for stage I/II non-small cell lung cancer. *Eur J Cardiothorac Surg* 2004;26:158–164.
14. Ohtsuka T, Nomori H, Horio H, et al. Is major pulmonary resection by video-assisted thoracic surgery an adequate procedure in clinical stage I lung cancer? *Chest* 2004;125:1742–1746.
15. Shiraishi T, Shirakusa T, Miyoshi T, et al. A completely thoracoscopic lobectomy/segmentectomy for primary lung cancer–technique, feasibility, and advantages. *Thorac Cardiovasc Surg* 2006;54:202–207.
16. Atkins BZ, Harpole DH Jr, Mangum JH, et al. Pulmonary segmentectomy by thoracotomy or thoracoscopy: reduced hospital length of stay with a minimally-invasive approach. *Annals Thorac Surg* 2007;84:1107–1112; discussion 12–13.
17. Schuchert MJ, Pettiford BL, Pennathur A, et al. Anatomic segmentectomy for stage I non-small-cell lung cancer: comparison of video-assisted thoracic surgery versus open approach. *J Thorac Cardiovasc Surg* 2009;138:1318–1325.
18. Kilic A, Schuchert MJ, Pettiford BL, et al. Anatomic segmentectomy for stage I non-small cell lung cancer in the elderly. *Ann Thorac Surg* 2009;87:1662–1666; discussion 7–8.
19. Leshnower BG, Miller DL, Fernandez FG, et al. Video-assisted thoracoscopic surgery segmentectomy: a safe and effective procedure. *Ann Thorac Surg* 2010;89:1571–1576.

20. Landreneau RJ, Hazelrigg SR, Mack MJ, et al. Postoperative pain-related morbidity: video-assisted thoracic surgery versus thoracotomy. *Ann Thorac Surg* 1993;56:1285–1289.
21. Alam N, Flores RM. Video-assisted thoracic surgery (VATS) lobectomy: the evidence base. *JSLS* 2007;11:368–374.
22. Demmy TL, Plante AJ, Nwogu CE, et al. Discharge independence with minimally invasive lobectomy. *Am J Surg* 2004;188:698–702.
23. Whitson BA, Andrade RS, Boettcher A, et al. Video-assisted thoracoscopic surgery is more favorable than thoracotomy for resection of clinical stage I non-small cell lung cancer. *Ann Thorac Surg* 2007;83:1965–1970.
24. Cattaneo SM, Park BJ, Wilton AS, et al. Use of video-assisted thoracic surgery for lobectomy in the elderly results in fewer complications. *Ann Thorac Surg* 2008;85:231–235; discussion 5–6.
25. Ceppa DP, Kosinski AS, Berry MF, et al. Thoracoscopic lobectomy has increasing benefit in patients with poor pulmonary function: a Society of Thoracic Surgeons Database analysis. *Ann Surg* 2012;256:487–493.
26. Burt BM, Kosinski AS, Shrager JB, et al. VATS lobectomy is not associated with prohibitive morbidity or mortality in patients with predicted postoperative FEV1 (ppoFEV1) less than 40% of normal: a Society of Thoracic Surgeons Database analysis. *J Thorac Cardiovasc Surg* 2014;148(1):19–28.
27. Pardolesi A, Park B, Petrella F, et al. Robotic anatomic segmentectomy of the lung: technical aspects and initial results. *Ann Thorac Surg* 2012;94:929–934.
28. Miyasaka Y, Oh S, Takahashi N, et al. Postoperative complications and respiratory function following segmentectomy of the lung–comparison of the methods of making an inter-segmental plane. *Int Cardiovasc Thorac Surg* 2011;12:426–429.
29. Fernando H, Landreneau RJ, Mandrekar S, et al. Impact of brachytherapy on local recurrence after sublobar resection: results from ACOSOG Z4032 (Alliance), a phase III randomized trial for high-risk operable non-small cell lung cancer (NSCLC). *JCO* 2014;32(23):2456–2462.
30. Higashiyama M, Kodama K, Takami K, et al. Intraoperative lavage cytologic analysis of surgical margins in patients undergoing limited surgery for lung cancer. *J Thorac Cardiovasc Surg* 2003;125:101–107.
31. Sawabata N, Matsumura A, Ohota M, et al. Cytologically malignant margins of wedge resected stage I non-small cell lung cancer. *Ann Thorac Surg* 2002;74:1953–1957.
32. El-Sherif A, Fernando HC, Santos R, et al. Margin and local recurrence after sublobar resection of non-small cell lung cancer. *Ann Surg Oncol* 2007;14:2400–2405.
33. Sienel W, Stremmel C, Kirschbaum A, et al. Frequency of local recurrence following segmentectomy of stage IA non-small cell lung cancer is influenced by segment localisation and width of resection margins–implications for patient selection for segmentectomy. *Eur J Cardiothorac Surg* 2007;31:522–527; discussion 7–8.
34. Sawabata N, Maeda H, Matsumura A, et al; Thoracic Surgery Study Group of Osaka University. Clinical implications of the margin cytology findings and margin/tumor size ratio in patients who underwent pulmonary excision for peripheral non-small cell lung cancer. *Surg Today* 2012;42:238–244.
35. Mohiuddin K, Haneuse S, Sofer T, et al. Relationship between margin distance and local recurrence among patients undergoing wedge resection for small (≤2 cm) non-small cell lung cancer. *J Thorac Cardiovasc Surg* 2014;147(4):1169–1175; discussion 1175–1177.

Segmentectomy: Key Question

In patients with stage I non–small cell lung cancer, what factors determine if segmentectomy should be abandoned for lobectomy?

INTRODUCTION

As detailed in the preceding section, lobectomy remains the gold standard for anatomical lung resection. However, some authors have demonstrated equivalent results to lobectomy in specific subsets of patients with early-stage lung cancer. Anatomic segmentectomy may be especially helpful to the patient with limited pulmonary reserve.

METHODOLOGY

We searched PubMed for English language articles published from 2005 through 2011 that were related to various factors that may influence the decision to abandon segmentectomy in favor of lobectomy in patients undergoing surgical resection for stage I NSCLC. Search terms were "non–small cell lung carcinoma" and "segmentectomy" and "lymph node involvement" or "lymphovascular invasion" or "CEA" or "SUV" or "visceral pleural invasion." In total, this search identified 583 potential abstracts. After excluding studies that contained insufficient patient numbers, included pathology other than NSCLC, focused on nonsurgical treatments for NSCLC, involved primarily advanced-stage NSCLC, or were descriptive technical papers, 70 abstracts were reviewed to identify articles addressing specific factors that may influence preoperative or intraoperative surgical decision making. After further excluding papers that involved additional intraoperative treatments (brachytherapy), we identified 26 publications (Table 10-2 and Fig. 10-2). These studies provided information about outcomes for anatomic segmentectomy for early-stage NSCLC; the prognostic significance of preoperative serum carcinoembryonic antigen (CEA) levels, SUVmax on positron emission tomography (PET)/computed tomography (CT), and visceral pleural invasion; and the significance of interlobar/hilar lymph node involvement on surgical resection outcomes of early-stage NSCLC.

FINDINGS

The decision to utilize anatomic segmentectomy rather than lobectomy for the definitive surgical management of stage IA NSCLC is affected by a number of preoperative diagnostic considerations and patient functional issues. Certainly, the patient's clinical early disease must be as accurately defined as possible using preoperative imaging studies (i.e., CT and/or PET) and minimally invasive interventions (i.e., mediastinoscopy and/or endobronchial ultrasonography). In spite of these preoperative measures to accurately identify stage I disease prior to surgical exploration, clinical disease stage and pathologic disease stage differ in 15% to 35% of patients.[1-3]

TABLE 10-2 Studies Examining Factors that May Influence When to Abort Segmentectomy in Favor of Lobectomy for Stage IA Non–Small Cell Lung Cancer

Author, Year	Study Design	No. of Patients	Main Objective	Key Finding	Potential for Bias
Schuchert et al, 2012[1]	Retrospective review of patients treated 2002–2010	785	Determine indications and perioperative outcomes for anatomic segmentectomy for stage IA NSCLC, IPN	59.6% of patients underwent VATS; the overall complication rate was 34.9%; the 30-day mortality rate was 1.1%; no differences in recurrence rates compared to lobectomy were noted.	
Shiono et al, 2013[2]	Retrospective study of prospectively collected data	183	Determine whether SUV index can be used to identify patients with clinical stage IA NSCLC who are appropriate for limited surgical resection	Disease was upstaged in 27% of patients; multivariate analysis revealed SUV index to be a significant predictor of recurrence ($P = .001$).	
Al-Sarraf et al, 2008[3]	Retrospective review of all patients who underwent surgical resection in a 30-month period	215	Examine the incidence, pattern, and predictors of occult mediastinal LN disease in patients with negative PET/CT findings	16% of patients had occult N2 disease; predictors of occult disease included centrally located tumors, right upper lobe tumors, and positive N1 nodes; patients with level 4 and 7 involvement had a high rate of occult mediastinal LN disease.	
Schuchert et al, 2007[4]	Retrospective review	428	Compare outcomes of segmentectomy to those of lobectomy in patients with stage I NSCLC	30-day mortality, total complications, disease-free recurrence, and survival were similar at 18 and 28.5 months; segmentectomy patients had shorter OR time and less blood loss; 32 (17.6%) segmentectomy patients had recurrences, of which 89% occurred in patients with surgical margins <2 cm at a mean time of 14 months.	

(continued)

TABLE 10-2 **Studies Examining Factors that May Influence When to Abort Segmentectomy in Favor of Lobectomy for Stage IA Non–Small Cell Lung Cancer** *(continued)*

Author, Year	Study Design	No. of Patients	Main Objective	Key Finding	Potential for Bias
Okada et al, 2005[5]	Retrospective review of all patients undergoing surgical resection for NSCLC	1,272	Examine the relationship between clinical/follow-up data and tumor dimension <10 mm, 10–20 mm, 21–30 mm, and >30 mm	Among patients with stage I disease <30 mm, the 5-year cancer-specific survival of those who underwent lobectomy was equivalent to that of those who underwent segmentectomy. Wedge resection was potentially acceptable in patients with tumors <20 mm only.	
Tsutani et al, 2013[6]	Retrospective review	481	Compare outcomes of lobectomy to those of segmentectomy in patients with clinical stage IA adenocarcinoma	There was no difference in recurrence-free or overall survival in 81 pairs of propensity score-matched patients.	Yes
Landreneau et al, 2014[7]	Retrospective propensity-matched review	420	Perform propensity-matched comparison of equal numbers of patients with stage IA NSCLC undergoing segmentectomy or lobectomy	Survival outcomes of lobectomy patients and segmentectomy patients were equivalent.	
Al-Sarraf et al, 2008[8]	Retrospective review	176	Assess the clinical implication of maximum SUV of primary tumor for patients with NSCLC	SUV >15 correlated with centrally located tumors, SCC, advanced T stage, advanced nodal stage, advanced AJCC, larger tumors	Yes
Inoue et al, 2006[9]	Retrospective review	143	Identify risk factors for peripheral NSCLC <2 cm that would favor more extensive resection	Increased preoperative serum CEA level, pleural invasion, and lymph node involvement increased the chances of poor prognosis.	

Study	Study type	N	Objective	Results
Stiles et al, 2013[10]	Retrospective review of patients who underwent surgical resection for NSCLC	530	Determine whether the ratio of SUVmax to tumor size has clinical implications for the surgical resection of NSCLC	Patients with ratios in the highest quartile had a higher rate of lymph node metastases and a lower rate of 3-year disease-free survival.
Li et al, 2013[11]	Retrospective review	80	Determine whether FDG uptake correlates with risk for lymph node metastasis	SUVmax of the primary tumor is significantly associated with pathologic N stage.
Bille et al, 2013[12]	Retrospective review	413	Determine the prognostic significance of SUVmax in surgically treated NSCLC patients	Multivariate analysis revealed that TNM stage, primary tumor grade, and primary tumor SUVmax were independent prognostic factors.
Chen et al, 2014[13]	Retrospective review	261	Determine the factors predicting locoregional recurrence in patients with stage IA NSCLC who underwent surgery	Tumor differentiation and serum CEA level were predictors of postoperative recurrence.
Kozu et al, 2013[14,15]	Retrospective review	467	Determine the clinicopathologic factors that may predict recurrence and poor survival in patients with pathologic stage I NSCLC	High serum CEA level and stage IB disease were independent risk factors for recurrence and poor survival.
Li et al, 2013[16]	Retrospective review	189	Determine the risk factors for occult nodal involvement in patients with clinical stage I disease as indicated by PET/CT findings who underwent surgical resection	Occult nodal metastases were found in 18% of patients; the SUVmax and size of the primary tumor were independent predictors of occult nodal metastases.

(continued)

TABLE 10-2 Studies Examining Factors that May Influence When to Abort Segmentectomy in Favor of Lobectomy for Stage IA Non–Small Cell Lung Cancer (continued)

Author, Year	Study Design	No. of Patients	Main Objective	Key Finding	Potential for Bias
Keenan et al, 2004[17]	Retrospective review	201	Determine whether segmentectomy or lobectomy confers more protection of lung function in patients undergoing resection for stage I NSCLC	Declines in FVC, FEV1, MVV, and DLCO were observed in lobectomy patients, whereas only a decline in DLCO was observed in segmentectomy patients. The groups had similar rates of 1- and 4-year survival.	
Kilic et al, 2009[18]	Retrospective review	184	Compare outcomes of lobectomy with those of segmentectomy in patients older than 75 years of age undergoing resection for stage I NSCLC	The operative mortality rates of the segmentectomy and lobectomy groups were 1.3% and 4.7%, respectively. The groups' 5-year disease-free survival rates (49.8% and 45.5%, respectively) did not differ significantly.	Yes; the lobectomy group had larger tumors, and the segmentectomy group had worse COPD.
Nomori et al, 2012[19]	Prospective single-arm study	195	Assess segmentectomy outcomes in patients with cT1N0M0 NSCLC	The 5-year overall survival rates were 94% for patients with tumors <2 cm and 81% for patients with tumors 2.1–3 cm. Only 9 recurrences (6 distant, 3 local) were reported. Postoperative pulmonary function was 90% that of preoperative levels.	Yes; selection bias
Smith et al, 2014[20]	Retrospective review of SEER data	577	Compare open surgery to VATS for segmental resection in elderly, propensity-matched patients	27% of patients underwent VATS. The VATS group had lower rates of postoperative complications and ICU admissions and shorter LOS. No significant difference in	

Study	Study type	No.	Objective	Findings	
Sawabata et al, 2013[21]	Review article		Assess locoregional recurrence rates following lobectomy or segmentectomy	12 lobectomy studies were included in the review; locoregional recurrence rates in these studies ranged from 1% to 9%. 14 segmentectomy studies were included; recurrence rates ranged from 0% to 13% overall but ranged from only 2% to 8% when T2 tumors were excluded.	
Schuchert et al, 2012[22]	Retrospective review	305	Assess the effect of age and stage IB status on survival following anatomic segmentectomy or lobectomy	Stage IB status, primarily owing to the presence of visceral pleural invasion, was a poor prognostic factor for the use of segmentectomy.	
Schuchert et al, 2011[23]	Retrospective review	524	Assess the effect of angiolymphatic invasion, visceral pleural invasion, and tumor inflammation on survival after lobectomy or segmentectomy	Angiolymphatic and visceral pleural invasion were associated with significantly decreased recurrence-free and overall survival.	
Okada et al, 2006[24]	Prospective, nonrandomized study of patients treated 1992–2001	305 seg, 262 lobe	Compare lobectomy to radical sublobar resection for stage IA NSCLC	The groups' recurrence rates and prognosis did not differ significantly. Patients who underwent radical sublobar resection had better postoperative lung function.	Yes
Tsutani et al, 2012[25]	Retrospective review	502	Identify predictors of pathologically node-negative stage IA adenocarcinoma	Solid tumor size <0.8 cm and SUVmax <1.5 were predictors of negative lymph node involvement.	Yes
Rena et al, 2014[26]	Retrospective review	124	Determine the significance of pN1 node positivity on prognosis	N1 node location affected 5-year overall survival, and survival decreased as the level of positive nodes increased.	

AJCC, American Joint Committee on Cancer; CEA, carcinoembryonic antigen; COPD, chronic obstructive pulmonary disease; CT, computed tomography; DLCO, diffusion capacity for carbon dioxide; FDG, fluorodeoxyglucose; FVC, forced vital capacity; ICU, intensive care unit; IPN, indeterminate pulmonary nodules; LN, lymph node; LOS, length of stay; MVV, maximum voluntary ventilation; NSCLC, non–small cell lung cancer; OR, operating room; PET, positron emission tomography; SCC, squamous cell carcinoma; SEER, Surveillance, Epidemiology, and End Results; SUV, standardized uptake value; TNM, tumor, node, metastasis; VATS, video-assisted thoracoscopic surgery.

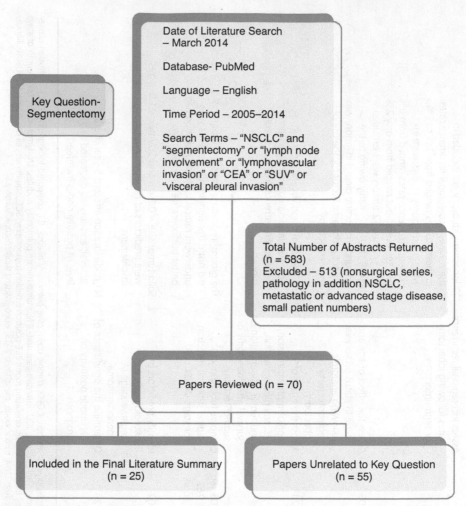

Date of Literature Search
– March 2014

Database- PubMed

Language – English

Time Period – 2005–2014

Search Terms – "NSCLC" and "segmentectomy" or "lymph node involvement" or "lymphovascular invasion" or "CEA" or "SUV" or "visceral pleural invasion"

Key Question- Segmentectomy

Total Number of Abstracts Returned (n = 583)
Excluded – 513 (nonsurgical series, pathology in addition NSCLC, metastatic or advanced stage disease, small patient numbers)

Papers Reviewed (n = 70)

Included in the Final Literature Summary (n = 25)

Papers Unrelated to Key Question (n = 55)

FIGURE 10-2 Flow diagram for literature review process to address key question of when segmentectomy should be abandoned for lobectomy.

Other preoperative findings to consider when deciding whether to perform segmentectomy or lobectomy relate to the size and anatomic location of the lesion as assessed by CT.[3-7] Because increased tumor metabolic activity is believed to be related to poorer prognosis, the intensity of the isotope uptake on PET as assessed by standardized uptake value (SUV) and the preoperative serum level of CEA are other factors to consider when determining the aggressiveness of resection.[8-16] Patient functionality and age are also preoperative considerations affecting the decision to perform segmentectomy or lobectomy for small peripheral lung cancers.[17-19]

Decisions made during surgery regarding the commitment to sublobar/anatomic segmentectomy as definitive surgical therapy for the target lung lesion are affected by a number of intraoperative findings. The intraoperative finding that the lesion crosses anatomic segmental boundaries, which effectively negates the validity of performing a "real" anatomic segmental resection, should lead the thoracic surgeon to convert to lobectomy as the definitive treatment. Although deeper lesions bridging the superior and basilar segments of the lower lobe are most commonly encountered, lesions in the left upper lobe bridging the boundary between the upper division and lingula are also a concern. This situation of tumors crossing the boundaries of a given segment poses an even greater concern when anatomic segmentectomy for right upper lobe lesions is considered. In all instances in which the lesion is found to bridge segmental boundaries, the size of the lesion affects the ability to effectively perform an anatomic segmentectomy with adequate surgical margins. This is precisely why most surgeons consider segmentectomy for only the small peripheral lung cancers confirmed to be within anatomic segmental boundaries.[1,4–7,21]

Another important factor to consider when performing segmentectomy is the intraoperative finding of visceral pleural invasion. More important than tumor size, the presence of visceral pleural invasion appears to be associated with poorer outcomes when anatomic segmentectomy, rather than lobectomy, is performed for stage IB NSCLCs.[9,22,23]

Perhaps most importantly, the intraoperative finding of disease involvement of the interlobar and/or hilar lymph nodes should prompt the thoracic surgeon to perform lobectomy instead of segmentectomy. Although a greater resection may not actually improve patient survival, it may result in better locoregional disease control than segmentectomy does in this setting.[23–26]

CONCLUSIONS

Segmentectomy should be abandoned in favor of anatomic lobectomy when the tumor is found to be crossing the anatomic segment boundaries, when interlobar and/or hilar lymph nodes are involved, or in the presence of visceral pleural invasion. High PET uptake and elevated CEA measurements should be taken into consideration.

REFERENCES

1. Schuchert MJ, Abbas G, Awais O, et al. Anatomic segmentectomy for the solitary pulmonary nodule and early-stage lung cancer. *Ann Thorac Surg* 2012;93:1780–1785.
2. Shiono S, Abiko M, Sato T. Limited resection for clinical stage IA non-small cell lung cancers based on a standardized-uptake value index. *Eur J Cardiothorac Surg* 2013;43(1):e7–e12.
3. Al-Sarraf N, Aziz R, Gately K, et al. Pattern and predictors of occult mediastinal lymph node involvement in non-small cell lung cancer patients with negative mediastinal uptake on positron emission tomography. *Eur J Cardiothorac Surg* 2008;33:104–109.
4. Schuchert MJ, Pettiford BL, Keeley S, et al. Anatomic segmentectomy in the treatment of non-small cell lung cancer. *Ann Thorac Surg* 2007;84:926–932.
5. Okada M, Nishio W, Sakamoto T, et al. Effect of tumor size on prognosis in patients with non-small cell lung cancer: the role of segmentectomy as a type of lesser resection. *J Thorac Cardiovasc Surg* 2005;129:87–93.
6. Tsutani Y, Miyata Y, Nakayama H, et al. Oncologic outcomes of segmentectomy compared with lobectomy for clinical stage IA lung adenocarcinoma: propensity sore-matched analysis in a multicenter study. *J Thorac Cardiovasc Surg* 2013;146(2):358–364.
7. Landreneau RJ, Normolle DP, Christie NA, et al. Recurrence and survival outcomes following anatomic segmentectomy vs. lobectomy for clinical stage I non-small cell cancer: a propensity-matched analysis. *J Clin Oncol* 2014;32(23):2449–2455.

8. Al-Sarraf N, Gately K, Lucey J, et al. Clinical implications and prognostic significance of standardized uptake values of primary non-small cell lung cancer on positron emission tomography: analysis of 176 cases. *Eur J Cardiothorac Surg* 2008;34:892–897.

9. Inoue M, Minami M, Shiono H, et al. Clinicopathologic study of resected, peripheral, small sized, non-small cell lung cancer tumors of 2 cm or less in diameter: pleural invasion and increased preoperative carcinoembryonic antigen levels as predictors of nodal involvement. *J Thorac Cardiovasc Surg* 2006;131:988–993.

10. Stiles BM, Nasar A, Mirza F, et al. Ratio of positron emission tomography uptake to tumor size in surgically resected non-small cell lung cancer. *Ann Thorac Surg* 2013;95(2):397–403.

11. Li M, Wu N, Zheng R, et al. Primary tumor PET/CT [18F]FDG uptake is an independent predictive factor for regional lymph node metastasis in patients with non-small cell lung cancer. *Cancer Imag* 2013;12:566–572.

12. Bille A, Okiror L, Skanjeti A, et al. The prognostic significance of maximum standardized uptake value of primary tumor in surgically treated non-small-cell lung cancer patients: analysis of 413 cases. *Clin Lung Cancer* 2013;14(2):149–156.

13. Chen Y, Huang T, Tsai W, et al. Risk factors of postoperative recurrences in patients with clinical stage I NSCLC. *World J Surg Oncol* 2014;12:10.

14. Kozu Y, Maniwa T, Takahashi S, et al. Prognostic significance of postoperative serum carcinoembryonic antigen levels in patients with completely resected pathological-stage I non-small cell lung cancer. *J Cardiothorac Surg* 2013;8(1):106.

15. Kozu Y, Maniwa T, Takahashi S, et al. Risk factors for both recurrence and survival in patients with pathological stage I non-small–cell lung cancer. *Eur J Cardiothoracic Surg* 2013;44(1): e53–e58.

16. Li L, Ren S, Zhang Y, et al. Risk factors for predicting the occult nodal metastasis in T1-2N0M0 NSCLC patients staged by PET/CT: potential value in the clinic. *Lung Cancer* 2013;81(2): 213–217.

17. Keenan RJ, Landreneau RJ, Maley RH Jr, et al. Segmental resection spares lung function in patients with stage I lung cancer. *Ann Thorac Surg* 2004;78:228–233.

18. Kilic A, Schuchert MJ, Pettiford BL, et al. Anatomic segmentectomy for stage I non-small cell lung cancer in the elderly. *Ann Thorac Surg* 2009;87:1662–1666.

19. Nomori H, Mori T, Ikeda K, et al. Segmentectomy for selected cT1N0M0 non-small cell lung cancer: a prospective study at a single institute. *J Thorac Cardiovasc Surg* 2012;144:87–93.

20. Smith CB, Kale M, Mhango G, et al. Comparative outcomes of elderly stage I lung cancer patients treated with segmentectomy via video-assisted thoracoscopic surgery versus open resection. *J Thorac Oncol* 2014;9:383–389.

21. Sawabata N. Locoregional recurrence after pulmonary sublobar resection of non-small cell lung cancer: can it be reduced by considering cancer cells at the surgical margin. *Gen Thorac Cardiovasc Surg* 2013;61:9–16.

22. Schuchert MJ, Awais O, Abbas G, et al. Influence of age and IB status after resection of node-negative non-small cell lung cancer. *Ann Thorac Surg* 2012;93:929–935.

23. Schuchert MJ, Schumacher L, Kilic A, et al. Impact of angiolymphatic invasion and pleural invasion on surgical outcomes for stage I non-small cell lung cancer. *Ann Thorac Surg* 2011;91: 105901065.

24. Okada M, Koike T, Higashiyama M, et al. Radical sublobar resection for small-sized non-small cell lung cancer: a multi-institutional study. *J Thorac Cardiovasc Surg* 2006;132:769–775.

25. Tsutani Y, Miyata Y, Nakayama H, et al. Prediction of pathologic node-negative clinical stage IA lung adenocarcinoma for optimal candidates undergoing sublobar resection. *J Thorac Cardiovasc Surg* 2012;144:1365–1371.

26. Rena O, Boldorini R, Papalia E, et al. Metastasis to subsegmental and segmental lymph nodes in patients resected for non-small cell lung cancer: prognostic impact. *Ann Thorac Surg* 2014;97(3):987–992.

CHAPTER 11

Lobectomy

CRITICAL ELEMENTS

- Patient Selection for Lobectomy
- Patient Selection for Bilobectomy or Other Advanced Lung Resection

1. PATIENT SELECTION FOR LOBECTOMY

Recommendation: Lobectomy is the preferred treatment for patients with resectable lung cancer.

Type of Data: Prospective.

Strength of Recommendation: Strong.

Rationale

Lobectomy remains the preferred surgery for the resection of lung cancer with curative intent, despite the fact that segmentectomy is increasingly being considered for such resection. Although its findings are being challenged in an ongoing major clinical trial, the original Lung Cancer Study Group trial demonstrated that the local recurrence rate of patients who underwent sublobar resection was three times that of patients who underwent lobectomy and that sublobar resection patients had a 50% higher rate of death with cancer compared with lobectomy patients.[1,2]

The primary contraindications to simple lobectomy are tumor and/or hilar nodal invasion at the origin of the lobar bronchus (Fig. 11-1), which precludes obtaining a negative surgical margin with bronchial division, and tumor and/or hilar nodal invasion of the lobar or main pulmonary arteries.

Bronchoscopy and careful review of contrast-enhanced chest computed tomography (CT) findings are imperative to identify central tumors that may involve major airway or vascular structures within the hilum and thus preclude lobectomy.

163

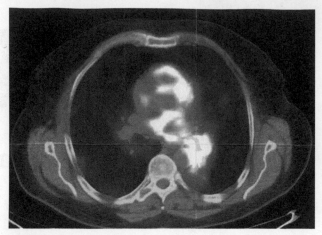

FIGURE 11-1 Positron emission tomography (PET)/CT image of proximal left hilar lung cancer with irregular bronchial mucosa. Bronchoscopically tumor is noted in the distal left main bronchus, precluding lobectomy and mandating pneumonectomy. (Courtesy of Linda Martin, MD, MPH.)

Intraoperative Technical Suggestions

Anatomic lobectomy is based on the individual dissection, ligation, and division of the lobar pulmonary arteries and venous branches to the lobe. The order in which these structures are divided often depends on the lobe being resected and/or the surgeon's preferred technique.

The branch points of the pulmonary artery offer an opportunity to meticulously dissect intra- and interlobar N1 nodal stations. Although published guidelines recommend that level 10 nodes be dissected, we believe that it is good practice to identify and separately dissect other N1 stations to more accurately stage the disease.[1,3] One recent study indicated that the presence of extralobar N1 disease (stations 10 and 11) predicts worse prognosis than does the presence of intralobar N1 disease (stations 12 to 14).[4] Dissecting the hilar lymph nodes (levels 10, 11, and 12), which exposes the hilar structures prior to their division, is extremely helpful during lobectomy. Following vascular division, the lobar bronchus or bronchi should be discreetly dissected, divided, and closed grossly free of tumor.

2. PATIENT SELECTION FOR BILOBECTOMY OR OTHER ADVANCED LUNG RESECTION

Recommendation: The parenchymal margin and bronchial margin should be evaluated to determine whether a bilobectomy or other advanced lung resection is required.

Rationale

The major and minor fissures of the lungs are often incomplete. In patients with incomplete lung fissures who are undergoing surgery for lung cancer, the lobes must be separated, and this is usually accomplished using a stapler-based technique. Interlobar venous anatomy may be used to distinguish the borders of the lobes. The location of a tumor relative to an incomplete fissure should be assessed to determine whether bilobectomy or other advanced lung resection is warranted. Bilobectomy may be considered for tumors that cross a fissure.

Although segmentectomy may be used for small tumors, >1 cm from the parenchymal margin, lobectomy should be performed for tumors ≤1 cm from the margin due to increased rates of locoregional failure.

The location of the tumor relative to the bronchial margin may also dictate the need for bilobectomy or advanced sleeve procedures. The findings of a preoperative bronchoscopic evaluation, especially for patients with more central tumors, or intraoperative frozen section analysis may indicate the need for a more advanced resection. Unless the tumor is small (i.e., T1 disease) or truly peripheral (Fig. 11-2A–D), intraoperative frozen section analysis should be used to assess the bronchial margin to determine whether a microscopically negative margin (R0 resection) has been

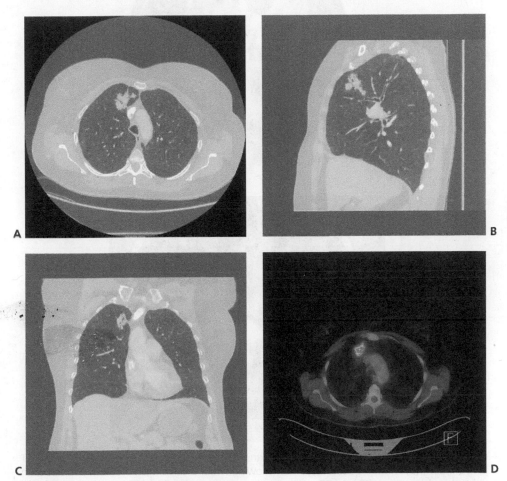

FIGURE 11-2 A: Axial, **(B)** sagittal, and **(C)** coronal CT images and **(D)** PET/CT image of a right upper lobe non–small cell lung cancer appropriate for anatomic right upper lobectomy. (Courtesy of Matthew Facktor, MD.)

obtained. If frozen section analysis reveals the bronchial margin to be positive for malignancy, the surgeon should either resect additional bronchial tissue or perform a sleeve lobectomy to achieve a microscopically negative bronchial margin.

If it is anatomically appropriate and likely to achieve negative surgical margins, lung-sparing anatomic resection (i.e., sleeve lobectomy) is preferable to pneumonectomy (Fig. 11-3A–D). Although pneumonectomy is a potentially safe curative-intent option in selected patients, the procedure is well known to impart a higher risk of short- and long-term morbidity and mortality.

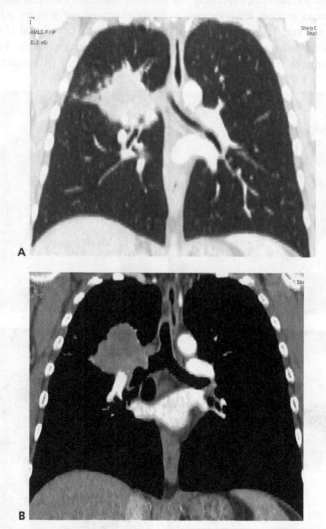

FIGURE 11-3 Right upper lobe malignancy extruding from right upper lobe orifice. **A:** Coronal CT lung window, **(B)** coronal CT soft tissue view showing tumor protruding into bronchial lumen from right upper lobe orifice, **(C)** axial CT soft tissue view showing proximity to main carina, and **(D)** axial CT lung window showing patent airways distal to the tumor. Right upper lobe sleeve resection was accomplished with negative margins. (Courtesy of Bryan Meyers, MD, MPH.)

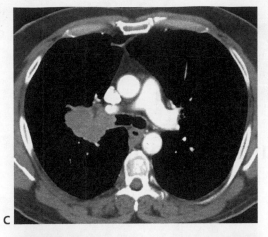

C

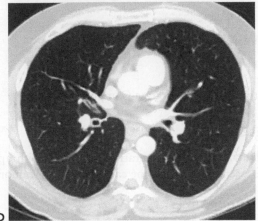

D

FIGURE 11-3 *(Continued).*

REFERENCES

1. National Comprehensive Cancer Network. Non-small cell lung cancer practice guidelines (version 3. 2014). http://www.nccn.org/professionals/physician_gls/f_guidelines_nojava.asp#site. Accessed March 25, 2015.
2. Ginsberg RJ, Rubinstein LV. Randomized trial of lobectomy versus limited resection for T1 N0 non-small cell lung cancer. Lung Cancer Study Group. *Ann Thorac Surg* 1995;60(3):615–622.
3. Osarogiagbon RU, Ogbata O, Yu X. Number of lymph nodes associated with maximal reduction of long-term mortality risk in pathologic node-negative non-small cell lung cancer. *Ann Thorac Surg* 2014;97:385–393.
4. Haney JC, Hanna JM, Berry MF, et al. Differential prognostic significance of extralobar and intralobar nodal metastases in patients with surgically resected stage II non-small cell lung cancer. *J Thorac Cardiovasc Surg* 2014;147(4):1164–1168.
5. Owen RM, Force SD, Gal AA, et al. Routine intraoperative frozen section analysis of bronchial margins is of limited utility in lung cancer resection. *Ann Thorac Surg* 2013;95(6):1859–1865.

CHAPTER 12

Pneumonectomy

CRITICAL ELEMENTS

- Patient Selection
- Technical Aspects
- Avoidance of Intra- and Postoperative Complications

1. PATIENT SELECTION

Recommendation: Proper preoperative evaluation with appropriate tests and imaging studies are essential to determine candidacy for pneumonectomy.

Type of Data: Retrospective.

Strength of Recommendation: Weak.

Rationale

Pneumonectomy is considered in patients who can physiologically tolerate the operation and whose disease cannot be cleared with lesser resections such as lobectomy, bilobectomy, or sleeve lobectomy. Patients for whom pneumonectomy is considered should first undergo careful evaluation to ensure that they can tolerate such an extensive lung resection. Preoperative pulmonary function tests, exercise testing, and room air arterial blood gas measurement, as well as imaging studies, can be used to assess a patient's candidacy for pneumonectomy.[1–4] In general, pneumonectomy is indicated for the resection of lung cancer that cannot be removed by lobectomy or sleeve resection. Examples include central tumors involving the main bronchus (Fig. 12-1) and central tumors that involve the proximal vasculature or interlobar vasculature or cross the fissure(s). Although many consider hilar lymph node involvement to be an indication for pneumonectomy, there is no survival advantage offered by pneumonectomy over sleeve lobectomy in this scenario.[5]

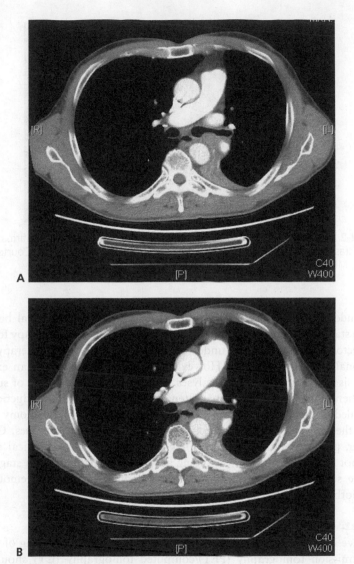

FIGURE 12-1 A,B: Axial CT images displaying proximal left main bronchus involvement by squamous cell cancer; left pneumonectomy was required for R0 resection. (Courtesy of Linda Martin, MD, MPH.)

The role of pneumonectomy in patients with N2 disease (Fig. 12-2) is controversial. Several authors presenting single-institution series have reported no overall increase in perioperative morbidity and mortality among patients undergoing induction therapy followed by pneumonectomy.[6–8] However, these same studies reported an increased incidence of postoperative morbidity and mortality for patients undergoing right pneumonectomy.[6,7]

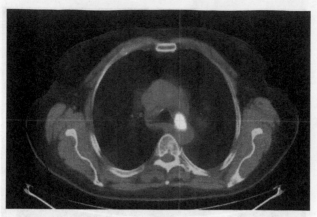

FIGURE 12-2   PET/CT image of malignant 4L lymph node, SUV of 4.9. "Confirmatory" endo-bronchial ultrasound biopsy of this node yielded squamous cell carcinoma. (Courtesy of Linda Martin, MD, MPH.)

One randomized multicenter study found no difference in survival between patients with stage III disease who underwent induction chemoradiotherapy followed by pneumonectomy and those who underwent induction chemoradiotherapy followed by additional radiation therapy.[9] However, these results were from an exploratory data analysis and not preplanned analyses. Another randomized trial of surgery versus radiotherapy in the setting of persistent N2 disease following induction chemotherapy failed to demonstrate any survival advantage for pneumonectomy patients.[10] However, these results were also the products of exploratory analyses. Given findings earlier, pneumonectomy can be safely performed from a technical standpoint but does not appear to offer an oncologic advantage in patients with stage IIIA disease in the setting of persistent N2 disease following induction chemotherapy or chemoradiotherapy.

Preoperative Imaging

Preoperative imaging should be used to assist the surgeon with staging of the tumor. Positron emission tomography (PET)/computed tomography (CT) should be performed to rule out distant metastatic disease such as liver, adrenal, and bone metastases.[11] For patients with proximal tumors, CT with intravenous contrast should be used to evaluate for tumor extension into vascular structures, including the pulmonary veins and main pulmonary artery. Tumor invasion into the proximal pulmonary vein may mandate intrapericardial dissection of the vessel at the time of surgery. Tumor invasion into the left atrium via the pulmonary vein indicates T4 disease. In some cases, cardiac magnetic resonance imaging (MRI) can be used to assess potential mediastinal or cardiac invasion if CT findings are equivocal. In addition, intraoperative transesophageal echocardiography can sometimes be helpful in assessing the degree of atrial involvement if visual inspection or palpation does not clearly demonstrate whether the tumor can be resected.

Bronchoscopic Evaluation of the Airway

Prior to or at the time of pneumonectomy, bronchoscopic evaluation of the airway is conducted. Although it should be performed before any kind of resection for lung cancer, this evaluation is especially important when pneumonectomy is being considered. The proximal location of the tumor in relation to both the mainstem bronchus and the carina should be noted to ensure that standard pneumonectomy is both necessary and feasible. In some patients with very proximal tumors, bronchoscopy may be optimally done on a date prior to the planned pneumonectomy to allow adequate time for pathologic analysis of bronchial and carinal biopsy samples to ensure that negative margins can be achieved with standard pneumonectomy. The surgeon should also take particular note of any anatomic abnormalities, such as a tracheal bronchus. Although they are uncommon,[12,13] such anomalies may alter the operative plan.

Evaluation of the Mediastinum

Prior to any exploration of the pleural space, the mediastinal lymph nodes should be thoroughly evaluated. In a center with reliable on-site frozen pathologic evaluation services, mediastinoscopy may be performed at the time of pneumonectomy and may be advantageous in terms of avoiding scar tissue or immobility of the mediastinum and hilum due to mediastinoscopy in a separate setting. The specifics of mediastinal nodal evaluation are discussed elsewhere in the manual.

Pneumonectomy versus Sleeve Lobectomy

Although no prospective randomized studies comparing pneumonectomy to sleeve resection have been performed, several studies have compared both the short- and long-term outcomes between the two techniques. Recent studies, including meta-analyses, have demonstrated that the two techniques are associated with similar rates of perioperative morbidity; importantly, however, sleeve lobectomy is associated with a lower rate of perioperative mortality.[14-17] From an oncologic perspective, the rates of locoregional recurrence in patients undergoing sleeve lobectomy are similar to those in patients undergoing pneumonectomy. However, patients undergoing sleeve lobectomy have higher rates of 5-year survival.

In addition, patients undergoing pneumonectomy appear to have worse postoperative and long-term quality of life outcomes than do patients undergoing sleeve resection. In the 12 months following surgical resection, pneumonectomy patients have significantly more dyspnea and pain than sleeve lobectomy or normal control patients.[18-20]

Given these considerations, surgeons should carefully consider whether complete oncologic resection can be achieved with sleeve resection, rather than pneumonectomy, in a patient who can physiologically tolerate either procedure. Whenever possible, sleeve resection is preferable to pneumonectomy. For example, although pneumonectomy may be considered for a centrally located right upper lobe tumor (see Fig. 11-3 in Chapter 11), this tumor was successfully removed by sleeve lobectomy.

Intraoperative Decisions

Certain intraoperative findings should prompt the surgeon to perform a pneumonectomy rather than a lesser resection. Such findings include involvement of the proximal pulmonary artery; the inability to separate the pulmonary veins, which would require more proximal resection; and disease extension into all parenchymal lobes. Surgeons should carefully consider the potential need for pneumonectomy before surgery in all patients with central tumors. Even if the need for pneumonectomy is believed to be unlikely, the surgeon should determine, before surgery, whether pneumonectomy would be physiologically feasible if more extensive or central disease is encountered at the time of resection.

2. TECHNICAL ASPECTS

Recommendation: Pneumonectomy can be performed via thoracotomy, thoracoscopically, or with robotic assistance, depending on the surgeon's experience and preference. (Please also see Chapter 9.)

Type of Data: Retrospective.

Strength of Recommendation: Weak.

Rationale

The sequence in which the vessels and bronchus are divided depends on tumor anatomy. In some cases, dividing the bronchus first may allow for better visualization and easier mobilization of the vessels. However, the priority should be minimizing the length of the bronchial stump to prevent postoperative secretion pooling and reduce the potential for postoperative pneumonia or bronchopleural fistula. If the bronchus is divided first to facilitate safer manipulation and isolation of the vascular structures, particularly the pulmonary artery, then the bronchial stump should be reassessed after the lung has been removed to ensure that the stump is optimally short. The method used to divide the vessels and bronchus—by use of a stapling device or by sharp division and oversewing—is chosen by the surgeon.

Pulmonary Veins

The pulmonary veins are gently palpated to determine the extent of the tumor. If the veins are clear of tumor, each vein is gently and circumferentially dissected and then divided. Intrapericardial dissection is considered if the tumor appears to extend into the vein. Although some surgeons theorize that dividing the pulmonary veins prior to the pulmonary artery minimizes the chance of tumor embolization during manipulation, others believe that controlling and dividing the pulmonary artery first minimizes the amount of bleeding during subsequent dissection. In general, however, the order in which the vessels are divided is dictated by the tumor itself. The most appropriate approach involves taking the vessels in an order that facilitates safe and complete resection and likely varies from case to case based on specific tumor location.

Pulmonary Artery

If the tumor does not involve it, the main pulmonary artery is gently and circumferentially dissected. For tumors encroaching onto the pulmonary artery, however, several maneuvers may be used to provide additional length for the dissection and division of the artery. On the right side, the superior vena cava can be mobilized medially to facilitate the dissection of the pulmonary artery. On the left side, the ligamentum arteriosum is divided to provide additional length for dissection; in this situation, care must be taken to avoid dividing the recurrent laryngeal nerve. Finally, intrapericardial dissection can also be performed to provide additional length for dissection and division. Pericardial defects, especially those on the right side, should be reapproximated or closed with a patch.

Bronchus

We recommend limiting the amount of dissection in the area of the proximal mainstem bronchus to preserve blood supply to the bronchial stump. However, complete clearing of the subcarinal mediastinal lymph nodes facilitates good visualization of the mainstem bronchus and thus an appropriate bronchial stump. Once the main bronchus has been circumferentially dissected, it is divided as close to the carina as possible to avoid leaving a long bronchial stump and its associated potential complications. If the bronchus is closed with suturing techniques, absorbable sutures are used to prevent the formation of suture granuloma. The resected bronchial margin is sent for frozen pathologic analysis to rule out microscopic disease. Despite the limited data in support of frozen sections of the bronchial margin, this may be the instance in which it is most helpful (refer to Chapter 9). Furthermore, we recommend testing the suture/staple line for air leaks using irrigation with saline or sterile water. The anesthesiologist is asked to perform a Valsalva maneuver to 30 cm H_2O airway pressure, and any leaks detected are closed with absorbable sutures. Finally, coverage of the bronchial stump with local soft tissue should be considered, especially on the right side. Although mediastinal tissue or mobilized pericardial fat can be useful in many cases, the use of an intercostal muscle flap or other autologous pedicled flap should be considered for patients who have been treated with induction therapy.[21]

3. AVOIDANCE OF INTRA- AND POSTOPERATIVE COMPLICATIONS

Recommendation: Close adherence to the proper technical aspects of the operation and careful postoperative care decreases morbidity and mortality.

Type of Data: Retrospective.

Strength of Recommendation: Weak.

Rationale

During pneumonectomy, several steps can be taken to prevent or reduce postoperative complications.

Hemostasis

Meticulous attention to hemostasis is especially important during pneumonectomy. The use of blood products should be avoided if possible, as transfusion has been found to be an independent risk factor for postoperative respiratory complications.[22] Significant bleeding from any of the major vascular structures, bronchial vessels, or the chest wall can occur. Although life-threatening bleeding is rare, it should be considered a possibility in patients with hilar tumor involvement; patients who have extensive inflammation or infection or who have received prior radiation; and patients who have undergone prior lung resection. In such patients, it may be beneficial to gain proximal control of the major vascular structures prior to intrapericardial dissection and/or control of the hilar vessels.

Hemorrhage after pneumonectomy is relatively rare, with only 1.5% of patients requiring reoperation for bleeding.[23] In these patients, bleeding is primarily from either the chest wall or bronchial vessels and not the major pulmonary structures. Regardless, hemostasis of the chest wall and pleura and diligent inspection for any bleeding after lung removal is critical to prevent unnecessary blood loss and avoid the need for reoperation. In addition, placing a chest tube after pneumonectomy in patients in whom hilar or pleural resection was difficult can help to identify postoperative bleeding before it destabilizes the patient.

Cardiac Tamponade and Herniation

Because pneumonectomy can have life-threatening mechanical cardiac complications requiring emergent reoperation, echocardiography should be considered in patients who have refractory hypotension after pneumonectomy. Pericardial tamponade caused by a bleeding intrapericardial bronchial vessel or a retracted pulmonary structure is rare but has been described. In addition, a defect created in the pericardium during pneumonectomy can give rise to cardiac herniation; pericardial repair with patching is required to prevent this complication. Large pericardiotomy or pericardiectomy may be tolerated after left pneumonectomy but should always be repaired after right pneumonectomy.[24] In cases of severe patient instability, the thoracotomy may have to be reopened prior to obtaining any studies so that hemodynamic stability can be restored as soon as possible. It should also be stressed that, owing to the large pneumonectomy space, chest compressions after pneumonectomy are very unlikely to generate adequate blood flow through the heart; therefore, in the event of cardiac arrest, the patient's chest should be reopened so that cardiac massage can be performed.

Pneumonia

Most patients have some degree of lung collapse after lung resection. Prevention of a subsequent pneumonia, which has a significant association with mortality, particularly in pneumonectomy patients, requires aggressive treatment with pain control, pulmonary hygiene, and physical therapy.[25,26] Frequent bronchoscopy and appropriate antibiotic therapy should be used in patients with poor respiration, excessive secretions, or radiographic or clinical features suspicious for persistent atelectasis or pneumonia. In addition, careful assessment of cough and vocal cord function should be performed before the patient transitions to a solid diet, as aspiration of food into the remaining lung can be a devastating postoperative event. Vocal cord dysfunction is more likely after left pneumonectomy given the location of the left recurrent nerve in the left chest near the lung hilum. Placement of a nasoenteric tube for nutrition and/or vocal cord injection should be considered for patients exhibiting signs and symptoms of aspiration.

Bronchopleural Fistula and Empyema

Postpneumonectomy empyema with or without bronchopleural fistula (BPF) can be a devastating complication with significant mortality.[27] Intraoperative techniques that decrease BPF risk include avoiding excessive dissection and devascularization of the bronchial stump, minimizing the bronchial stump length to prevent secretion pooling and subsequent stump breakdown, and reinforcing the bronchial stump with muscle or a pleural flap.[28,29] BPF should be suspected in patients who have fever, empyema, aspiration pneumonia, an excessively productive cough, or an increasing air leak or amount of pleural air after lung resection. Evaluation for BPF should include bronchoscopy and possibly CT in stable patients. Acute management of BPF focuses on controlling life-threatening conditions and includes postural drainage with the affected lung positioned downward in cases of airway flooding, early pleural drainage to prevent sepsis and aspiration pneumonia, and appropriate antibiotic therapy. Adequate nutrition is critical. Successful BPF treatment ultimately requires closure of the fistula, adequate drainage, and eventual obliteration of the chest cavity.

Postpneumonectomy Pulmonary Edema

Postpneumonectomy pulmonary edema is a syndrome of rapidly progressive dyspnea and hypoxemia requiring mechanical ventilation, with radiologic studies showing diffuse interstitial edema in the remaining lung and no identifiable cause such as heart failure, pulmonary embolism, pneumonia, or BPF.[30] This complication typically develops 2 or 3 days postoperatively, occurs in 1.1% to 4.5% of pneumonectomy patients, and has a mortality rate of 40% to 100%.[25,28,30,31] Some studies have identified perioperative fluid overload and right-sided pneumonectomy as risk factors. Prophylaxis against this complication includes the use of a balanced pleural drainage system, treatment of perioperative hypotension and low urine output with vasopressor or inotropic agents, and diuretic therapy with minimal fluid administration. Treatment is supportive.

REFERENCES

1. Bousamra M II, Presberg KW, Chammas JH, et al. Early and late morbidity in patients undergoing pulmonary resection with low diffusion capacity. *Ann Thorac Surg* 1996;62(4):968–974; discussion 974–975.
2. Ferguson MK, Little L, Rizzo L, et al. Diffusing capacity predicts morbidity and mortality after pulmonary resection. *J Thorac Cardiovasc Surg* 1988;96(6):894–900.
3. Morice RC, Peters EJ, Ryan MB, et al. Exercise testing in the evaluation of patients at high risk for complications from lung resection. *Chest* 1992;101(2):356–361.
4. Walsh GL, Morice RC, Putnam JB Jr, et al. Resection of lung cancer is justified in high-risk patients selected by exercise oxygen consumption. *Ann Thorac Surg* 1994;58(3):704–710; discussion 711.
5. Berry MF, Worni M, Wang X, et al. Sleeve lobectomy for non-small cell lung cancer with N1 nodal disease does not compromise survival. *Ann Thorac Surg* 2014;97(1):230–235.
6. Gaissert HA, Keum DY, Wright CD, et al. POINT: operative risk of pneumonectomy–influence of preoperative induction therapy. *J Thorac Cardiovasc Surg* 2009;138(2):289–294.
7. Mansour Z, Kochetkova EA, Ducrocq X, et al. Induction chemotherapy does not increase the operative risk of pneumonectomy! *Eur J Cardiothorac Surg* 2007;31(2):181–185.
8. Weder W, Collaud S, Eberhardt WE, et al. Pneumonectomy is a valuable treatment option after neoadjuvant therapy for stage III non-small-cell lung cancer. *J Thorac Cardiovasc Surg* 2010;139(6):1424–1430.

9. Albain KS, Swann RS, Rusch VW, et al. Radiotherapy plus chemotherapy with or without surgical resection for stage III non-small-cell lung cancer: a phase III randomised controlled trial. *Lancet* 2009;374(9687):379–386.

10. van Meerbeeck JP, Kramer GW, Van Schil PE, et al. Randomized controlled trial of resection versus radiotherapy after induction chemotherapy in stage IIIA-N2 non-small-cell lung cancer. *J Natl Cancer Inst* 2007;99(6):442–450.

11. Qu X, Huang X, Yan W, et al. A meta-analysis of (1)(8)FDG-PET-CT, (1)(8)FDG-PET, MRI and bone scintigraphy for diagnosis of bone metastases in patients with lung cancer. *Eur J Radiol* 2012;81(5):1007–1015.

12. Inada K, Kishimoto S. An anomalous tracheal bronchus to the right upper lobe; report of two cases. *Dis Chest* 1957;31(1):109–112.

13. Ritsema GH. Ectopic right bronchus: indication for bronchography. *AJR Am J Roentgenol* 1983;140(4):671–674.

14. Ma Z, Dong A, Fan J, et al. Does sleeve lobectomy concomitant with or without pulmonary artery reconstruction (double sleeve) have favorable results for non-small cell lung cancer compared with pneumonectomy? A meta-analysis. *Eur J Cardiothorac Surg* 2007;32(1):20–28.

15. Ferguson MK, Lehman AG. Sleeve lobectomy or pneumonectomy: optimal management strategy using decision analysis techniques. *Ann Thorac Surg* 2003;76(6):1782–1728.

16. Shi W, Zhang W, Sun H, et al. Sleeve lobectomy versus pneumonectomy for non-small cell lung cancer: a meta-analysis. *World J Surg Oncol* 2012;10:265.

17. Deslauriers J, Gregoire J, Jacques LF, et al. Sleeve lobectomy versus pneumonectomy for lung cancer: a comparative analysis of survival and sites or recurrences. *Ann Thorac Surg* 2004;77(4):1152–1156; discussion 1156.

18. Balduyck B, Hendriks J, Lauwers P, et al. Quality of life after lung cancer surgery: a prospective pilot study comparing bronchial sleeve lobectomy with pneumonectomy. *J Thorac Oncol* 2008;3(6):604–608.

19. Ilonen IK, Räsänen JV, Sihvo EI, et al. Pneumonectomy: post-operative quality of life and lung function. *Lung Cancer* 2007;58(3):397–402.

20. Bryant AS, Cerfolio RJ, Minnich DJ. Survival and quality of life at least 1 year after pneumonectomy. *J Thorac Cardiovasc Surg* 2012;144(5):1139–1145.

21. Cerfolio RJ, Bryant AS, Jones VL, et al. Pulmonary resection after concurrent chemotherapy and high dose (60Gy) radiation for non-small cell lung cancer is safe and may provide increased survival. *Eur J Cardiothorac Surg* 2009;35(4):718–723; discussion 723.

22. Blank RS, Hucklenbruch C, Gurka KK, et al. Intraoperative factors and the risk of respiratory complications after pneumonectomy. *Ann Thorac Surg* 2011;92(4):1188–1194.

23. Shapiro M, Swanson SJ, Wright CD, et al. Predictors of major morbidity and mortality after pneumonectomy utilizing the Society for Thoracic Surgeons General Thoracic Surgery Database. *Ann Thorac Surg* 2010;90(3):927–934; discussion 934–935.

24. Grillo HC, Shepard JA, Mathisen DJ, et al. Postpneumonectomy syndrome: diagnosis, management, and results. *Ann Thorac Surg* 1992;54(4):638–650; discussion 650–651.

25. Licker M, Spiliopoulos A, Frey JG, et al. Risk factors for early mortality and major complications following pneumonectomy for non-small cell carcinoma of the lung. *Chest* 2002;121(6): 1890–1897.

26. Patel RL, Townsend ER, Fountain SW. Elective pneumonectomy: factors associated with morbidity and operative mortality. *Ann Thorac Surg* 1992;54(1):84–88.

27. Hollaus PH, Lax F, el-Nashef BB, et al. Natural history of bronchopleural fistula after pneumonectomy: a review of 96 cases. *Ann Thorac Surg* 1997;63(5):1391–1396; discussion 1396–1397.

28. Bernard A, Deschamps C, Allen MS, et al. Pneumonectomy for malignant disease: factors affecting early morbidity and mortality. *J Thorac Cardiovasc Surg* 2001;121(6):1076–1082.

29. Deschamps C, Bernard A, Nichols FC III, et al. Empyema and bronchopleural fistula after pneumonectomy: factors affecting incidence. *Ann Thorac Surg* 2001;72(1):243–247; discussion 248.

30. Deslauriers J, Aucoin A, Gregoire J. Postpneumonectomy pulmonary edema. *Chest Surg Clin N Am* 1998;8(3):611–631, ix.

31. Turnage WS, Lunn JJ. Postpneumonectomy pulmonary edema. A retrospective analysis of associated variables. *Chest* 1993;103(6):1646–1650.

As the first comprehensive, evidence-based evaluation of standardized surgical practices for several key malignancies, this manual represents a critically important initiative. The lung section, written by expert contributors in our field, describes numerous important principles for the optimal conduct of lung cancer surgery and will serve as a premiere guide to operative management of our lung cancer patients.

As highlighted in the "Introduction" chapter of the "Lung" section, lung cancer remains an enormous public health problem. It is currently the number one cause of cancer-related mortality in the United States for both men and women. Accounting for more predicted deaths than malignancies of the breast, prostate, colon and rectum, and pancreas combined, lung cancer continues to take an enormous toll—in terms of both health care expenses and lives lost. Our ability to provide broad curative therapy for this disease is significantly limited by the preponderance of advanced and inoperable lung cancer at the time of presentation. For this reason, extensive efforts have been put forth in recent years to identify early staged lung cancer through improved screening and to expand our treatment options for those with advanced disease, utilizing novel therapeutic agents and targeted therapy.

For those patients with early staged non–small cell lung cancer (NSCLC), complete surgical resection remains the standard of care. However, despite the efficacy of surgical therapy for early-stage disease, there exists significant variability in overall and disease-free survival following surgical resection. We, as surgeons, should be driven to ensure that those patients who are fortunate enough to receive surgical therapy all undergo optimal oncologic procedures, with minimal variability in postoperative outcome.

There may be a number of reasons contributing to variability in surgical outcomes. From our perspective, there are several key parameters. Although it is not specifically addressed in the chapters that follow, surgeon training and expertise are of critical importance. There is ample evidence that resections for lung cancer performed by fully trained and board-certified thoracic surgeons are associated with better outcomes and reduced cost. Patient selection must be thoughtful, appropriate, and conducted with full consideration of the range of multimodality therapies available and their relative risks and benefits for each patient. Staging must be accurate in the preoperative, operative, and pathologic settings. Resections should be precisely stage-specific and complete. Finally, but of significant importance, in order to minimize variability in outcomes and optimize survival for our patients, regardless of the operating surgeon and institution, a key set of standardized, clearly defined operative procedures must be utilized. In providing a standardized approach to operative management of patients with lung cancer, these chapters serve as an informative guide to the practicing thoracic surgeon, the surgical trainee, and all professionals clinically involved in lung cancer care.

This manual was created utilizing input from some of the most experienced experts in our field, with meticulous attention to evidence-based best practices. Critical elements are presented in great detail, with additional attention directed

177

toward addressing areas of controversy that merit further investigation and ongoing evaluation through clinical trials. As a key collaborative effort between the American College of Surgeons and the National Cancer Institute, the value of this publication in standardizing practices cannot be overstated. This manual should serve as a living document as we move into the future, amenable to change as new data and techniques become available. In conjunction with further efforts to standardize cancer care for our patients, these chapters help us, as surgeons, take a huge leap toward providing consistent cancer care.

Mara B. Antonoff, MD
Department of Thoracic and Cardiovascular Surgery
University of Texas MD Anderson Cancer Center
Houston, TX

G. Alexander Patterson, MD
Division of Cardiothoracic Surgery
Washington University School of Medicine
St. Louis, MO

Lung Cancer Critical Elements of Synoptic

Preresection Staging

None
EBUS
EUS
Cervical mediastinoscopy
VATS/thoracotomy
Chamberlain

Preresection Nodal Staging (with Diagnostic Lymphoid Tissue)

N/A	
Right nodal stations	Left nodal stations
2	2
4	4
7	5
8	6
9	7
10	8
Other N1	9
	10
	Other N1

Nodal Evaluation at Time of Resection

Systematic sampling   Nodal dissection

Nodal Stations Examined at Time of Resection

N/A	
Right nodal stations	Left nodal stations
2	2
4	4
7	5
8	6
9	7
10	8
Other N1	9
	10
	Other N1

Method of Lung Resection

VATS   Thoracotomy   Robot assisted

Extent of Lung Resection

Segmentectomy   Lobectomy   Pneumonectomy   Wedge resection

Component of
non-anatomic resection as   yes   no
part of anatomic resection

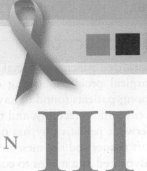

SECTION III

PANCREAS

INTRODUCTION

Localized pancreatic ductal adenocarcinoma (PDAC) was once considered a uniquely surgical problem. Staging of PDAC was routinely accomplished in the operating room; patients found to have technically removable tumors upon exploration underwent pancreatectomy, and those who were not found to have removable tumors underwent palliative bypass operations. Radical resections involving wide clearance of soft tissues and the mesenteric vasculature[1] and/or total pancreatectomy[2] were often advocated as a means to control local recurrence and distant progression. Perioperative mortality was common,[3] and adjuvant therapy was not routine.[4] Although long-term survival was distinctly rare, it was never observed in the absence of a potentially curative pancreatectomy.[5] Therefore, despite generally discouraging results, surgery became accepted as the only potentially curative therapy for patients with an otherwise uniformly fatal disease.

Although PDAC remains a considerable clinical problem, the perioperative management of patients with localized disease has changed significantly over the past 35 years. Advances in multidisciplinary treatment programs that emphasize high-quality pretreatment staging, meticulous surgical care, and perioperative adjuvant therapies have collectively provided a basis for optimism; now, as many as one-quarter of patients who receive combination therapy with chemotherapy with or without chemoradiation and pancreatectomy can expect to live 5 years or longer.[6] However, among the treatments administered as part of these multimodality programs, surgery remains the only one that is potentially curative on its own. Therefore, although localized PDAC is no longer considered a uniquely surgical condition, resection of the primary pancreatic tumor and regional lymph nodes remains as important today as it was 35 years ago.

Staging

In the 1970s and 1980s, accurate pretreatment staging of PDAC was impossible because only low-resolution cross-sectional imaging technologies were available at that time. Discrimination between localized and disseminated disease and between resectable and nonresectable primary tumors was therefore largely made in the operating room at exploratory surgery. Cross-sectional imaging has now improved to the point at which the primary tumor's anatomy and relationship to the mesenteric vasculature can be determined radiographically with great precision, and metastatic disease can be safely ruled out in the majority of patients. Furthermore, studies correlating radiographic findings to surgical outcomes have led to the establishment of objective staging designations that reflect the surgeon's likelihood of achieving a margin-negative resection.

Pretreatment staging with computed tomography or magnetic resonance imaging is now used to help optimize and individualize the treatment of patients with localized PDAC (Table I-1 and Fig. I-1).[7–10] Locally advanced disease is represented radiographically as the cancer's extensive involvement of the mesenteric vasculature. Complete resection of the primary cancer to microscopically clear margins (R0 resection) is rarely feasible for patients with this stage of disease, and attempts to use neoadjuvant therapy to reduce the size or anatomic extent of such cancers and thus improve the surgeon's ability to remove them have been unsuccessful.[11] Therefore, patients with locally advanced cancers are typically treated with chemotherapy

TABLE I-1   Staging Designations Used for Patients with Localized Pancreatic Cancer

| | Staging Designation | | |
Vessel	Potentially Resectable	Borderline Resectable	Locally Advanced
SMV-PV	No interface or interface between the tumor and vessel measuring <180° of the circumference of the vessel wall	Interface between the tumor and vessel measuring ≥180° of the circumference of the vessel wall and/or reconstructible occlusion	Unreconstructable occlusion of the vessel by the tumor
SMA	No interface	Interface between the tumor and vessel measuring <180° of the circumference of the vessel wall	Interface between the tumor and vessel measuring ≥180° of the circumference of the vessel wall
CHA	No interface	Reconstructible, short-segment interface between the tumor and vessel of any degree	Unreconstructable interface between the tumor and vessel
Celiac trunk	No interface	Interface between the tumor and vessel measuring <180° of the circumference of the vessel wall	Interface between the tumor and vessel measuring ≥180° of the circumference of the vessel wall

CHA, common hepatic artery; SMA, superior mesenteric artery; SMV-PV, superior mesenteric vein–portal vein.
From Katz MH, Marsh R, Herman JM, et al. Borderline resectable pancreatic cancer: need for standardization and methods for optimal clinical trial design. *Ann Surg Oncol* 2013;20(8):2787–2795, with permission.

and/or chemoradiation. At the other end of the spectrum, potentially resectable cancers on computed tomography scans appear to be separate from the mesenteric vasculature or approximate the vessels only minimally, and such tumors can routinely be resected safely to negative margins, so surgery is generally recommended as the initial therapeutic approach.[12] Finally, borderline resectable tumors radiographically appear to approximate the mesenteric vasculature to a limited degree. Patients with these tumors are at high risk for at least microscopically incomplete (R1) resection.[10]

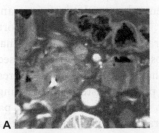 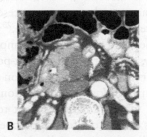 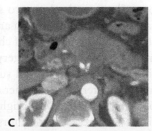

A   **B**   **C**

FIGURE I-1 Radiographic examples of resectable **(A)**, borderline resectable **(B)**, and locally advanced **(C)** primary tumors. **A:** The primary tumor (T) is separated from the superior mesenteric vein, superior mesenteric artery, and aorta by a plane of fat. **B:** The primary tumor has an interface with the superior mesenteric artery measuring <180° of the circumference of the vessel wall. **C:** The primary tumor has interfaces with the splenic artery, common hepatic artery, and celiac trunk that each measure ≥180° of the circumferences of the respective vessels' walls.

Preoperative therapy is therefore recommended for patients with borderline resectable cancers prior to planned surgical resection.[7] Because the initial treatment recommended to each patient with localized PDAC depends on the radiographic stage of the primary tumor, precise preoperative imaging and its accurate clinical interpretation by the surgeon, preferably in the context of a multidisciplinary conference or clinic, now represents the primary objective of the pretreatment workup.[13]

Operative Management and Outcomes

The fundamental technical elements of pancreatoduodenectomy and distal pancreatectomy for cancer are essentially identical to those employed in operations performed in the first part of the 20th century.[14,15] Nonetheless, patients who undergo pancreatic resection today benefit from improvements in perioperative management that have occurred in high-volume centers over the past 3 decades.[16] The bases for these improvements are many and include, but certainly are not limited to, better patient selection for surgery, better surgical training, centralization of care to high-volume surgeons and hospitals, improvements in the ability to rescue from perioperative complications, and advances in perioperative anesthesia and medicine.[17–19] The reduction in perioperative morbidity and mortality is all the more notable as surgeons attempt increasingly complex operations requiring venous and even arterial resection and reconstruction, thereby expanding the role of potentially curative therapy to patients previously considered to have unresectable—and therefore incurable—disease.[20] Furthermore, recent major advances in minimally invasive surgical techniques and equipment now facilitate the complex surgical maneuvers required as part of pancreatoduodenectomy and distal pancreatectomy to be performed without the morbidity of a major abdominal incision, which may translate into further reductions in surgical morbidity and mortality and increases in quality and quantity of life.[21]

Adjuvant and Neoadjuvant Therapy

Although the propensity for PDAC to recur both locally and systemically—even following R0 resection of a node-negative tumor—has been recognized as long as operations for PDAC have been performed, the results of the first major trial of postoperative therapy for pancreatic cancer were only published in 1985.[22] Systemic chemotherapy following potentially curative resection, which offers better progression-free and overall survival relative to surgery alone, now represents the standard of care, and rates of its administration are increasing nationwide.[23,24] Favorable anecdotal reports that the administration of chemotherapy and/or chemoradiation prior to surgery may improve selection for surgery, reduce rates of margin-positive and node-positive resection, and prolong overall survival following resection have led to increasing interest in administering chemotherapy and/or chemoradiation prior to, instead of following, pancreatectomy.[25] Although many remain resistant to using this approach for patients with resectable tumors owing to a fear of preoperative disease progression that would eliminate the possibility for potentially curative surgery, neoadjuvant treatment strategies are now the preferred approach for patients with borderline resectable cancers.[26] Furthermore, the recent approval of two novel chemotherapeutic regimens, FOLFIRINOX (folinic acid, fluorouracil, irinotecan, oxaliplatin)[27] and gemcitabine–nab-paclitaxel,[28] have given hope that the relatively favorable results observed with these regimens in patients with advanced disease may translate into improvements in the adjuvant and/or neoadjuvant setting. Ongoing trials of both neoadjuvant and adjuvant strategies are necessary to improve results following surgery alone.

Objectives of This Section

Despite the rapidly evolving multidisciplinary care programs that have improved the survival of patients with localized PDAC over the past 35 years, important clinical questions and opportunities for improvement clearly remain. It is interesting and perhaps surprising that many of these questions relate to the technical performance of operations that have not changed significantly for 100 years. Indeed, the specific surgical elements that comprise a pancreatectomy, the only component of care that has ever been proven to be potentially curative, remain largely nonstandardized within and among surgical centers in the United States.[29] For this reason, the potential influence of many of these technical components of surgery on oncologic outcome has not been established. Precisely which lymph node basins should be resected at pancreatoduodenectomy? Within which surgical plane should the deep dissection of distal pancreatectomy be routinely performed? How should the superior mesenteric artery margin of resection be managed surgically, and how should it be evaluated pathologically and reported? Ambiguity with regard to the answers to these and many other technical questions, as well as consequent variability with which both pancreatoduodenectomy and pancreatectomy for cancer are performed, may be responsible for the high rates of margin-positive and node-positive resections and suboptimal surgical outcomes that are often reported.[30,31]

Within this section, we present the specific "critical elements" of distal pancreatectomy and pancreatoduodenectomy for cancer that have been catalogued by high-volume pancreatic surgeons and pathologists from both academic and community centers. Recommendations for the performance of each technical element presumed to have a significant association with oncologic outcome, achieved through consensus based on available data, are also presented. Components of surgical therapy believed to represent a "key question" are reviewed in greater depth, with a recommendation generated following a rigorous literature review. Finally, the oncologically significant aspects of surgical care that might be included in a synoptic operative report are proposed. It is hoped that the concepts outlined in this section will be used not only to improve the technical performance of and outcomes associated with pancreatectomy but also to identify opportunities for clinical studies and standardize surgical approaches for clinical protocols.

REFERENCES

1. Fortner JG, Kim DK, Cubilla A, et al. Regional pancreatectomy: en bloc pancreatic, portal vein and lymph node resection. *Ann Surg* 1977;186(1):42–50.
2. Moossa AR, Lewis MH, Mackie CR. Surgical treatment of pancreatic cancer. *Mayo Clin Proc* 1979;54(7):468–474.
3. Beall MS, Dyer GA, Stephenson HE Jr. Disappointments in the management of patients with malignancy of pancreas, duodenum, and common bile duct. *Arch Surg* 1970;101(4):461–465.
4. Bilimoria KY, Bentrem DJ, Ko CY, et al. Multimodality therapy for pancreatic cancer in the U.S.: utilization, outcomes, and the effect of hospital volume. *Cancer* 2007;110(6):1227–1234.
5. Morrow M, Hilaris B, Brennan MF. Comparison of conventional surgical resection, radioactive implantation, and bypass procedures for exocrine carcinoma of the pancreas 1975-1980. *Ann Surg* 1984;199(1):1–5.

6. Katz MH, Wang H, Fleming JB, et al. Long-term survival after multidisciplinary management of resected pancreatic adenocarcinoma. *Ann Surg Oncol* 2009;16(4):836–847.
7. Callery MP, Chang KJ, Fishman EK, et al. Pretreatment assessment of resectable and border-line resectable pancreatic cancer: expert consensus statement. *Ann Surg Oncol* 2009;16(7): 1727–1733.
8. Varadhachary GR, Tamm EP, Abbruzzese JL, et al. Borderline resectable pancreatic cancer: defi-nitions, management, and role of preoperative therapy. *Ann Surg Oncol* 2006;13(8):1035–1046.
9. Exocrine and endocrine pancreas. In: Edge SB, Byrd DR, Compton CC, eds. *AJCC Cancer Staging Manual*. 7th ed. Chicago: Springer; 2010.
10. Katz MH, Marsh R, Herman JM, et al. Borderline resectable pancreatic cancer: need for standard-ization and methods for optimal clinical trial design. *Ann Surg Oncol* 2013;20(8):2787–2795.
11. Kim HJ, Czischke K, Brennan MF, et al. Does neoadjuvant chemoradiation downstage locally advanced pancreatic cancer? *J Gastr Surg* 2002;6(5):763–769.
12. Tamm EP, Loyer EM, Faria S, et al. Staging of pancreatic cancer with multidetector CT in the setting of preoperative chemoradiation therapy. *Abdom Imaging* 2006;31(5):568–574.
13. Pawlik TM, Laheru D, Hruban RH, et al. Evaluating the impact of a single-day multidisciplinary clinic on the management of pancreatic cancer. *Ann Surg Oncol* 2008;15(8):2081–2088.
14. Specht G, Stinshoff K. Walther Kausch (1867–1928) and his significance in pancreatic surgery [article in German]. *Zentralblatt fur Chirurgie* 2001;126(6):479–481.
15. McClusky DA III, Skandalakis LJ, Colborn GL, et al. Harbinger or hermit? Pancreatic anatomy and surgery through the ages–part 3. *World J Surg* 2002;26(12):1512–1524.
16. Winter JM, Cameron JL, Campbell KA, et al. 1423 pancreaticoduodenectomies for pancreatic cancer: a single-institution experience. *J Gastr Surg* 2006;10(9):1199–1210; discussion 1191–1210.
17. Tseng JF, Pisters PW, Lee JE, et al. The learning curve in pancreatic surgery. *Surgery* 2007;141(5): 694–701.
18. Eppsteiner RW, Csikesz NG, McPhee JT, et al. Surgeon volume impacts hospital mortality for pancreatic resection. *Ann Surg* 2009;249(4):635–640.
19. Reames BN, Ghaferi AA, Birkmeyer JD, et al. Hospital volume and operative mortality in the modern era. *Ann Surg* 2014;260(2):244–251.
20. Gurusamy KS, Kumar S, Davidson BR, et al. Resection versus other treatments for locally ad-vanced pancreatic cancer. *Cochrane Database Syst Rev* 2014;2:CD010244.
21. Kendrick ML. Laparoscopic and robotic resection for pancreatic cancer. *Cancer J* 2012;18(6): 571–576.
22. Kalser MH, Ellenberg SS. Pancreatic cancer. Adjuvant combined radiation and chemotherapy following curative resection. *Arch Surg* 1985;120(8):899–903.
23. Simons JP, Ng SC, McDade TP, et al. Progress for resectable pancreatic [corrected] cancer?: a population-based assessment of US practices. *Cancer* 2010;116(7):1681–1690.
24. Oettle H, Post S, Neuhaus P, et al. Adjuvant chemotherapy with gemcitabine vs observation in patients undergoing curative-intent resection of pancreatic cancer: a randomized controlled trial. *JAMA* 2007;297(3):267–277.
25. Crane CH, Varadhachary G, Wolff RA, et al. The argument for pre-operative chemoradiation for localized, radiographically resectable pancreatic cancer. Best practice & research. *Clin Gastr* 2006;20(2):365–382.
26. Evans DB, Farnell MB, Lillemoe KD, et al. Surgical treatment of resectable and borderline resect-able pancreas cancer: expert consensus statement. *Ann Surg Oncol* 2009;16(7):1736–1744.
27. Conroy T, Desseigne F, Ychou M, et al. FOLFIRINOX versus gemcitabine for metastatic pancre-atic cancer. *N Engl J Med* 2011;364(19):1817–1825.
28. Von Hoff DD, Ervin T, Arena FP, et al. Increased survival in pancreatic cancer with nab-paclitaxel plus gemcitabine. *N Engl J Med* 2013;369(18):1691–1703.
29. Katz MH, Merchant NB, Brower S, et al. Standardization of surgical and pathologic variables is needed in multicenter trials of adjuvant therapy for pancreatic cancer: results from the ACOSOG Z5031 trial. *Ann Surg Oncol* 2011;18(2):337–344.
30. Merkow RP, Bilimoria KY, Bentrem DJ, et al. National assessment of margin status as a quality indicator after pancreatic cancer surgery. *Ann Surg Oncol* 2014;21(4):1067–1074.
31. Schwarz RE, Smith DD. Extent of lymph node retrieval and pancreatic cancer survival: informa-tion from a large US population database. *Ann Surg Oncol* 2006;13(9):1189–1200.

CHAPTER 13

Pancreatic Surgery

CRITICAL ELEMENTS

- Evaluation for Extrapancreatic Disease and Assessment of Locoregional Tumor Anatomy
- Pathologic Examination of the Surgical Specimen

1. EVALUATION FOR EXTRAPANCREATIC DISEASE AND ASSESSMENT OF LOCOREGIONAL TUMOR ANATOMY

Recommendation: Staging laparoscopy should be performed prior to laparotomy to exclude radiographically occult metastatic disease. If no such disease is identified, a thorough, open exploration to identify local infiltration or metastases not revealed during laparoscopy should be conducted before tumor resection.

Type of Data: Primarily retrospective, low-level evidence.

Strength of Recommendation: Strong.

Rationale

Pancreatic adenocarcinoma has a high malignant potential, and the majority of patients have metastases at diagnosis. Pancreatectomy is not associated with a survival benefit in these patients.[1,2] Pancreatic cancers may also infiltrate locally into the retroperitoneum and root of the mesentery to involve the superior mesenteric artery (SMA), aorta, and/or celiac trunk, and such involvement precludes a safe and effective margin-negative resection. Unfortunately, even the most advanced cross-sectional imaging and echoendoscopy tests do not have the capacity to detect all low-volume metastatic disease. Therefore, for patients with ostensibly localized pancreatic cancer, rigorous operative staging is critical.

187

Staging Laparoscopy

The evolution of multidetector row computed tomography and advanced magnetic resonance imaging has increased the accuracy with which the anatomic extent of the primary cancer can be determined. However, the capacity of these modalities to identify small (<1 cm) metastases to the liver or peritoneum remains limited.[3] Therefore, a thorough examination of all visceral and parietal surfaces before tumor resection is mandatory. Historically, this examination was accomplished via laparotomy, and patients found to have radiographically occult metastases or unresectable locoregional disease would undergo surgical biliary and enteric bypass to palliative or prevent symptoms of biliary or gastric outlet obstruction.

Steady advances in endoscopic and laparoscopic techniques have substantially reduced the need for open palliative operations, thereby limiting the role of exploratory surgery to staging alone. Staging laparoscopy was first used as a minimally invasive technique to identify occult metastatic pancreatic ductal adenocarcinoma (PDAC) lesions in 1978, obviating the need for nontherapeutic staging laparotomy and its associated morbidity, costs, and delay of definitive oncologic therapy (Fig. 13-1).[4] When the procedure was first introduced, some voiced concerns about its possible association with trocar site disease and peritoneal dissemination, but subsequent studies did not support these concerns, so the use of staging laparoscopy became more widespread.[5] Many now advocate laparoscopic staging for all patients with potentially resectable pancreatic cancer prior to open exploration and resection.[6–9] When utilized liberally, staging laparoscopy radiographically may identify occult metastases in 14% to 37% of patients.

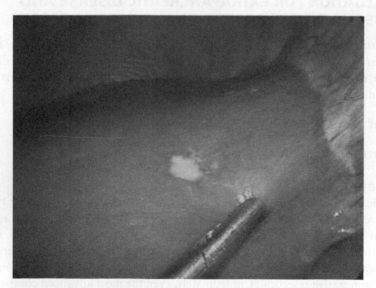

FIGURE 13-1 Radiographically occult lesion on the surface of segment IV of the liver that was identified in a patient with potentially resectable pancreatic cancer upon staging laparoscopy. A tissue biopsy was acquired laparoscopically and immediate histopathologic analysis confirmed metastatic adenocarcinoma. The planned pancreatoduodenectomy was aborted.

Selective Laparoscopy

Staging laparoscopy is most cost-effective when its findings redirect patients with unresectable disease from unnecessary open operative exploration to nonsurgical palliation. Staging laparoscopy becomes increasingly less cost-effective when yield decreases as preoperative imaging improves or as tumor biology becomes increasingly favorable and the risk of metastatic disease decreases. Thus, staging laparoscopy is most cost-effective when it is utilized selectively in patients whose primary cancers are located in the pancreatic body or tail, are large or anatomically extensive, are associated with a high cancer antigen 19-9 level, are associated with equivocal computed tomography findings of metastasis, and/or are associated with clinical findings suggesting advanced disease, such as marked weight loss.[10-16] In these scenarios, the use of staging laparoscopy is particularly encouraged.[17,18]

Advanced/Extended Staging Laparoscopy

Although laparoscopy facilitates the detection of small, superficial metastases on the liver and in the peritoneum that are easily missed using radiologic staging techniques, a simple laparoscopic survey of the abdomen may not detect locally advanced disease and vessel encasement that would also represent a contraindication to resection.[19] Modifications to improve the accuracy of laparoscopic staging have included the use of extensive wider laparoscopic dissections and laparoscopic ultrasonography to more thoroughly inspect vascular structures and evaluate occult intrahepatic lesions, extra-anatomic lymph node involvement, and extrapancreatic tumor extension.[8,9] Although retrospective analyses have shown that all these techniques have added benefits, their detection yield has diminished as significant improvements in preoperative imaging have been made.[15,16] In general, advanced laparoscopy appears to have limited capacity to detect unresectable locoregional tumor extension in patients who have no radiographic evidence of locally advanced disease.

Peritoneal Lavage

Because pancreatic tumors shed malignant cells into the peritoneum, laparoscopic lavage has been proposed as an additional index of resectability. Several early studies showed that patients with positive peritoneal washings developed metastasis earlier and had shorter survival durations after resection than did patients with negative peritoneal washings.[20-22] The results of subsequent investigations have suggested that positive peritoneal cytology alone (without other visible evidence of metastatic disease) should not necessarily preclude resection in pancreatic cancer patients whose tumors would otherwise be considered resectable, as these patients may still achieve long-term survival.[23,24] Regardless, until additional high-level evidence is found to support its widespread use, routine use of peritoneal lavage cannot be recommended at present. It may be used selectively for patients at high risk for surgery to provide support for a nonoperative therapeutic approach.

Timing of Laparoscopy

Staging laparoscopy should typically be performed at the time of the planned resection. Staged procedures to allow time for biopsy specimen analysis, particularly those utilizing peritoneal cytology results as a determinant for proceeding to resection, have been described; however, because these procedures carry additional costs and require additional resources, their routine use in the absence of other obvious indications is not recommended.

Technical Aspects

Technique of Staging Laparoscopic Exploration

Camera port incisions can be made along the proposed lines of the laparotomy incision or (most commonly) periumbilically. Following carbon dioxide insufflation, an angled ($\geq 30°$) laparoscope is used to visually inspect the abdominal cavity, including the peritoneal, diaphragmatic, and hepatic surfaces and the porta hepatis, for evidence of occult metastases. Additional trocars may be placed to elevate the liver lobes and mobilize viscera to facilitate a more thorough evaluation of the pelvis for drop deposits specifically and the mesenteric root for evidence of tumor extension or matted nodes. Abnormal lesions, which may vary in size and morphology but typically appear firm and have evidence of microvasculature, should be biopsied, and the samples should be sent for frozen section pathologic evaluation.

Beyond simple laparoscopic maneuvers for visual evaluation of the peritoneal and visceral surfaces, additional extensive laparoscopic maneuvers are not considered standard. Such maneuvers include elevating the omentum from the transverse colon to access the omental bursa, performing a partial kocherization and evaluating the aortocaval nodes, and dividing the gastrohepatic ligament and examining the caudate lobe surface and celiac axis. At some centers, laparoscopic exploration is performed in conjunction with laparoscopic ultrasonography. These types of advanced laparoscopic evaluations of the extent of locoregional disease may be best reserved for patients undergoing planned minimally invasive resections, in which laparoscopic palliative procedures can be performed without formally converting to laparotomy.

Technique of Open Exploration for Staging

Formal laparotomy is reserved primarily for potentially curative operations. If no evidence of obvious unresectability is identified at laparoscopy, conversion to open exploration is performed. The incision used for open exploration depends on surgeon preference and abdominal anatomical considerations and is typically a midline, or bilateral, subcostal incision. The surgical field is then thoroughly examined to identify any other occult disease not easily visualized by laparoscopy and to assess extrapancreatic extension and locoregional resectability. The omental bursa is accessed by dividing the gastrocolic ligament and elevating the omentum from the mesocolon. For lesions in the pancreatic body or tail, the dissection is extended sufficiently to the left to facilitate full visualization of the pancreas to its tail and the hilum of the spleen. For proximal lesions, the hepatic flexure is mobilized inferiorly by dissecting in the avascular plane between the hepatic flexure and the duodenum and performing an extended Kocher maneuver to free the third portion of the duodenum from the colonic mesentery. The gastrocolic venous trunk or middle colic vein is used as landmark to identify the superior mesenteric vein (SMV) inferior to the neck of the pancreas, where the SMV is assessed for direct tumor involvement. Tumor involvement of the

SMA is classically assessed by placing one's hand posterior to the pancreatic head after kocherization; however, SMA involvement should be readily apparent if high-quality preoperative imaging studies have been performed and skillfully interpreted, and any discrepancy between imaging and intraoperative findings should be met with caution. The porta hepatis is assessed for direct tumor infiltration, and the root of the mesentery should be evaluated to rule out nodal disease outside the surgical field. Once locoregional extent has been thoroughly evaluated, formal dissection to resect the tumor and involved tissues begins.

Conclusion

Despite improvements in modern radiographic imaging studies and the use of these studies' findings to predict locoregional unresectability, cross-sectional imaging studies and echoendoscopy remain relatively nonspecific tests for predicting resectability owing to radiographically occult peritoneal metastases and/or liver metastases in a significant proportion of patients with seemingly localized pancreatic cancer. Minimally invasive procedures and thorough intraoperative evaluation continue to have important roles in staging pancreatic cancers prior to resection with curative intent.

2. PATHOLOGIC EXAMINATION OF THE SURGICAL SPECIMEN

Recommendation: Communication between surgeons and pathologists is essential for the accurate reporting of margin status following pancreatectomy. A standard nomenclature should be used to describe surgical margins. For pancreatoduodenectomy specimens, the status of the pancreatic neck margin, bile duct margin, anterior surface, posterior surface, portal vein/SMV groove, and SMA/uncinate margin should be described. For distal pancreatectomy specimens, the anterior surface, posterior surface, and pancreatic transection margins should be described.

Type of Data: Primarily retrospective, low-level evidence.

Strength of Recommendation: Strong.

Rationale

The oncologic status of the surgical margins (R status) is generally—but not uniformly—regarded as a critical prognostic factor following pancreatectomy and is the most important such factor under the direct influence of the surgeon. For these reasons, the presence or absence of cancer cells at the surgical margins of transection is commonly reported as a primary metric with which the technical success of an individual operation is communicated to patients and other health care providers. The reported association between surgical margins and survival has led to the use of R status as a measure of surgical quality,[25,26] an indicator of technical proficiency,[27] a surrogate marker of the effect associated with preoperative treatment,[28] and a key factor used to stratify patients enrolled in clinical trials of adjuvant therapies.[29]

Historically, cancer cells have been identified at the inked margins of 20% to 40% of surgical specimens resected from patients treated at single institutions[30,31] and within the context of major clinical trials.[32] However, recent investigations that have used meticulous histopathologic protocols to critically evaluate pancreatectomy margins have demonstrated that cancer cells can be identified at one or more surgical margins in close to 90% of resected specimens, a rate that can more easily be reconciled with the reality that as many as 80% of patients who undergo curative resection for pancreatic cancer die with local recurrence.[33,34] Therefore, whether a curative operation is *reported* as microscopically complete (R0) or incomplete (R1) may depend as much on the surgical pathologist as on the surgeon.

Differences in the methods used to handle and process surgical specimens and to interpret and report pathologic findings may contribute to significant variability in R1 resection rates across populations.[35] Because an inaccurate assessment of the surgical margins may alter the purported relationship between margin status and outcome, the utility of R status both as a robust technical metric and as a prognostic variable has been questioned. Furthermore, such variability may adversely influence the accuracy of assessments of patients' eligibility for clinical trials of adjuvant therapies, the interpretation of the results of such trials, and ultimately oncologic outcomes. A discussion of the precise histopathologic protocols pathologists use to evaluate the status of pancreatectomy margins is beyond the scope of this book. However, surgeons play a critical role in certain aspects of the pathologic analysis of the surgical specimen, and these aspects are reviewed here.

Surgical Margins and Terminology

The seventh edition of the American Joint Committee on Cancer (AJCC) *Cancer Staging Manual* references the College of American Pathologists (CAP) Checklist for Exocrine Pancreatic Tumors as the standard document that should be used to guide pathologic evaluation of pancreatic resection specimens in the United States.[36,37] This document does not specifically address differences between the handling or processing of pancreatoduodenectomy and distal pancreatectomy specimens. Rather, it lists the following margins and surfaces as important to evaluate when appropriate: the proximal (gastric or duodenal) and distal (jejunal) enteric margins, the pancreatic neck transection and bile duct margins, the deep retroperitoneal posterior surface, and the nonperitonealized surface of the uncinate process that lies adjacent to the SMA.

Among these anatomic components, the nonperitonealized uncinate surface of pancreatoduodenectomy specimens is emphasized by both the AJCC and CAP as having particular oncologic significance, as it is the most commonly positive margin following potentially curative resection and is the site of most local recurrences following the resection of cancers in the pancreatic head. Although the CAP guidelines refer to the corresponding tissue margin as the "uncinate process (retroperitoneal) margin," the AJCC refers to it as the "SMA margin." This inconsistency has further complicated the already confusing nomenclature used to describe the margin(s) that lie adjacent to the SMA and SMV, which have also been variably described as the "radial," "deep," and "posterior" margin(s), among other terms, by high-volume pancreatic cancer treatment centers.[35]

Furthermore, guidelines published by the Royal College of Pathologists promote a different nomenclature that is used by pancreatic surgeons and pathologists in

Europe.[34,38,39] In this system, the anterior and posterior surfaces of the pancreato-duodenectomy specimen flank a medial "circumferential resection margin" (also described as the "vascular" or "superior mesenteric vessel" margin), which is composed of both an SMV groove margin and an SMA margin. As opposed to those published by the CAP, these guidelines describe in greater detail the important anatomic components of distal pancreatectomy specimens (e.g., inking the anterior and posterior surfaces is recommended specifically) and vein segments removed at pancreatectomy (e.g., examination of the proximal and distal ends of the resected vein is recommended). This lexicon and its accompanying analysis protocol were recently utilized in the first multicenter study to prospectively analyze margin involvement in pancreatectomy specimens.[40]

A standard terminology should be adopted and utilized in both the operative and pathologic reports to reduce confusion and promote standardization. For pancreato-duodenectomy specimens, the status of the pancreatic neck margin, bile duct margin, anterior surface, posterior surface, portal vein/SMV groove, and SMA/uncinate margin should be described (Fig. 13-2). For distal pancreatectomy specimens, the anterior surface, posterior surface, and pancreatic transection margins should be described (Fig. 13-3).

Specimen Orientation

Although the histopathologic analysis of surgical margins is ultimately performed by the pathologist, the surgeon plays a crucial role in helping the pathologist accurately assess surgical margins. Several obstacles may prevent the isolated pathologist from accurately assessing surgical margins. First, characterized by multiple sites of transection and multiple surfaces, the anatomy of the pancreatectomy specimen is extraordinarily complex, making orientation of the specimen difficult following its removal, particularly for less experienced surgical pathologists.[41] In particular, the oncologically important uncinate process is less well-defined as a distinct structure *ex vivo* than it may appear either on cross-sectional images or in the operating room because its anatomy is based on its relationship to the mesenteric vessels. Second, the pathologist cannot reliably determine R status on the basis of the resected specimen alone. Specifically, although the histopathologic techniques the pathologist uses are required to differentiate a microscopically negative (R0) margin from a microscopically positive (R1) margin, only the surgeon, who can view gross residual disease in the abdomen, is in a position to reliably distinguish an R1 margin from a macroscopically positive (R2) margin.

Given these obstacles, the surgeon must be an active participant in the orientation of the surgical specimen. Of particular importance is the surgeon's identification of structures that may have been resected *en bloc*, such as a segment of the SMV or portal vein or another organ (e.g., colon, adrenal gland). Although some surgeons prefer to ink or mark the margins in the operating room, surgical pathologists generally prefer to ink the specimen themselves in collaboration with the surgeon. Similarly, although some surgeons cut pancreatic neck or bile duct margins for immediate histopathologic analysis, experienced surgical pathologists generally frown upon this practice because it may introduce confusion or even diagnostic ambiguity if the margin

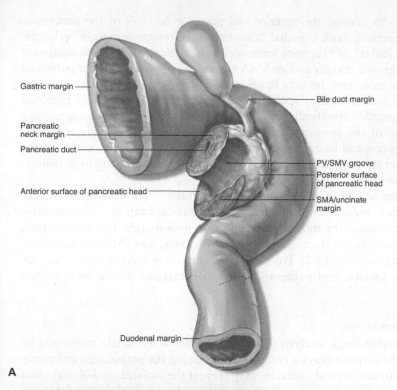

Gastric margin

Bile duct margin

Pancreatic neck margin

Pancreatic duct

PV/SMV groove

Posterior surface of pancreatic head

Anterior surface of pancreatic head

SMA/uncinate margin

Duodenal margin

A

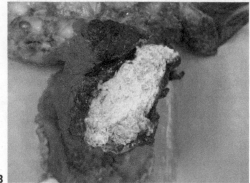

B

FIGURE 13-2 A: Posterior view of the pancreatoduodenectomy specimen. **B:** Lateral view of the inked pancreatoduodenectomy specimen depicting the anterior surface (*red*), pancreatic neck margin (*black*), portal vein/SMV groove (*blue*), and SMA/uncinate margin (*yellow*).

proper is artifactually altered. The CAP guidelines recommend that the pathologist ink the posterior surface and the SMA/uncinate margin, bile duct margin, and pancreatic neck margin of pancreatoduodenectomy specimens, working with the surgeon when necessary. However, given the aforementioned recommendations, it would seem reasonable to also ink the anterior surface and portal vein/SMV groove (Fig. 13-2B). For distal pancreatectomy specimens, the anterior and posterior surfaces and the pancreatic transection margin should be inked (Fig. 13-3B,D).

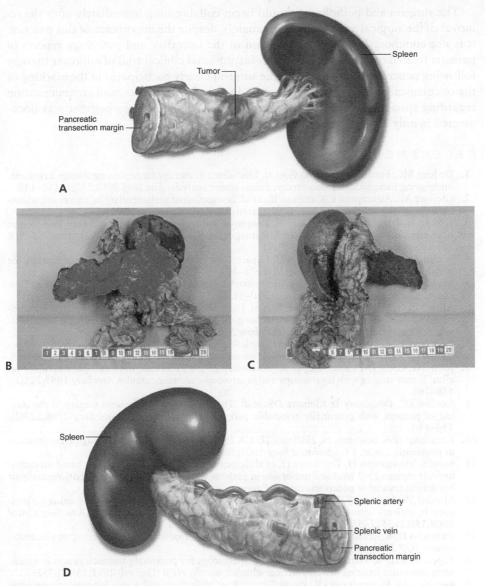

FIGURE 13-3   A,B: Anterior and **(C,D)** posterior surfaces of the distal pancreatectomy with en bloc splenectomy specimen.

The surgeon and pathologist should begin collaborating immediately after the removal of the surgical specimen. Unfortunately, despite the importance of this practice, it is not common. In a recent evaluation of the operative and pathology reports of patients treated on a prospective, multi-institutional clinical trial of adjuvant therapy following pancreatoduodenectomy, the surgeon clearly participated in the marking of the oncologically important SMA margin in only 25% of cases, and communication regarding specimen orientation between the surgeon and the pathologist was documented in only 15% of cases.[35]

REFERENCES

1. De Jong MC, Farnell MB, Sclabas G, et al. Liver-directed therapy for hepatic metastases in patients undergoing pancreaticoduodenectomy: a dual-center analysis. *Ann Surg* 2010;252(1):142–148.
2. Gleisner AL, Assumpcao L, Cameron JL, et al. Is resection of periampullary or pancreatic adenocarcinoma with synchronous hepatic metastasis justified? *Cancer* 2007;110(11):2484–2492.
3. Schima W, Fugger R, Schober E, et al. Diagnosis and staging of pancreatic cancer: comparison of mangafodipir trisodium-enhanced MR imaging and contrast-enhanced helical hydro-CT. *AJR Am J Roentgenol* 2002;179(3):717–724.
4. Warshaw AL, Tepper JE, Shipley WU. Laparoscopy in the staging and planning of therapy for pancreatic cancer. *Am J Surg* 1986;151(1):76–80.
5. Velanovich V. The effects of staging laparoscopy on trocar site and peritoneal recurrence of pancreatic cancer. *Surg Endosc* 2004;18(2):310–313.
6. Allen VB, Gurusamy KS, Takwoingi Y, et al. Diagnostic accuracy of laparoscopy following computed tomography (CT) scanning for assessing the resectability with curative intent in pancreatic and periampullary cancer. *Cochrane Database Syst Rev* 2013;11:CD009323.
7. Contreras CM, Stanelle EJ, Mansour J, et al. Staging laparoscopy enhances the detection of occult metastases in patients with pancreatic adenocarcinoma. *J Surg Oncol* 2009;100(8):663–669.
8. John TG, Greig JD, Carter DC, et al. Carcinoma of the pancreatic head and periampullary region. Tumor staging with laparoscopy and laparoscopic ultrasonography. *Ann Surg* 1995;221(2):156–164.
9. Conlon KC, Dougherty E, Klimstra DS, et al. The value of minimal access surgery in the staging of patients with potentially resectable peripancreatic malignancy. *Ann Surg* 1996;223(2):134–140.
10. Karachristos A, Scarmeas N, Hoffman JP. CA 19-9 levels predict results of staging laparoscopy in pancreatic cancer. *J Gastrointest Surg* 2005;9(9):1286–1292.
11. Satoi S, Yanagimoto H, Toyokawa H, et al. Selective use of staging laparoscopy based on carbohydrate antigen 19-9 level and tumor size in patients with radiographically defined potentially or borderline resectable pancreatic cancer. *Pancreas* 2011;40(3):426–432.
12. Maithel SK, Maloney S, Winston C, et al. Preoperative CA 19-9 and the yield of staging laparoscopy in patients with radiographically resectable pancreatic adenocarcinoma. *Ann Surg Oncol* 2008;15(12):3512–3520.
13. Camacho D, Reichenbach D, Duerr GD, et al. Value of laparoscopy in the staging of pancreatic cancer. *JOP* 2005;6(6):552–561.
14. Tapper E, Kalb B, Martin DR, et al. Staging laparoscopy for proximal pancreatic cancer in a magnetic resonance imaging-driven practice: what's it worth? *HPB (Oxford)* 2011;13(10):732–737.
15. Barabino M, Santambrogio R, Pisani Ceretti A, et al. Is there still a role for laparoscopy combined with laparoscopic ultrasonography in the staging of pancreatic cancer? *Surg Endosc* 2011;25(1):160–165.
16. Pisters PW, Lee JE, Vauthey JN, et al. Laparoscopy in the staging of pancreatic cancer. *Br J Surg* 2001;88(3):325–337.
17. Ellsmere J, Mortele K, Sahani D, et al. Does multidetector-row CT eliminate the role of diagnostic laparoscopy in assessing the resectability of pancreatic head adenocarcinoma? *Surg Endosc* 2005;19(3):369–373.
18. Slaar A, Eshuis WJ, van der Gaag NA, et al. Predicting distant metastasis in patients with suspected pancreatic and periampullary tumors for selective use of staging laparoscopy. *World J Surg* 2011;35(11):2528–2534.
19. Ahmed SI, Bochkarev V, Oleynikov D, et al. Patients with pancreatic adenocarcinoma benefit from staging laparoscopy. *J Laparoendosc Adv Surg Tech A* 2006;16(5):458–463.

20. Warshaw AL. Implications of peritoneal cytology for staging of early pancreatic cancer. *Am J Surg* 1991;161(1):26–29; discussion 29–30.
21. Leach SD, Rose JA, Lowy AM, et al. Significance of peritoneal cytology in patients with potentially resectable adenocarcinoma of the pancreatic head. *Surgery* 1995;118(3):472–478.
22. Merchant NB, Conlon KC, Saigo P, et al. Positive peritoneal cytology predicts unresectability of pancreatic adenocarcinoma. *J Am Coll Surg* 1999;188(4):421–426.
23. Yoshioka R, Saiura A, Koga R, et al. The implications of positive peritoneal lavage cytology in potentially resectable pancreatic cancer. *World J Surg* 2012;36(9):2187–2191.
24. Meszoely IM, Lee JS, Watson JC, et al. Peritoneal cytology in patients with potentially resectable adenocarcinoma of the pancreas. *Am Surg* 2004;70(3):208–213; discussion 213–214.
25. Bilimoria KY, Bentrem DJ, Lillemoe KD, et al. Assessment of pancreatic cancer care in the United States based on formally developed quality indicators. *J Natl Cancer Inst* 2009;101(12):848–859.
26. Sabater L, García-Granero A, Escrig-Sos J, et al. Outcome quality standards in pancreatic oncologic surgery. *Ann Surg Oncol* 2014;21:1138–1146.
27. Tseng JF, Pisters PW, Lee JE, et al. The learning curve in pancreatic surgery. *Surgery* 2007;141(5):694–701.
28. Gillen S, Schuster T, Meyer zum Büschenfelde C, et al. Preoperative/neoadjuvant therapy in pancreatic cancer: a systematic review and meta-analysis of response and resection percentages. *PLoS Med* 2010;7(4):e1000267.
29. Neoptolemos JP, Stocken DD, Dunn JA, et al. Influence of resection margins on survival for patients with pancreatic cancer treated by adjuvant chemoradiation and/or chemotherapy in the ESPAC-1 randomized controlled trial. *Ann Surg* 2001;234(6):758–768.
30. Raut CP, Tseng JF, Sun CC, et al. Impact of resection status on pattern of failure and survival after pancreaticoduodenectomy for pancreatic adenocarcinoma. *Ann Surg* 2007;246(1):52–60.
31. Sohn TA, Yeo CJ, Cameron JL, et al. Resected adenocarcinoma of the pancreas-616 patients: results, outcomes, and prognostic indicators. *J Gastrointest Surg* 2000;4(6):567–579.
32. Butturini G, Stocken DD, Wente MN, et al. Influence of resection margins and treatment on survival in patients with pancreatic cancer: meta-analysis of randomized controlled trials. *Arch Surg* 2008;143(1):75–83; discussion 83.
33. Iacobuzio-Donahue CA, Fu B, Yachida S, et al. DPC4 gene status of the primary carcinoma correlates with patterns of failure in patients with pancreatic cancer. *J Clin Oncol* 2009;27(11):1806–1813.
34. Verbeke CS, Leitch D, Menon KV, et al. Redefining the R1 resection in pancreatic cancer. *Br J Surg* 2006;93(10):1232–1237.
35. Katz MH, Merchant NB, Brower S, et al. Standardization of surgical and pathologic variables is needed in multicenter trials of adjuvant therapy for pancreatic cancer: results from the ACOSOG Z5031 trial. *Ann Surg Oncol* 2011;18(2):337–344.
36. Exocrine and endocrine pancreas. In: Edge SB, Byrd DR, Compton CC, et al, eds. *AJCC Cancer Staging Manual*. 7th ed. New York, NY: Springer; 2010:241–249.
37. Washington K, Berlin J, Branton P, et al. Protocol for the examination of specimens from patients with carcinoma of the exocrine pancreas. 2011. http://www.cap.org/apps/docs/committees/cancer/cancer_protocols/2011/PancreasExo_11protocol.pdf. Accessed February 6, 2015.
38. Verbeke CS, Menon KV. Redefining resection margin status in pancreatic cancer. *HPB (Oxford)* 2009;11(4):282–289.
39. Campbell F, Foulis AK, Verbeke CS. Dataset for the histopathological reporting of carcinomas of the pancreas, ampulla of Vater and common bile duct. 2010. http://www.rcpath.org/Resources/RCPath/Migrated%20Resources/Documents/D/datasethistopathologicalreportingcarcinomas may10.pdf.
40. Delpero JR, Bachellier P, Regenet N, et al. Pancreaticoduodenectomy for pancreatic ductal adenocarcinoma: a French multicentre prospective evaluation of resection margins in 150 evaluable specimens. *HPB (Oxford)* 2014;16(1):20–33.
41. Adsay NV, Basturk O, Saka B, et al. Whipple made simple for surgical pathologists: orientation, dissection, and sampling of pancreaticoduodenectomy specimens for a more practical and accurate evaluation of pancreatic, distal common bile duct, and ampullary tumors. *Am J Surg Pathol* 2014;38(4):480–493.

Pancreatic Surgery: Key Question

Among patients who have resectable pancreatic adenocarcinoma with venous or arterial involvement, does performing a pancreatectomy with vascular resection and reconstruction result in better survival outcomes than performing an R2 resection or aborting surgery?

INTRODUCTION

First described in 1951[1] and later conceptualized as an "extended Whipple procedure,"[2,3] vascular resection and reconstruction (VR) at pancreatectomy for cancer has been an area of considerable interest. Authors of single- and multiple-institution reports and of large database analyses have described a significant experience with pancreatectomy with and without resection of the portal vein, superior mesenteric vein, hepatic artery, and occasionally superior mesenteric artery. Despite these studies, the extent to which VR at pancreatectomy improves survival outcomes in patients who have resectable pancreatic adenocarcinoma with venous or arterial involvement remains unknown. The current review seeks to answer the following question, to the extent that the data can be extracted from the literature and compared: Among patients who have resectable pancreatic adenocarcinoma with venous or arterial involvement, does performing a pancreatectomy VR/reconstruction result in better survival outcomes than performing an R2 resection or aborting surgery?

For clarity and comparability, we have focused on survival as the oncologic metric of interest. Other important metrics include margin status, perioperative morbidity, and the ability to receive adjuvant therapy, insofar as they are associated with overall survival. Although they are beyond the scope of the review, performance status and quality of life, which are increasingly studied outcome measures, may also add additional insight to future investigations and are particularly important in the design of clinical trials. Other issues that are related to the care of patients undergoing planned pancreatectomy, such as whether adjuvant treatments should be given before or after surgery, are beyond the scope of this review but are important considerations when determining whether patients with pancreatic adenocarcinoma with apparent vascular involvement are candidates for pancreatectomy.

METHODOLOGY

Two authors independently performed an organized search of PubMed for English language articles with abstracts published from January 1990 through March 2014. Keyword combinations included "vascular resection" plus "pancreatectomy"; "vascular resection" plus "pancreatic cancer"; ("margin status" or "positive margin" or "R1" or "R2") plus "pancreatic cancer" plus "survival"; and ("locally unresectable" or "borderline") plus "pancreatic cancer" plus "survival."

The initial search yielded 1,045 unique articles. Of these articles, 849 review articles, duplicate series, and technique-focused papers were excluded based on a review of the title and brief review of the abstract because they did not meet the inclusion criteria. The remaining 196 abstracts were reviewed in detail by both authors independently, and an additional 164 abstracts were excluded because the study did not address the clinical question of interest. Thus, both investigators reviewed 32 full-text articles independently. Of these 32 articles, 16 were excluded because they were small series, had inadequate survival data, had no data for patients who did or did not undergo VR at pancreatectomy, or had inadequate follow-up; the final 16 articles were then selected that were used for the complete review of the data (Fig. 13-4).[4–19] Each article was

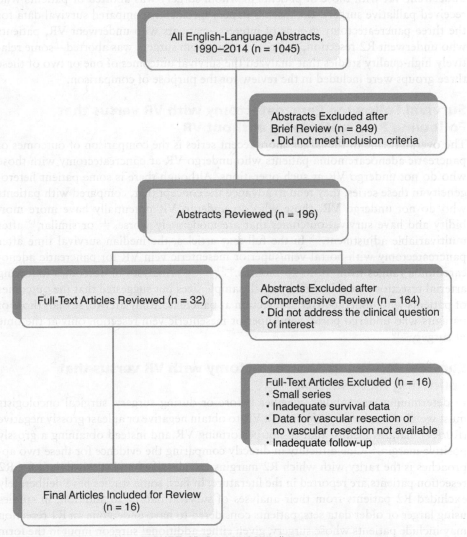

FIGURE 13-4 CONSORT diagram.

then reviewed by both authors and assigned a strength of recommendation based on the Grades of Recommendation, Assessment, Development, and Evaluation system.[20]

FINDINGS

The reviewed papers are listed in Table 13-1. No randomized studies have compared survival outcomes in patients with vascular involvement by tumor following pancreatectomy with and without VR. Most of the reviewed articles are retrospective reports describing one institution's experience with pancreatectomy with VR over time; some of these articles include comparison groups of patients who underwent non-VR pancreatectomies. A few studies compared the outcomes of patients who underwent VR with those of patients in whom surgery was aborted or patients who received palliative surgery. Because no papers specifically compared survival data for the three pancreatectomy groups of interest—patients who underwent VR, patients who underwent R2 resection, and patients in whom surgery was aborted—some relatively high-quality studies that analyzed the survival outcomes of one or two of these three groups were included in the review for the purpose of comparison.

Survival Following Pancreatectomy with VR versus that Following Pancreatectomy without VR

The overall theme of the larger, more recent series is the comparison of outcomes of pancreatic adenocarcinoma patients who undergo VR at pancreatectomy with those who do not undergo VR at such operations. Although there is some patient heterogeneity in these series, they tend to advance the concept that, compared with patients who do not undergo VR, those who do undergo VR potentially have more morbidity and have survival outcomes that are moderately worse,[9,13] or similar,[15] after multivariable adjustment.[5,8] In the full-text articles, the median survival time after pancreatectomy with portal vein/superior mesenteric vein VR for pancreatic adenocarcinoma ranges from 10 to 23 months.[4-11,13-15,18] Analyses of outcomes following arterial resections were limited by small sample sizes but suggested that the outcomes of patients who undergo arterial resection at pancreatectomy are worse than those of patients who undergo portal vein/superior mesenteric vein resection only at the time of surgery.[4,10]

Survival Following Pancreatectomy with VR versus that Following R2 Resection

In determining resectability, whether before or during surgery, surgical oncologists must weigh the value of performing a VR to obtain negative or at least grossly negative (R0/R1) margins against that of not performing VR and instead obtaining a grossly positive margin.[21] One difficulty in directly comparing the evidence for these two approaches is the rarity with which R2 margins are identified and survival data for R2 resection patients are reported in the literature. In fact, some studies have deliberately excluded R2 patients from their analyses of survival data.[14] In addition, in studies using larger or older data sets, patients considered to have undergone an R1 resection may include patients whose surgery, given either additional surgeon input in the form

TABLE 13-1 Studies Assessing Overall Survival of Pancreatic Adenocarcinoma Patients Technically Undergoing Pancreatectomy with or without Vascular Resection

Author, Year	Study Design	No. of Patients	Survival After VR	Survival After R1/R2 Resection	Survival After Palliative or Aborted Surgery	Evidence Grade	Comments
Bachellier et al, 2001	Retrospective	87 (21 VR [PV/SMV], 66 no VR)	1-year OS rate, 53.6%; 2-year OS rate, 21.5%	2-year survival rate, 0%	N/A	1C	
Tseng et al, 2004	Retrospective	291 (110 VR [100 PV/SMV, including 3 HA and 1 IVC; 8 HA only; 2 IVC only]; 181 no VR)	Median OS duration, 23.4 months	Median OS duration, 21.4 months (R1 only)	N/A	1C	70%–75% of patients received neoadjuvant therapy.
Nakoa et al, 2006	Retrospective	289 (201 VR [186 PV only])	Median OS duration, ~10 months	N/A	Median OS duration, ~4 months	2C	KM curves were used for survival estimates.
Shimada et al, 2006	Retrospective	149 (86 VR [PV])	Median OS duration, 14 months	Median OS duration, 12 months (R1 only)	N/A	2C	
Yekebas et al, 2008	Retrospective	482 (100 VR [92 PV, including 5 HA; 8 HA only], 382 no VR)	Median OS duration, 15 months (histopath+); 2-year OS rate, 33.7% (histopath+), 41.1% (histopath +/–)	N/A	N/A	2C	Survival stratified by histopathologic venous invasion.

(continued)

TABLE 13-1 Studies Assessing Overall Survival of Pancreatic Adenocarcinoma Patients Technically Undergoing Pancreatectomy with or without Vascular Resection *(continued)*

Author, Year	Study Design	No. of Patients	Survival After VR	Survival After R1/R2 Resection	Survival After Palliative or Aborted Surgery	Evidence Grade	Comments
Abramson et al, 2008	Literature review	Pooled analysis of studies reviewing a total of 1324 patients undergoing PD with VR	1-year OS rate, 55% (DA model), 53%–62% (weighted in lit review)	1-year OS, 39% (DA model), 34% (weighted in lit review)	N/A	N/A	This was a literature review and DA only; no primary data were available.
Bilimoria et al, 2008	Retrospective; NCDB	N/A	N/A	5-year OS rate, 17.0% (R0), 7.7% (R1), 7.1% (R2); median OS duration, 16.7 months (R0), 12.3 months (R1), 11.9 months (R2)	N/A	N/A	This study included background data for survival after R1 or R2 resection.
Muller et al, 2009	Retrospective	488 (110 VR [PV/SMV])	Median OS duration, 14.5 months; 1-, 2-, and 3-year OS rates, 55.2%, 23.1%, and 14.4%, respectively	No survival difference R0 vs. R1 (P = .26)	N/A	2C	

Study	Type	n (VR)	Outcomes			Level	Comments
Toomey et al, 2009	Retrospective	220 (48 VR [PV/SMV])	Median OS duration, 18 months (R0, 20 months)	Median OS duration, 15 months (VR), 13 months (no VR; R1 only)	N/A	2C	
Kaneoka et al, 2009	Retrospective	84 (42 VR [PV/SMV])	Median OS duration, 12 months (20 with R0 VR); 5-year OS rate, 17% (23% with R0 VR)		R2 excluded	2C	This was a small study; the average number of PDs performed per year for cancer was 8.6. R1 survival data were not separately assessed.
Ouaissi et al, 2010	Retrospective	149 (67 VR [59 PV/SMV; 8 HA])	Median OS duration, 17.5 months (PV), 11.4 months (HA); 5-year OS rate, 11% (PV), 0% (HA)		N/A	2C	R1 survival data were not separately assessed.
Fatima et al, 2010	Retrospective	617 (99 VR [PV/SMV])	Median OS duration, 19 months (R0 en bloc), 18 months (R0 non–en bloc), 15 months (R1), 10 months (R2)	VR and no VR data were not separately assessed	N/A	2C	The analysis was not tailored to VR survival. Multivariate analysis revealed that the HR for death was significant for R2 resection (HR = 2.15, $P = .002$) but not R1 resection (HR = 1.26, $P = .08$).

(continued)

TABLE 13-1 **Studies Assessing Overall Survival of Pancreatic Adenocarcinoma Patients Technically Undergoing Pancreatectomy with or without Vascular Resection** (*continued*)

Author, Year	Study Design	No. of Patients	Survival After VR	Survival After R1/R2 Resection	Survival After Palliative or Aborted Surgery	Evidence Grade	Comments
Konstantinidis et al, 2013		1084 (38 VR [PV/SMV] of 460 PD patients)	Median OS duration, 35 months (R0 "wide" [>1 mm]), 16 months (R0 "close" [<1 mm]; *P* <.001)	Median OS duration, 14 months (R1)	Median OS 11 months (locally advanced disease), 7 months (metastatic disease)	2C	554 patients underwent resection (397 with R0 margins and 157 with R1 margins). The study investigated margin status vs. locally unresectable disease; VR was not the focus.
Ravikumar et al, 2014	Retrospective; multi-institution	1488 (230 borderline PDAC)	Median OS duration, 18.2 months (VR), 18 months (no VR)	No difference in R1 rate for VR (62.9%) and no VR (51.6%, *P* >.05)	Median OS duration, 8 months (surgical bypass)	1C	

DA, decision analysis; DFS, disease free survival; HA, hepatic artery; HR, hazard ratio; IVC, inferior vena cava; KM, Kaplan Meyer; NCDB, National Cancer Database; OS, overall survival; PDAC, pancreatic cancer; PD, pancreatoduodenectomy; PV/SMV, portal vein/superior mesenteric vein; VR, vascular resection.

of a more oncologically detailed operative note or consistent pathologic methods, would be designated an R2 resection.

Using the National Cancer Database, composed of patient data from Commission on Cancer–accredited hospitals, Bilimoria et al[17] stratified patient survival according to surgical margin status. The median overall survival durations of patients who underwent R0, R1, or R2 pancreatectomies were 16.7 months, 12.3 months, and 7.1 months, respectively. Although the study was limited by its use of administrative data, its findings suggest that the survival outcomes of patients who undergo margin-negative resections and those who undergo margin-positive resections differ substantially. Fatima et al,[16] from the Mayo Clinic, also assessed patients' survival according to their margin status following resection. Patients with R0 resections had a median survival duration of 18 to 19 months, depending on whether *en bloc* resection was performed; patients with R1 resections had a median survival duration of 15 months; and patients with R2 resections had a median survival duration of 10 months. Although the Mayo Clinic study included 99 patients who underwent pancreatectomy with VR, it did not directly compare the survival outcomes of patients who underwent pancreatectomy with VR to those who underwent an R2 resection. The hazard ratio for death was significant for patients with R2 resection (HR = 2.15, $P = .002$) but not those with R1 resection (HR = 1.26, $P = .08$). Finally, Konstantinidis et al[12] published the Massachusetts General Hospital experience, in which patients who had "wide" R0 surgical margins (>1 mm) had a median survival duration of 35 months, whereas patients who had "close" R0 surgical margins (≤1 mm) had a median survival duration of 16 months, which was similar to that of patients who underwent R1 resection (14 months).

Survival Following Pancreatectomy with VR versus that Following Aborted Surgery

Data from studies directly comparing outcomes following pancreatectomy with PD with those following aborted or palliative procedures are analogously limited. However, data from an article detailing the Massachusetts General Hospital experience with VR suggest that patients with locally advanced disease who undergo palliative surgery or in whom surgery is aborted have a median survival duration of 11 months.[12] One recent multicenter series from the United Kingdom demonstrated that patients who did or did not undergo VR had similar median survival times (18.2 months and 18 months, respectively); in both groups, >50% of patients had R1 margins. In contrast, surgical bypass patients had a median survival duration of 8 months.[8]

CONCLUSION

Published data are generally from high-volume centers and may not be generalizable to smaller centers. This limitation notwithstanding, available data suggest that patients who undergo pancreatectomy with VR have a longer overall survival time than those undergoing R2 resections or aborted operations. The data for venous reconstructions are more robust than those for arterial reconstructions. Accurate preoperative staging using high quality imaging, and judicious use of preoperative therapies to select those patients most likely benefit from these aggressive operations, are both critical.

REFERENCES

1. Moore GE, Sako Y, Thomas LB. Radical pancreatoduodenectomy with resection and reanastomosis of the superior mesenteric vein. *Surgery* 1951;30:550–553.
2. Asada S, Itaya H, Nakamura K, et al. Radical pancreatoduodenectomy and portal vein resection. Report of two successful cases with transplantation of portal vein. *Arch Surg* 1963;87:609–613.
3. Fortner JG. Regional resection of cancer of the pancreas: a new surgical approach. *Surgery* 1973;73:307–320.
4. Yekebas EF, Bogoevski D, Cataldegirmen G, et al. En bloc vascular resection for locally advanced pancreatic malignancies infiltrating major blood vessels: perioperative outcome and long-term survival in 136 patients. *Ann Surg* 2008;247:300–309.
5. Tseng JF, Raut CP, Lee JE, et al. Pancreaticoduodenectomy with vascular resection: margin status and survival duration. *J Gastrointest Surg* 2004;8:935–949.
6. Toomey P, Hernandez J, Morton C, et al. Resection of portovenous structures to obtain microscopically negative margins during pancreaticoduodenectomy for pancreatic adenocarcinoma is worthwhile. *Am Surg* 2009;75:804–809; discussion 809–810.
7. Shimada K, Sano T, Sakamoto Y, et al. Clinical implications of combined portal vein resection as a palliative procedure in patients undergoing pancreaticoduodenectomy for pancreatic head carcinoma. *Ann Surg Oncol* 2006;13:1569–1578.
8. Ravikumar R, Sabin C, Abu Hilal M, et al. Portal vein resection in borderline resectable pancreatic cancer: a United Kingdom multicenter study. *J Am Coll Surg* 2014;218:401–411.
9. Ouaissi M, Hubert C, Verhelst R, et al. Vascular reconstruction during pancreatoduodenectomy for ductal adenocarcinoma of the pancreas improves resectability but does not achieve cure. *World J Surg* 2010;34:2648–2661.
10. Nakao A, Takeda S, Inoue S, et al. Indications and techniques of extended resection for pancreatic cancer. *World J Surg* 2006;30:976–982; discussion 983–974.
11. Muller SA, Hartel M, Mehrabi A, et al. Vascular resection in pancreatic cancer surgery: survival determinants. *J Gastrointest Surg* 2009;13:784–792.
12. Konstantinidis IT, Warshaw AL, Allen JN, et al. Pancreatic ductal adenocarcinoma: is there a survival difference for R1 resections versus locally advanced unresectable tumors? What is a "true" R0 resection? *Ann Surg* 2013;257:731–736.
13. Kelly KJ, Winslow E, Kooby D, et al. Vein involvement during pancreaticoduodenectomy: is there a need for redefinition of "borderline resectable disease"? *J Gastrointest Surg* 2013;17:1209–1217; discussion 1217.
14. Kaneoka Y, Yamaguchi A, Isogai M. Portal or superior mesenteric vein resection for pancreatic head adenocarcinoma: prognostic value of the length of venous resection. *Surgery* 2009;145:417–425.
15. Hristov B, Reddy S, Lin SH, et al. Outcomes of adjuvant chemoradiation after pancreaticoduodenectomy with mesenterico-portal vein resection for adenocarcinoma of the pancreas. *Int J Radiat Oncol* 2010;76:176–180.
16. Fatima J, Schnelldorfer T, Barton J, et al. Pancreatoduodenectomy for ductal adenocarcinoma: implications of positive margin on survival. *Arch Surg* 2010;145:167–172.
17. Bilimoria KY, Talamonti MS, Sener SF, et al. Effect of hospital volume on margin status after pancreaticoduodenectomy for cancer. *J Am Coll Surg* 2008;207:510–519.
18. Bachellier P, Nakano H, Oussoultzoglou PD, et al. Is pancreaticoduodenectomy with mesentericoportal venous resection safe and worthwhile? *Am J Surg* 2001;182:120–129.
19. Abramson MA, Swanson EW, Whang EE. Surgical resection versus palliative chemoradiotherapy for the management of pancreatic cancer with local venous invasion: a decision analysis. *J Gastrointest Surg* 2009;13:26–34.
20. Guyatt G, Gutterman D, Baumann MH, et al. Grading strength of recommendations and quality of evidence in clinical guidelines: report from an american college of chest physicians task force. *Chest* 2006;129:174–181.
21. Raut CP, Tseng JF, Sun CC, et al. Impact of resection status on pattern of failure and survival after pancreaticoduodenectomy for pancreatic adenocarcinoma. *Ann Surg* 2007;246:52–60.

CHAPTER 14

Pancreatoduodenectomy

CRITICAL ELEMENTS

- Division of the Uncinate Process from the Superior Mesenteric Artery
- Radical Lymphadenectomy
- Resection and Reconstruction of the Superior Mesenteric Vein/Portal Vein to Obtain Negative Margins
- Resection to Negative Margins at the Pancreatic Neck and Bile Duct

1. DIVISION OF THE UNCINATE PROCESS FROM THE SUPERIOR MESENTERIC ARTERY

Recommendation: The uncinate process of the pancreas should be dissected from the SMA along the periadventitial plane of the vessel. The right lateral aspect of the vessel should be skeletonized from the level of the first jejunal branch of the superior mesenteric vein (SMV) to the takeoff of the SMA from the aorta.

Type of Data: Primarily retrospective, low-level evidence.

Strength of Recommendation: Strong.

Rationale

The SMA courses from the aorta just to the left of the uncinate process as it enters the root of the small bowel mesentery. Thus, the vessel lies, at most, within millimeters of primary tumors of the proximal pancreas, and these tumors may infiltrate through the peripancreatic soft tissues into the perineural and lymphatic plexus surrounding the vessel. Resection and reconstruction of the SMA at the time of pancreatoduodenectomy is associated with unfavorable survival rates and is not recommended, even when it is performed in an attempt to clear the tissues around it of cancer and achieve a margin-negative resection.[1] Furthermore, access to and dissection of the soft tissues

207

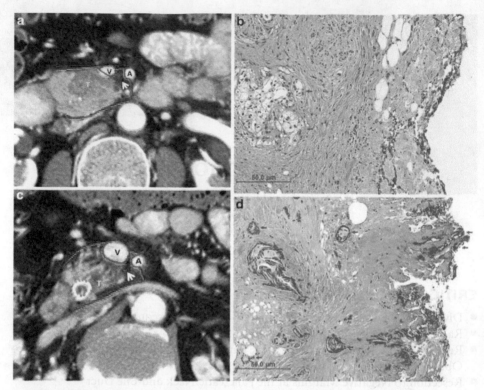

FIGURE 14-1 Meticulous dissection of the retroperitoneal tissues in a patient with a well-staged primary tumor should maximize the opportunity for, but not guarantee, an R0 resection. **A,B:** A patient with a negative SMA/uncinate margin but tumor cells (*arrows*) within 1 mm of the inked margin despite a radiographically resectable cancer and the performance of a periadventitial dissection of the SMA. Tangential resection with saphenous vein reconstruction of the SMV-PV was performed as part of the procedure. **C,D:** A patient with a positive SMA margin. From Katz MH, Wang H, Balachandran A, et al. Effect of neoadjuvant chemoradiation and surgical technique on recurrence of localized pancreatic cancer. *J Gastrointest Surg* 2012;16(1):68–78; discussion 78–79, with permission.

adjacent to the SMA are impeded by the venous confluence and pancreatic neck, both of which lie directly anterior to the artery. Therefore, meticulous dissection of the uncinate process from the SMA is simultaneously the most oncologically critical and technically challenging aspect of pancreatoduodenectomy.

Tumor cells are found at the surgical margins in close to 90% of pancreatoduodenectomy specimens subjected to a rigorous pathologic protocol.[2] The tissue between the uncinate process and SMA is the most likely anatomic location for a microscopically positive (R1) margin.[3] Because meticulous dissection of the retropancreatic complex to the right of the SMA can minimize the amount of residual tissue on the artery, this technique may decrease, but not eliminate, the possibility of an R1 resection in well-staged patients (Fig. 14-1).[4] The retropancreatic complex, which contains fatty tissue, lymphatics, and nerves—described as a "mesopancreas" by some[3]—can be resected in its entirety by skeletonizing the right lateral aspect of the SMA from the level

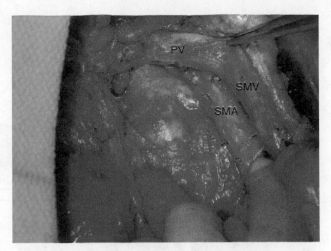

FIGURE 14-2 Operative field following removal of the pancreatoduodenectomy specimen. The superior mesenteric vein is retracted to the patient's left, exposing the right lateral aspect of the superior mesenteric artery. The artery has been dissected in its periadventitial plane. PV, portal vein; SMA, superior mesenteric artery; SMV, superior mesenteric vein.

of the aorta to the level of the first jejunal branch of the SMV (Fig. 14-2). R0 resection rates achieved using this approach have not been directly compared with R0 rates achieved using a less radical dissection of the uncinate. However, no data suggests that this approach increases morbidity, and in fact the opposite may be true because the relevant vascular anatomy can be more fully appreciated using this meticulous technique.[5] Routine dissection in this manner is therefore strongly recommended.

Some continue to advocate using a stapler to divide the uncinate from the SMA. In a small study in which 19 patients who underwent resection using a stapler were compared to 20 patients who underwent a more formal resection, neither group had a positive resection margin. However, the median number of lymph nodes retrieved and evaluated in each group (6.1 and 5.9 nodes, respectively) was low relative to that recommended by the American Joint Committee on Cancer (AJCC), suggesting that the histopathologic evaluation of the specimens had been suboptimal.[6] Further, an anatomic study of cadavers revealed that the application of a surgical stapler to divide the uncinate from the SMA left up to 43% of the alveolar and lymphatic tissue on the SMA.[5] Therefore, optimal dissection and skeletonization of the SMA requires the use of sharp, ultrasonic (harmonic scalpel), or thermal (LigaSure or Enseal) dissectors. The stapler must be avoided (Fig. 14-3).

Technical Aspects

Because the proximal SMA typically lies directly posterior to the SMV-portal vein (PV) confluence, the confluence must be completely mobilized to access the right lateral aspect of the SMA. For smaller tumors that minimally disturb the anatomy of this region, little dissection may be needed to retract the confluence to the left to expose the SMA. However, tumors that are in close proximity to either the SMV or PV often

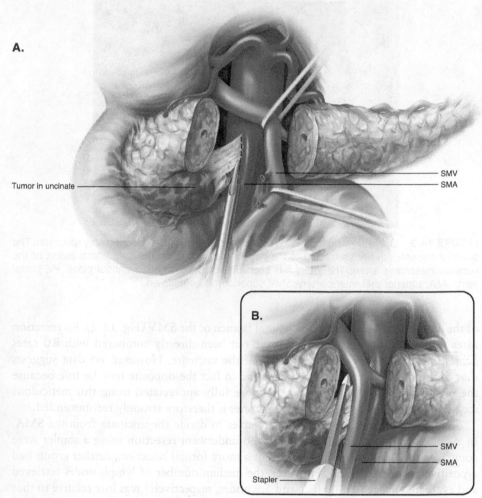

A.

Tumor in uncinate ———————

SMV
SMA

B.

SMV
SMA

Stapler ———————

FIGURE 14-3 **A:** Proper and **(B)** improper surgical technique employed for dissection of the superior mesenteric artery. Exposure of the proximal SMA is required for a safe periadventitial dissection, here performed with the ultrasonic dissector, of the right lateral aspect of the artery. This method ensures all tissues to the right of the SMA are removed with the surgical specimen.

require meticulous dissection to separate the vein from the pancreas. If the SMV or PV is inseparable from the head of the pancreas, vein resection may be necessary.

If the SMV-PV confluence can be easily mobilized from the uncinate process, the specimen is gently retracted to the right, and the SMV-PV confluence is then swept to the left. This exposes the retropancreatic connective tissue. Meticulous dissection of the SMA proceeds either superiorly from the level of the first jejunal branch of the SMV or inferiorly from the takeoff of the SMA from the aorta (see Fig. 14-3). Although the caudal-to-cranial approach is more commonly described in the literature, a working knowledge of both techniques is necessary to safely deliver the specimen.

If the tumor is inseparable from the venous confluence, division of the pancreatic neck and leftward retraction of the confluence may be impossible. In this case, the pancreas may be divided to facilitate the exposure of the SMA; ligation of the splenic vein (SV) may also be performed to facilitate the rightward retraction of the confluence with the surgical specimen.[7] Alternatively, dissection of the SMA may be performed using a posterior approach.[8] No individual technical maneuver is mandatory; a combination of several maneuvers may be required for a safe, complete resection.

Once the SMA is completely exposed, all lymphatic, nervous, and adipose tissue lateral to the vessel is dissected to the right, and the inferior pancreaticoduodenal artery and branches are individually ligated. The relatively bloodless, periadventitial plane should be used for the dissection; circumferential dissection of the SMA is avoided to preserve the surrounding sympathetic plexus and minimize arterial injury. Skeletonization of the lateral, anterior, and posterior borders of the SMA to the level of the adventitia maximizes the yield of soft tissue adjacent to the SMA and presumably the likelihood of a margin-negative resection at this location.

CONCLUSION

The division of the uncinate process from the SMA is one of the most challenging operative components of pancreatoduodenectomy. A thorough working knowledge of the regional anatomy and its variations is key to performing a safe dissection. Complete mobilization of the SMV-PV confluence and dissection of the SMA margin along its periadventitial plane should maximize uncinate yield and thereby decrease the risk of an R1 resection.

2. RADICAL LYMPHADENECTOMY

Recommendation: A standard lymphadenectomy that includes the resection of nodes along the common bile duct, common hepatic artery, portal vein (PV), posterior and anterior pancreaticoduodenal arcades, superior mesenteric vein (SMV), and right lateral wall of the superior mesenteric artery (SMA) should be performed routinely at pancreatoduodenectomy.

Type of Data: Prospective, randomized (albeit flawed) studies, moderate-level evidence.

Strength of Recommendation: Strong.

Rationale

Pancreatic ductal adenocarcinoma (PDAC) has an extremely high propensity for both locoregional infiltration and systemic metastasis. The majority of tumors that appear localized on current state-of-the-art imaging are found to have regional lymph node involvement at the time of resection. Even among node-negative tumors, involvement of extrapancreatic lymphatic pathways within the retroperitoneal soft tissues is common.[9,10]

Lymphatic involvement is the most dominant pathologic prognostic factor for localized PDAC, and the quality of pathologic staging correlates strongly with the number of lymph nodes evaluated in the pathologic examination.[11] Indeed, the primary purpose of lymphadenectomy at the time of pancreatoduodenectomy is to obtain staging information. Current American Joint Committee on Cancer staging guidelines recommend that a minimum of 12 lymph nodes be analyzed, but others have argued that the examination of a minimum of 15 nodes is optimal for staging.[12,13] Although higher lymph node counts have been correlated with better survival outcomes[11] and one may postulate that lymphadenectomy impacts survival, the likelihood that extensive regional clearance significantly enhances survival is low given the propensity of PDAC toward early systemic dissemination.[14] Nevertheless, it is sensible to perform a standard lymphadenectomy as part of pancreatoduodenectomy both to provide precise staging information and to optimize local control.

Standard Lymphadenectomy

Most peripancreatic lymph nodes are not visible intraoperatively, as they tend to be embedded within retroperitoneal adipose tissue. Thus, lymphadenectomy at the time of pancreatoduodenectomy conceptually is not a resective procedure guided by visible lymphatic anatomy; its extent is instead defined by vascular and visceral anatomic structures. The regional lymph node basins that are included in standard lymphadenectomy at the resection of tumors located in the pancreatic head and neck include nodes along the common bile duct, common hepatic artery, PV, posterior and anterior pancreaticoduodenal arcades, SMV, and right lateral wall of the SMA.[13,15] The anatomy of the basins and their corresponding Japanese nomenclature are reported in Table 14-1 and depicted in Figure 14-4. The anatomic division of regional lymph nodes within the specimen is not necessary, but any nodes the surgeon separately submits for pathologic analysis should be reported as labeled by the surgeon.[13] Completion of a standard lymphadenectomy should lead to acceptable lymph node counts (median, 13 to 17 nodes),[16–21] provided that the surgical specimen is subjected to comprehensive pathologic analysis.

TABLE 14-1   Peripancreatic Lymph node stations

Station Number	Anatomic Area
5	Suprapyloric
6	Infrapyloric
8	(a) Anterior and (p) posterior common hepatic artery
9	Celiac artery
10	Splenic hilum
11	(p) Proximal and (d) distal splenic artery
12	(a1, a2) Proper hepatic artery; (b1, b2) common bile duct and hepatic duct; (p1, p2) portal vein; (c) gallbladder, (h) liver hilum
13	(a) Posterosuperior and (b) posteroinferior head of pancreas
14	(a–d) superior mesenteric artery
16	Para-aortic
17	(a) Anterosuperior and (b) anteroinferior head of pancreas
18	Superior margin of pancreas

Adapted from Japan Pancreas Society as reported in Harisinghani MG, ed. *Atlas of Lymph Node Anatomy.* New York, NY: Springer Science + Business Media; 2013. doi:10.1007/978-1-4419-9767-8_3.

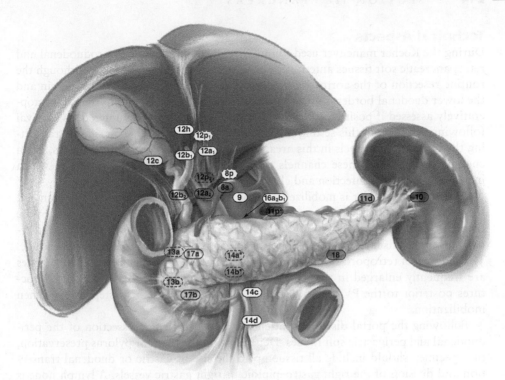

FIGURE 14-4 Lymph node basins that should be resected as part of a standard pancreato-duodenectomy (*yellow*) or distal pancreatectomy with en bloc splenectomy (*blue*). •, station 11p should be dissected only for tumors in the proximal body; *, only the right lateral aspect of stations 14a and 14b should be dissected; stations enclosed in *dotted lines* are posterior.

Standard versus Extended Lymphadenectomy

Five randomized studies have now evaluated the possible benefits associated with extended lymphadenectomy over standard lymphadenectomy. These trials were performed in response to concerns that a more limited resection might leave residual cancer that could lead to local failure and poor survival, as well as in response to several prior retrospective studies that reported that a more extended lymphadenectomy offered a survival advantage over standard lymphatic dissection. These five studies' designs differed to some degree, and the studies were inconsistent in terms of both the lymph node basins considered to comprise an extended lymphadenectomy and the technical methods used to perform the resections. Furthermore, each of the first four studies that were performed has been individually characterized as being underpowered. These limitations notwithstanding, none of the five studies showed that extended lymphadenectomy offered a clear benefit over standard lymphadenectomy in terms of long-term survival.[16-21] Furthermore, associated quality of life analyses revealed that postoperative diarrhea occurred more frequently in patients who underwent extended lymphadenectomy than in patients who underwent standard lymphadenectomy. On the basis of these results, routine extended lymphadenectomy cannot be advocated.

Technical Aspects

During the Kocher maneuver used to mobilize the duodenum, the retroduodenal and retropancreatic soft tissues anterior to the vena cava are also mobilized. Although the routine resection of the aortocaval nodes between the level of the left renal vein and the lower duodenal border is not advocated, these nodes can be sampled and intraoperatively assessed if positive aortocaval lymphadenopathy is encountered, as survival following resection in this setting is particularly poor.[22] Rather than simply transecting the lymphatic channels in this area, the surgeon should use clips, ligatures, or an energy device to seal these channels to prevent postoperative fluid buildup, which increases the risk for infection and chylous ascites.

After the gallbladder is mobilized en bloc to within the hepatoduodenal ligament, the pericholedochal tissues are resected below the level of the transection site of the common hepatic or bile duct; in addition, all soft tissues adjacent to the proper hepatic artery at this level and those anterior and lateral to the PV are removed en bloc. The removal of retroportal lymph nodes poses a special challenge because these nodes are frequently enlarged in the setting of biliary stenting or cholangitis; these structures posterior to the PV may best be left in place until the final steps of specimen mobilization.

Following the portal dissection, attention is turned to the dissection of the periduodenal and perigastric soft tissues. Depending on the plan for pylorus preservation, the specimen should include all tissue up to the site of gastric or duodenal transection and division of the right gastroepiploic or right gastric vessels. A lymph node is frequently encountered proximal to the origin of the gastroduodenal artery from the common hepatic artery, and this node marks well a transection plane within the soft tissue towards the pancreatic neck. Specific dissection of hepatic artery lymph nodes more proximal to this point is not routinely performed. In select cases, intraoperative sampling of the node may provide important prognostic information, as tumor involvement of this node is a poor prognostic factor for survival.[23]

After the pancreas neck is transected anterior to the PV and the distal duodenum and proximal jejunum are transected and mobilized, dissection continues along the SMV-PV confluence. All surrounding soft tissues are dissected, and small vascular branches are divided. This dissection exposes the soft tissues of the mesenteric root that surround the SMA. Unless the presence of tumor extension requires a different approach to be taken, the periarterial tissue is divided anterior to the artery course, and all soft tissues to the right lateral aspect of the SMA are mobilized with the specimen. The goal of this maneuver is to remove 180° of periarterial tissue to the level of the adventitia and to control small branches close to their origin. This facilitates the complete removal of the uncinate process parenchyma, the creation of the best possible margin clearance at the SMA, and the removal of all relevant lymph nodes in this area. This dissection should not be continued beyond the first jejunal branch of the SMA unless specific abnormalities of nodes within the mesenteric root are encountered. Similarly, transverse mesocolon nodes are not routinely resected unless specific findings suggest tumor involvement. The retropancreatic dissection is then completed from the SMA origin towards the liver hilus, and the retroportal lymph nodes can then be removed if necessary. Unless tumor encases it, any replaced right hepatic artery originating from the SMA can usually be preserved even after the surrounding lymphoareolar and adipose tissues have been completely dissected. Final hemostatic maneuvers in all divided soft tissue areas complete the regional dissection.

3. RESECTION AND RECONSTRUCTION OF THE SUPERIOR MESENTERIC VEIN/PORTAL VEIN TO OBTAIN NEGATIVE MARGINS

Recommendation: The SMV, PV, or its confluence should be resected and reconstructed at pancreatoduodenectomy if the primary tumor is inseparable from the vessel and vascular involvement is all that impedes the performance of a margin-negative resection.

Type of Data: Primarily retrospective, low-level evidence and meta-analyses thereof.

Strength of Recommendation: Strong.

Rationale

During pancreatoduodenectomy for PDAC, vascular involvement of the tumor poses additional technical challenges to an already complex procedure. Preoperative planning for pancreatoduodenectomy must include high-quality pancreas protocol computed tomography with three-dimensional vascular reconstruction, which enables the surgeon to anticipate the need for venous resection and facilitates adequate preoperative preparation for vascular reconstruction. A review of the imaging should focus on assessing not only the relationship between the tumor and the surrounding major vessels, including the SMV and its first-order tributaries, but also the vascular anatomy itself, including evaluation for the presence of any anatomic variations, such as a replaced right hepatic artery.

The PV courses posterior to the neck of the pancreas and arises from the confluence of the SMV and SV. The SMV originates from the confluence of the jejunal and ileal tributaries, which are adjacent to the uncinate process of the pancreas. Given the proximity of the vessels to tumors in the head, uncinate process, and neck of the pancreas, neoplastic involvement of these vessels is common (Fig. 14-5A,B). Attempts to skeletonize a primary tumor that is densely adherent to the vein may lead to vascular injury and/or macroscopically positive surgical margins (R2 resection). Although pancreatectomy with resection of the major mesenteric arteries carries five times the risk of perioperative mortality and twice the risk of death at 1 year compared with pancreatectomy without arterial resection, pancreatectomy with vein resection, when performed by surgeons experienced with the techniques required, results in morbidity and mortality equivalent to that of standard pancreatectomy.[1,24–26] A recent meta-analysis of 19 previous studies estimated 1-, 3-, and 5-year overall survival rates of 61%, 19%, and 12%, respectively, for patients who underwent pancreatoduodenectomy with vein resection and 62%, 27%, and 17%, respectively, for patients who underwent standard pancreatoduodenectomy. This and other meta-analyses included heterogenous, nonrandomized studies; thus, the overall level of evidence is low. Regardless, pancreatoduodenectomy with vein resection and reconstruction should be

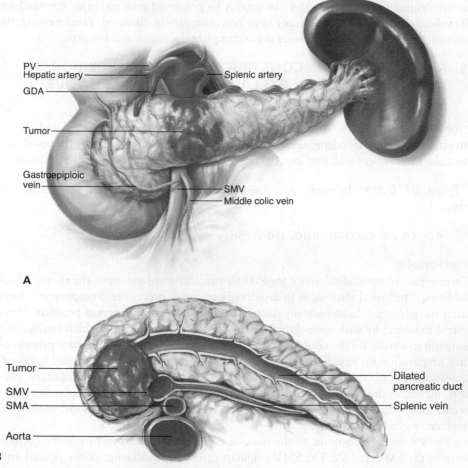

FIGURE 14-5 Due to the proximity of the head and uncinate process of the pancreas to the portal and superior mesenteric veins, tumor infiltration into these vessels is common. **A:** Coronal view, and **(B)** axial view.

considered standard practice for nonmetastatic PDAC involving the SMV-PV confluence, provided that adequate inflow and outflow veins are present, the tumor does not involve the SMA or hepatic artery, and an R0/R1 resection can be reasonably expected.[27] However, vein resection has no role as part of a "regional pancreatectomy," initially described in the 1970s and 1980s, in which a greater amount of grossly uninvolved regional soft tissues is cleared in an attempt to improve outcomes.[28,29]

Intraoperative Margin Evaluation

Among patients who undergo venous resection for PDAC, patients with histologic tumor involvement of the resected vein have a poorer prognosis than patients without tumor involvement.[30] However, the clinical significance of a positive venous transection margin (either tangential or segmental) is unclear. Given the logistical difficulties associated with performing an intraoperative assessment of the vein margin while the portal system is cross-clamped, routine intraoperative analysis of the vein is therefore not recommended at present. The vein should be resected to grossly clear margins. Resecting clinically uninvolved vein is discouraged because doing so increases the likelihood that a simple lateral venorrhaphy or end-to-end vascular reconstruction must be converted to a more complex reconstruction involving a patch or interposition graft.

Technical Aspects

In cases in which the pancreas can be transected at the neck, the extent of venous involvement may be appreciated as the head and uncinate process are separated from the SMV and PV by dividing the small venous tributaries from the pancreas. If the extent of tumor involvement is more pronounced, transection of the pancreas at the neck may not be possible; in such cases, the pancreas should be divided further to the left of the SMV (superficial to the SV) to prepare for segmental venous resection. The specimen is then separated to fully mobilize the SMV-PV confluence to identify the SMA over its entire proximal course. It may be advantageous to mobilize the specimen from the left side of the vein, separating it from the SMA following acquisition of adequate vascular control proximal and distal to the area of venous involvement. Regardless, it is best to defer final resection and reconstruction of SMV/PV until the entire specimen has been completely resected from all surrounding structures, including the SMA. This allows for better vascular control and minimizes the time needed for venous occlusion.

Options for SMV and/or PV resection and reconstruction depend on the site and extent of tumor involvement. If only a small portion of the lateral or posterior aspect of the SMV or PV is involved, the uninvolved uncinate process is separated from the vein, and a Satinsky clamp may be used to gain vascular control of the involved segment; after sharp transection of the involved vein, a primary repair with a 6-0 polypropylene suture can be performed if the lumen of the vessel is not compromised. If a primary repair would create significant narrowing of the venous lumen, a vein patch may be used to repair the SMV or PV (Fig. 14-6A).

If a short segment (≤2 cm) of the PV must be resected, a primary end-to-end anastomosis of the PV should be performed with preservation of the SV and inferior mesenteric vein (IMV) if possible (Fig. 14-6B). Additional PV length for a primary anastomosis can be gained by performing a complete Cattell–Braasch maneuver with mobilization of the retroperitoneal attachments of the small bowel and right colon mesentery up to the ligament of Treitz, which allows cephalad retraction of the root of the mesentery and the first-order SMV tributaries; division of the middle colic vein may also allow further mobilization of the SMV. In addition, easing the tension of a primary end-to-end PV anastomosis can be achieved by completely dissecting the falciform ligament and right triangular ligament and placing laparotomy pads above the liver, which allows for the caudal displacement of the proximal PV stump. Primary anastomosis of the SMV-PV confluence is usually not possible if the tumor involves the SMV below the level of the SV-PV confluence, as the SV prevents the caudal mobilization of the PV. Therefore, the resection of an SMV segment ≥2 cm with SV preservation generally requires an interposition graft (Fig. 14-6C). Autologous grafts created from the left internal jugular vein,[31] superficial femoral vein,[32] and left renal

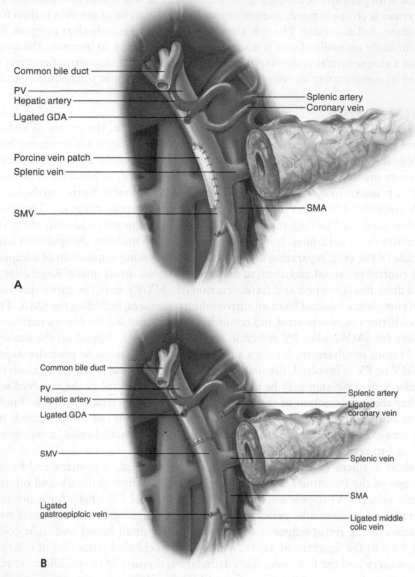

FIGURE 14-6 Venous reconstruction following resection of a primary cancer of the head of the pancreas with involvement of the portal vein and/or superior mesenteric vein. **A:** A defect of the right lateral wall of the vein may best be managed by patch venoplasty. Reconstruction of the vessel following removal of a segment of vein may be accomplished without **(B)** or with **(C)** an interposition graft. If the splenic vein has been ligated **(C)** and signs of sinistral portal hypertension develop, implantation into the graft **(D)** is an option; more straightforwardly, the splenic vein can be implanted into the left renal vein or inferior mesenteric vein to provide venous outflow from the stomach and spleen.

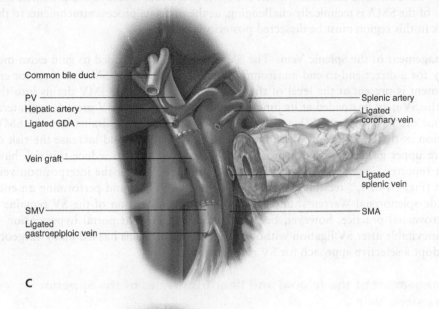

Common bile duct

PV
Hepatic artery
Ligated GDA

Vein graft

SMV
Ligated
gastroepiploic vein

Splenic artery
Ligated
coronary vein

Ligated
splenic vein

SMA

C

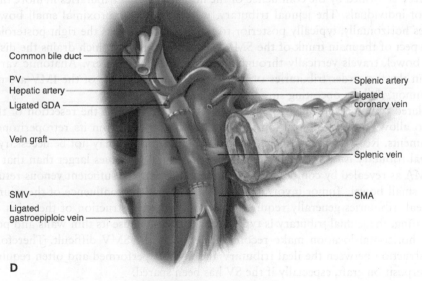

Common bile duct

PV
Hepatic artery
Ligated GDA

Vein graft

SMV
Ligated
gastroepiploic vein

Splenic artery
Ligated
coronary vein

Splenic vein

SMA

D

FIGURE 14-6 (Continued).

vein[33] have all been described. When the SV is preserved, access to the proximal 3 to 4 cm of the SMA is technically challenging, as the uncinate process attachments to the SMA in this region must be dissected posteriorly.

Management of the Splenic Vein. The SV may have to be divided to gain extra mobility for a direct end-to-end anastomosis between the PV and SMV or if tumor encasement is present at the level of the SV-PV confluence. If the IMV drains into the SV, the SV may be divided at its junction with the PV, as the IMV provides collateral venous drainage of the SV (Fig. 14-6D). However, if the IMV drains into the SMV, ligation of the SV can result in sinistral portal hypertension and increase the risk of future upper gastrointestinal hemorrhage. Various methods to reduce this risk have been reported, including reimplanting the SV into the side of the interposition vein graft (Fig. 14-6D),[32] reimplanting the IMV into the SV,[34,35] and performing an end-to-side splenorenal Warren shunt.[36] Mandatory reconstruction of the SV remains a controversial practice, however, because studies suggest that portal hypertension is not inevitable after SV ligation without reconstruction.[35] This has led many surgeons to adopt a selective approach for SV reconstruction.[34,35]

Management of the Jejunal and Ileal Tributaries of the Superior Mesenteric Vein

The SMV is formed by the confluence of the ileal and jejunal tributaries in more than 90% of individuals. The jejunal tributary, which drains the proximal small bowel, courses horizontally, typically posterior to the SMA, and enters the right posterolateral aspect of the main trunk of the SMV. The ileal tributary, which drains the distal small bowel, travels vertically through the small bowel mesentery. Anatomic variations in the first-order tributaries of the SMV and the drainage of the IMV are not uncommon, and the operating surgeon must be aware of these.

Isolated tumor involvement of the jejunal tributary requires the resection of this vein to allow for the mobilization of the uncinate process from its retroperitoneal attachments. Reconstruction of the resected jejunal tributary may not be necessary if the ileal tributary is of adequate diameter (i.e., around 1.5 times larger than that of the SMA as revealed by computed tomography[37]) to provide sufficient venous return to the small bowel. Tumor involvement of the SMV at the confluence of the jejunal and ileal tributaries generally requires resection and reconstruction of the veins. In this setting, the jejunal tributary is typically sacrificed because its thin walls and posterior, horizontal location make reconstructing it to the SMV difficult. Therefore, reconstruction between the ileal tributary and SMV is performed and often requires an interposition graft, especially if the SV has been spared.

Resection and Reconstruction

If possible, the specimen should be completely resected from all surrounding attachments, including the SMA, before resection and reconstruction of the SMV/PV. After the specimen has been removed, systemic anticoagulation is induced with 2,500 to 5,000 U of intravenous heparin. Complete vascular control is obtained by placing vascular clamps proximal and distal to the involved segment of vein and by clamping the SV, IMV, and/or jejunal branches if necessary. Subsequent biliary and pancreatic reconstruction can be made less difficult by applying a Rummel tourniquet or soft bulldog clamp to the SMA to prevent inflow to reduce small bowel edema. The anterior walls of the SMV and PV and the interposition graft (when used) are inked proximally and distally with a marker to help orient the vein during reconstruction. The vein is transected, and the tumor is removed en bloc. The vein is then reconstructed using an interrupted or running 5-0 or 6-0 polypropylene suture with care taken to keep the inked walls aligned. Tying the running suture loosely is generally advocated, and when a graft is used, it is typically easier to complete the distal anastomosis first.

4. RESECTION TO NEGATIVE MARGINS AT THE PANCREATIC NECK AND BILE DUCT

Recommendation: The pancreas should be divided at the neck of the gland or, if that is not possible, to the left of the neck. The bile duct should be divided close to the junction of the common bile duct and hepatic duct. In both pancreas division and bile duct division, transection should occur through grossly normal tissue in an attempt to achieve negative margins. Intraoperative evaluation of the status of these margins and re-resection, if positive, may be considered but are not obligatory, particularly if they are likely to result in the sacrifice of a significant amount of normal duct or pancreatic parenchyma.

Type of Data: Primarily retrospective data, low-level evidence.

Strength of Recommendation: Weak.

Rationale

It is reasonably well-established that prognosis following potentially curative pancreatoduodenectomy is associated with the status of the surgical transection margins. In most cases of margin-positive resection, the residual tumor cells are found within the soft tissue adjacent to the SMA. Although they are less commonly found to be positive on histopathologic analysis, the bile duct and pancreatic neck are two other anatomic sites at which residual tumor cells are commonly found following tissue transection.[38,39] In a recent analysis of the pathology reports for patients enrolled on a multi-institutional trial of adjuvant therapy following pancreatoduodenectomy, the SMA, pancreatic neck, and bile duct margins were positive in 38%, 15%, and 3% of evaluated specimens, respectively.[40]

Unfortunately, few studies have reported the status of individual surgical margins separately or have evaluated the influence of the status of these individual margins on survival. Furthermore, because specimen analysis is not standardized, comparisons between studies are difficult. Thus, the extent to which residual cells at the bile duct or pancreatic neck margins influence either recurrence or survival is unclear.

Owing to its anatomic location immediately adjacent to the unresectable SMA, the SMA-uncinate margin, if dissected properly, cannot be re-resected in an attempt to clear the margin of malignant tissue if an intraoperative evaluation shows residual

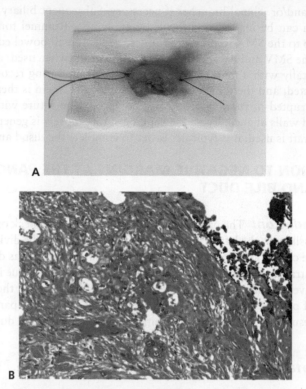

FIGURE 14-7   Immediate histopathologic analysis of the margin at the pancreatic neck by frozen section should be considered but whether re-resection of a positive margin to a negative one improves survival is unclear. **A:** If taken, the margin should be properly oriented to direct analysis of the "true" margin. **B:** In this example, cancer cells were identified at the pancreatic neck margin so additional pancreatic parenchyma was resected prior to reconstruction.

disease. In contrast, the pancreatic neck and bile duct can be re-resected if the initial margin is positive for cancer (Fig. 14-7).[41] Surprisingly, however, the data that would substantiate re-resection of the margins in this clinical scenario are conflicting, and so the role of intraoperative evaluation of these margins is the subject of significant debate. One recent single-center study found that the survival of patients in whom an intraoperative extension of the pancreatic resection was performed to convert a microscopically positive pancreatic neck margin was significantly poorer than that of patients who underwent R0 resection initially.[42] Similarly, another analysis found that (often multiple) re-resections of the pancreatic parenchyma or bile ducts in patients who initially had positive margins did not improve survival.[43] These studies' findings imply that a margin-positive resection is a reflection of aggressive tumor biology, not simple anatomy or surgical technique. However, their results must be interpreted cautiously; other studies have found the exact opposite (i.e., that margin-positive resection reflects anatomy or surgical technique) and suggest that margins should be re-resected until they are negative.[44,45] One of these studies even suggested that total pancreatectomy, given that it was associated with more favorable overall survival, is preferable to pancreatoduodenectomy with a positive neck margin.[45]

Given current knowledge, surgeons should clearly attempt to resect to negative margins at the initial transection of the bile duct or pancreatic parenchyma. However, although intraoperative evaluation of those margins should be considered, re-resection should not be pursued to attain negative margins at the expense of significant amounts of otherwise normal-appearing bile duct or pancreatic parenchyma.

Technical Aspects

After a wide Kocher maneuver and cholecystectomy are performed, dissection of the hepatoduodenal ligament can be initiated. Soft tissue anterior to the porta hepatis is divided at approximately the level of the cystic duct stump. Whether arterial (left) or biliary (right) structures are dissected initially is a matter of preference. The clearance of all soft tissues surrounding the portal structures is followed by the isolation of the proper hepatic artery and common hepatic artery and then the ligation of the gastro-duodenal artery. Division of the gastroduodenal artery allows for the cephalic retraction of the common hepatic artery and more effective soft tissue clearance, which is achieved by developing a plane of dissection anterior to the PV and extending this plane caudally toward the inferior neck of the pancreas. Lymphadenectomy combined with the clearance of soft tissue directly in contact with the neck of the pancreas is extended to the left as far as needed for transection of the pancreas.

REFERENCES

1. Mollberg N, Rahbari NN, Koch M, et al. Arterial resection during pancreatectomy for pancreatic cancer: a systematic review and meta-analysis. *Ann Surg* 2011;254(6):882–893.
2. Verbeke CS, Menon KV. Redefining the R1 resection in pancreatic cancer. *Br J Surg* 2006; 93(10):1232–1237.
3. Gaedcke J, Gunawan B, Grade M, et al. The mesopancreas is the primary site for R1 resection in pancreatic head cancer: relevance for clinical trials. *Langenbecks Arch Surg* 2010;395(4):451–458.
4. Katz MH, Wang H, Balachandran A, et al. Effect of neoadjuvant chemoradiation and surgical technique on recurrence of localized pancreatic cancer. *J Gastrointest Surg* 2012;16(1):68–78; discussion 78–79.
5. Baqué P, Iannelli A, Delotte J, et al. Division of the right posterior attachments of the head of the pancreas with a linear stapler during pancreaticoduodenectomy: vascular and oncological considerations based on an anatomical cadaver-based study. *Surg Radiol Anat* 2009;31(1):13–17.
6. D'Souza MA, Singh K, Hawaldar RV, et al. The vascular stapler in uncinate process division during pancreaticoduodenectomy: technical considerations and results. *Dig Surg* 2010;27(3):175–181.
7. Katz MH, Lee JE, Pisters PW, et al. Retroperitoneal dissection in patients with borderline resectable pancreatic cancer: operative principles and techniques. *J Am Coll Surg* 2012;215(2): e11–e18.
8. Dumitrascu T, David L, Popescu I. Posterior versus standard approach in pancreatoduodenectomy: a case-match study. *Langenbecks Arch Surg* 2010;395(6):677–684.
9. Hatzaras I, George N, Muscarella P, et al. Predictors of survival in periampullary cancers following pancreaticoduodenectomy. *Ann Surg Oncol* 2010;17(4):991–997.
10. Chen JW, Bhandari M, Astill DS, et al. Predicting patient survival after pancreaticoduodenectomy for malignancy: histopathological criteria based on perineural infiltration and lymphovascular invasion. *HPB (Oxford)* 2010;12(2):101–108.
11. Schwarz RE, Smith DD. Extent of lymph node retrieval and pancreatic cancer survival: information from a large US population database. *Ann Surg Oncol* 2006;13(9):1189–1200.
12. Tomlinson JS, Jain S, Bentrem DJ, et al. Accuracy of staging node-negative pancreas cancer: a potential quality measure. *Arch Surg* 2007;142(8):767–723; discussion 773–774.
13. Edge SB, Byrd DR, Compton CC, et al, eds; American Joint Committee on Cancer. *AJCC Cancer Staging Manual.* 7th ed. New York, NY: Springer; 2010.

14. Pawlik TM, Abdalla EK, Barnett CC, et al. Feasibility of a randomized trial of extended lymphadenectomy for pancreatic cancer. *Arch Surg* 2005;140(6):584–589; discussion 589–591.

15. Pedrazzoli S, Günther Beger H, Obertop H, et al. A surgical and pathological based classification of resective treatment of pancreatic cancer. Summary of an international workshop on surgical procedures in pancreatic cancer. *Dig Surg* 1999;16(4):337–345.

16. Farnell MB, Aranha GV, Nimura Y, et al. The role of extended lymphadenectomy for adenocarcinoma of the head of the pancreas: strength of the evidence. *J Gastrointest Surg* 2008;12(4): 651–656.

17. Michalski CW, Kleeff J, Wente MN, et al. Systematic review and meta-analysis of standard and extended lymphadenectomy in pancreaticoduodenectomy for pancreatic cancer. *Br J Surg* 2007;94(3):265–273.

18. Pedrazzoli S, DiCarlo V, Dionigi R, et al. Standard versus extended lymphadenectomy associated with pancreatoduodenectomy in the surgical treatment of adenocarcinoma of the head of the pancreas: a multicenter, prospective, randomized study. Lymphadenectomy Study Group. *Ann Surg* 1998;228(4):508–517.

19. Yeo CJ, Cameron JL, Lillemoe KD, et al. Pancreaticoduodenectomy with or without distal gastrectomy and extended retroperitoneal lymphadenectomy for periampullary adenocarcinoma, part 2: randomized controlled trial evaluating survival, morbidity, and mortality. *Ann Surg* 2002;236(3):355–366; discussion 366–368.

20. Farnell MB, Pearson RK, Sarr MG, et al. A prospective randomized trial comparing standard pancreatoduodenectomy with pancreatoduodenectomy with extended lymphadenectomy in resectable pancreatic head adenocarcinoma. *Surgery* 2005;138(4):618–628; discussion 628–630.

21. Jang JY, Kang MJ, Heo JS, et al. A prospective randomized controlled study comparing outcomes of standard resection and extended resection, including dissection of the nerve plexus and various lymph nodes, in patients with pancreatic head cancer. *Ann Surg* 2014;259(4):656–664.

22. Shimada K, Sakamoto Y, Sano T, et al. The role of paraaortic lymph node involvement on early recurrence and survival after macroscopic curative resection with extended lymphadenectomy for pancreatic carcinoma. *J Am Coll Surg* 2006;203(3):345–352.

23. LaFemina J, Chou JF, Gönen M, et al. Hepatic arterial nodal metastases in pancreatic cancer: is this the node of importance? *J Gastrointest Surg* 2013;17(6):1092–1097.

24. Chua TC, Saxena A. Extended pancreaticoduodenectomy with vascular resection for pancreatic cancer: a systematic review. *J Gastrointest Surg* 2010;14(9):1442–1452.

25. Yu XZ, Li LJ, Fu DL, et al. Benefit from synchronous portal-superior mesenteric vein resection during pancreaticoduodenectomy for cancer: a meta-analysis. *Eur J Surg Oncol* 2014;40(4):371–378.

26. Zhou Y, Zhang Z, Liu Y, et al. Pancreatectomy combined with superior mesenteric vein-portal vein resection for pancreatic cancer: a meta-analysis. *World J Surg* 2012;36(4):884–891.

27. Callery MP, Chang KJ, Fishman EK, et al. Pretreatment assessment of resectable and borderline resectable pancreatic cancer: expert consensus statement. *Ann Surg Oncol* 2009;16(7): 1727–1733.

28. Fortner JG. Regional resection of cancer of the pancreas: a new surgical approach. *Surgery* 1973;73(2):307–320.

29. Fortner JG, Kim DK, Cubilla A, et al. Regional pancreatectomy: en bloc pancreatic, portal vein and lymph node resection. *Ann Surg* 1977;186(1):42–50.

30. Wang J, Estrella JS, Peng L, et al. Histologic tumor involvement of superior mesenteric vein/portal vein predicts poor prognosis in patients with stage II pancreatic adenocarcinoma treated with neoadjuvant chemoradiation. *Cancer* 2012;118(15):3801–3811.

31. Tseng JF, Raut CP, Lee JE, et al. Pancreaticoduodenectomy with vascular resection: margin status and survival duration. *J Gastrointest Surg* 2004;8(8):935–949; discussion 949–950.

32. Fleming JB, Barnett CC, Clagett GP. Superficial femoral vein as a conduit for portal vein reconstruction during pancreaticoduodenectomy. *Arch Surg* 2005;140(7):698–701.

33. Smoot RL, Christein JD, Farnell MB. An innovative option for venous reconstruction after pancreaticoduodenectomy: the left renal vein. *J Gastrointest Surg* 2007;11(4):425–431.

34. Ferreira N, Oussoultzoglou E, Fuchshuber P, et al. Splenic vein-inferior mesenteric vein anastomosis to lessen left-sided portal hypertension after pancreaticoduodenectomy with concomitant vascular resection. *Arch Surg* 2011;146(12):1375–1381.

35. Strasberg SM, Bhalla S, Sanchez LA, et al. Pattern of venous collateral development after splenic vein occlusion in an extended Whipple procedure: comparison with collateral vein pattern in cases of sinistral portal hypertension. *J Gastrointest Surg* 2011;15(11):2070–2079.

36. Christians KK, Tsai S, Tolat PP, et al. Critical steps for pancreaticoduodenectomy in the setting of pancreatic adenocarcinoma. *J Surg Oncol* 2013;107(1):33–38.

37. Katz MH, Fleming JB, Pisters PWT, et al. Anatomy of the superior mesenteric vein with special reference to the surgical management of first-order branch involvement at pancreaticoduodenectomy. *Ann Surg* 2008;248(6):1098–1102.

38. Gnerlich JL, Luka SR, Deshpande AD, et al. Microscopic margins and patterns of treatment failure in resected pancreatic adenocarcinoma. *Arch Surg* 2012;147(8):753–760.

39. Raut CP, Tseng JF, Sun CC, et al. Impact of resection status on pattern of failure and survival after pancreaticoduodenectomy for pancreatic adenocarcinoma. *Ann Surg* 2007;246(1):52–60.

40. Katz MH, Merchant NB, Brower S, et al. Standardization of surgical and pathologic variables is needed in multicenter trials of adjuvant therapy for pancreatic cancer: results from the ACOSOG Z5031 trial. *Ann Surg Oncol* 2011;18(2):337–344.

41. Dillhoff M, Yates R, Wall K, et al. Intraoperative assessment of pancreatic neck margin at the time of pancreaticoduodenectomy increases likelihood of margin-negative resection in patients with pancreatic cancer. *J Gastrointest Surg* 2009;13(5):825–830.

42. Lad NL, Squires MH, Maithel SK, et al. Is it time to stop checking frozen section neck margins during pancreaticoduodenectomy? *Ann Surg Oncol* 2013;20(11):3626–3633.

43. Hernandez J, Mullinax J, Clark W, et al. Survival after pancreaticoduodenectomy is not improved by extending resections to achieve negative margins. *Ann Surg* 2009;250(1):76–80.

44. Fatima J, Schnelldorfer T, Barton J, et al. Pancreaticoduodenectomy for ductal adenocarcinoma: implications of positive margin on survival. *Arch Surg* 2010;145(2):167–172.

45. Schmidt CM, Glant J, Winter JM, et al. Total pancreatectomy (R0 resection) improves survival over subtotal pancreatectomy in isolated neck margin positive pancreatic adenocarcinoma. *Surgery* 2007;142(4):572–578; discussion 578–580.

Pancreatoduodenectomy: Key Question

In patients with resectable adenocarcinoma of the pancreatic head, should a periadventitial dissection of the superior mesenteric artery (i.e., total mesopancreas excision) be performed at the time of pancreatoduodenectomy?

INTRODUCTION

Pancreatic ductal adenocarcinoma (PDAC) is the fourth leading cause of cancer-related death in the United States and the eighth worldwide. Despite advances in medical therapy, the median survival duration of patients diagnosed with PDAC is only 4 to 6 months. However, for the 10% to 20% of PDAC patients who are candidates for pancreatoduodenectomy (PD) at the time of diagnosis, the 5-year overall survival rate approaches 25%, and the median survival duration is 20 to 22 months. Among patients who undergo resection, multiple clinical variables have been determined to be associated with postoperative prognosis. Of these, margin status appears to be one of the most important.

The American Joint Committee on Cancer staging guidelines have attempted to standardize the pathologic evaluation of PD specimens to facilitate margin assessment.[1] According to these guidelines, PD specimen margins that should be evaluated by the pathologist include the pancreatic neck, bile duct, duodenum, and stomach margins, as well as the superior mesenteric artery (SMA) margin. The last of these margins, referred to in this book as the SMA/uncinate margin, is specifically emphasized. The SMA/uncinate margin comprises the tissue that connects the uncinate process to the right lateral border of the proximal 3 to 4 cm of the SMA. PDAC has a propensity to spread through this tissue along the perineural autonomic plexus that surrounds the artery. However, the SMA cannot be removed and reconstructed at surgery in the absence of considerable morbidity. Many surgeons therefore strongly recommend that a periadventitial dissection of the SMA be performed at PD to skeletonize the right lateral aspect of the vessel from the uncinate process and adjacent tissues to maximize the likelihood of obtaining a negative margin in the retroperitoneum.

Although this recommendation is commonly made, the association between the status of the SMA/uncinate margin and oncologic outcomes is unclear. Indeed, the incidence of a positive SMA/uncinate margin and any association between margin status and outcome may reflect "tumor biology" rather than surgical approach or technical skill.[2,3] The contribution of this specific surgical technique to postoperative outcome is therefore incompletely understood. Herein, we describe our review of the literature to determine the effect of performing a periadventitial dissection of the SMA during PD.

METHODOLOGY

We searched Medline and PubMed for English language articles published from January 1990 through January 2014 that addressed the effect of margin status on survival and recurrence following PD. Combinations of the following keywords were used: "pancreas," "retroperitoneal margin," "pancreaticoduodenectomy," "Whipple," "margin," "SMA dissection," "mesopancreas," "retroperitoneal dissection," "morbidity," and "uncinate dissection." Our initial search yielded 520 unique articles. Of these articles, 66 were selected for further review following review of the abstract. The articles selected for analysis focused specifically on pancreatic cancer, commented on margin status following PD, and reported outcomes related to PD and/or margin status. Directed searches of embedded references from the selected articles yielded an additional 16 articles, providing a total of 82 articles for review. Among these, 43 were selected for further analysis.

Of the 43 articles selected, 5 were prospective trials; the others were retrospective reviews of institutional databases (37 articles) or national registry data (1 article). Articles selected for the analysis were specifically scrutinized for standardization of the surgical technique for SMA dissection, pathologic evaluation of the retroperitoneal margin, and margin status–related outcomes, including local recurrence and overall survival. All articles were then reviewed by two members of the group and assigned a strength of recommendation using the GRADE (Grades of Recommendation, Assessment, Development, and Evaluation) system.

FINDINGS

The margin that is or more most often positive following PD is the SMA/uncinate margin. It is positive in 10% or more of resected specimens.[3,4] This is related to the close proximity of the tumor to the perineural plexus surrounding the SMA and the inability to resect additional tissue when the surgeon is confronted with a positive margin along the artery.

Retrospective Studies of Margin Status, Survival, and Local Recurrence

Thirty-eight retrospective studies meeting the eligibility criteria were evaluated (Table 14-2). The incidence of positive (R1) resections reported in these 38 studies ranged widely from 16% to 79%. Only 16 studies reported the status of different margins individually. The SMA margin was the most frequently positive margin. The incidence of a positive SMA margin in these studies ranged from 10% to 88%. None specifically evaluated the potential effect of periadventitial SMA dissection on margin status, local recurrence, or survival.

Among these 38 retrospective studies, 33 concluded that a positive resection margin (any margin) correlated with poorer overall survival, whereas five reported that margin positivity did not influence survival. Only five studies commented on the influence of margin status on local recurrence. Three studies found that margin status had no effect on the incidence of local recurrence, and two found that the local recurrence rates of patients with positive resection margins were higher than those of patients with negative resection margins.

Several methodologic flaws inherent in these retrospective studies are worthy of discussion. First, a standardized surgical technique used to clear the margins (e.g., whether

TABLE 14-2 Summary of Retrospective Studies Commenting on the Relationship between Margin Status and Overall Survival and Local Recurrence in Patients Undergoing Pancreatoduodenectomy*

Author, Year	No. of Patients	R0 Definition	R1, %	SMA+, %	Effect of Margin Status on Survival	Effect of Margin Status on LR
Willett et al, 1993[8]	72	n/s	51	73	+ (KM)	+
Nitecki et al, 1995[9]	174	n/s	16	n/s	+ (KM)	n/s
Nishimura et al, 1997[10]	105	n/s	45	n/s	+ (mva)	n/s
Millikan et al, 1999[11]	60	n/s	29	n/s	+ (uva only)	n/s
Benassai et al, 2000[12]	75	n/s	20	n/s	+ (mva)	n/s
Bouvet et al, 2000[13]	71	n/s	35	n/s	+ (mva)	n/s
Sohn et al, 2000[14]	526	n/s	30	n/s	+ (uva)/–(mva)	n/s
Ahmad et al, 2001[15]	116	n/s	24	n/s	– (mva)	n/s
Pingpank et al, 2001[16]	100	>1 mm	62	50	+ (mva)	n/s
Richter et al, 2003[17]	194	n/s	37	n/s	+ (KM)	n/s
Wagner et al, 2004[18]	164	0 cm	24	n/s	+-(KM)	n/s
Kuhlmann et al, 2004[19]	160	0 mm	50	46	+ (mva)	n/s
Jarufe et al, 2004[20]	251	0 mm	49	n/s	+ (mva)	n/s
Winter et al, 2006[21]	1,423	n/s	42	n/s	+ (mva)	n/s
Moon et al, 2006[22]	71	n/s	24	n/s	+ (mva)	n/s
Han et al, 2006[23]	100	n/s	24	n/s	+ (mva)	n/s
Howard et al, 2006[24]	204	0 mm	30	n/s	+ (mva)	n/s
Verbeke et al, 2006[25]	102	>1 mm	53	39	+(uva)/–(mva)	n/s
Raut et al, 2007[3]	360	0 mm	17	88	– (mva)	–
Murakami et al, 2008[26]	61	0 mm	56	n/s	– (mva)	n/s
Schnelldorfer et al, 2008[27]	357	n/s	23	n/s	+ (log)/–(mva)	n/s
Fusai et al, 2008[28]	67	n/s	60	n/s	– (KM)	n/s

	n					
Westgaard et al, 2008[29]	114	>1 mm	35	80	+ (mva)	n/s
Kinsella et al, 2008[30]	59	>1 mm	49	64	+ (mva)	n/s
Bilimoria et al, 2008[31]	12,101	0 mm	24	n/s	+ (mva)	n/s
Ueda et al, 2009[32]	103	n/s	31	n/s	+ (uva)/– (mva)	n/s
Van den Broeck et al, 2009[33]	121	0 mm	19	63	+ (KM)	–
Campbell et al, 2009[4]	163	>1 mm	79	54	+ (uva)/–(mva)	n/s
Hernandez et al, 2009[34]	202	0 mm	21	n/s	+ (KM)	n/s
Chang et al, 2009[35]	295	0 mm	36	58	+ (mva)	n/s
Jamieson et al, 2010[36]	161	>1 mm	74	46	+ (mva)	n/s
Fatima et al, 2010[37]	617	0 mm	21	78	+ (mva)	n/s
Hartwig et al, 2011[38]	1,071	0 mm (<2005)/ >1 mm (>2005)	64	n/s	+ (mva)	n/s
Gnerlich et al, 2012[39]	285	>1 mm	34	38	+ (KM)	n/s
Sugiura et al, 2013[40]	164	0 mm	35	55	–	+
Tummalu et al, 2013[41]	128	0 mm	32	n/s	+ (mva)	n/s
Jamieson et al, 2013[42]	217	>1 mm	72	47	+ (mva)	–
Kimbrough et al, 2013[43]	283	0 mm	27	n/s	+ (uva)/–(mva)	n/s

KM, Kaplan–Meier; LR, local recurrence; mva, multivariate analysis; n/s, not stated; SMA, superior mesenteric artery; uva, univariate analysis.
*The grade of evidence of all papers is 2C.

a periadventitial dissection of the SMA was performed in all cases) was not routinely reported. Furthermore, the definitions of "R0" and "R1" were not applied consistently: 16 studies did not provide a specific definition of an R0 resection, 14 reports defined R0 as the microscopic absence of any tumor cells at the margin, and eight reports, mostly from European investigators, defined an R0 resection as no tumor cells >1 mm from the cut edge of the specimen. Not surprisingly, investigators who applied more stringent definitions of R0 resection (i.e., a clear margin >1 mm) reported higher rates of R1 resection. A standardized system for naming, processing, and evaluating the surgical margins was not applied consistently. Finally, many studies used both univariate and multivariate analyses to assess the association between margin status and survival. In some of these studies, the univariate analysis, but not the multivariate analysis, revealed that margin status significantly affected survival. In other studies, the effect of margin status on survival was evaluated by comparing Kaplan–Meier survival curves for margin-negative patients to those of margin-positive patients (e.g., by log-rank analysis).

Prospective Studies of Margin Status, Survival, and Local Recurrence

Since 1990, only five prospective randomized studies from Europe and North America have investigated the influence of resection margins on survival and local recurrence following PD (Table 14-3). The margin-positive rates in these series ranged from 17% to 34%. None of these studies specifically addressed the potential association of periadvential dissection of the SMA during PD with either survival or local recurrence.

Three of the five studies did not mandate that a standard surgical technique be used or a pathologic review be performed, and only two of the studies specifically excluded patients with R2 resections. None of the studies reported the oncologic status of the SMA margin independently or evaluated its relationship to survival or local recurrence. As an example, the Charité Oncologie 001 study[5,6] randomized 354 patients to surgery followed by observation or adjuvant gemcitabine. The authors reported an overall margin-positive rate of 17% and found that gemcitabine improved survival following either margin-positive or margin-negative resection but seemed to

TABLE 14-3 Summary of Prospective Studies Commenting on the Relationship between Margin Status and Overall Survival and Local Recurrence Following Pancreatoduodenectomy + Positive Association

Author, Year	No. of Patients	Patients with Margin-Positive Resection, %	Effect of Margin Status on Survival	Grade of Evidence
Klinkenbijl et al, 1999[44]	218	22	NA	2C
Neoptolemos et al, 2004[7]	289	18	+	2A
Regine et al, 2008[45]	451	34	+	2A
Oettle H et al, 2013[5]	368	17	+	2A
Delpero et al, 2014[46]	150	10	+	2C

offer more benefit following margin-positive resection. However, no specific information about the SMA margin or its association with either survival or patterns of recurrence was provided.

Neoptolemos et al[7] reported the results of the ESPAC study in which patients were randomized to surgery alone, surgery followed by chemoradiation, surgery followed by chemotherapy, or surgery followed by both chemoradiation and chemotherapy. The overall rate of margin-positive resection in this study was 18%. In a separate follow-up analysis of this study,[2] Neoptolemos et al[7] found that resection margin status was a prognostic factor for survival; the median survival duration of patients with R1 margins (10.9 months) was much shorter than that of patients with R0 margins (16.9 months). Resection margin status remained an independent factor in a

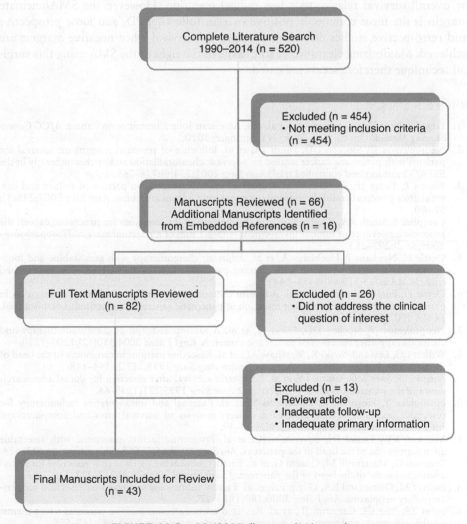

FIGURE 14-8   CONSORT diagram: SMA margin.

Cox proportional hazards model only in the absence of tumor grade and nodal status, suggesting that R1 margin positivity was a reflection of biologic phenotype and not surgical technique. Among patients with R0 margins, those who received chemotherapy had longer survival times than those who did not receive chemotherapy. The authors did not report the rate of SMA margin positivity or its relationship to local or systemic recurrence.

CONCLUSION

Although a periadventitial dissection of the right lateral aspect of the SMA is commonly advocated as a critical technical aspect of PD, no existing studies specifically address the impact of this technique on rates of margin positivity, local recurrence, or overall survival relative to a less radical resection. However, the SMA/uncinate margin is the most commonly positive margin following PD, and most prospective and retrospective studies demonstrate improved survival when negative margins are achieved. Maximizing clearance of soft tissue to the right of the SMA using this surgical technique therefore seems indicated.

REFERENCES

1. Edge SB, Byrd DR, Compton CC, et al, eds; American Joint Committee on Cancer. *AJCC Cancer Staging Manual*. 7th ed. New York, NY: Springer; 2010.
2. Neoptolemos JP, Stocken DD, Dunn JA, et al. Influence of resection margins on survival for patients with pancreatic cancer treated by adjuvant chemoradiation and/or chemotherapy in the ESPAC-1 randomized controlled trial. *Ann Surg* 2001;234(6):758–768.
3. Raut CP, Tseng JF, Sun CC, et al. Impact of resection status on pattern of failure and survival after pancreaticoduodenectomy for pancreatic adenocarcinoma. *Ann Surg* 2007;246(1): 52–60.
4. Campbell F, Smith RA, Whelan P, et al. Classification of R1 resections for pancreatic cancer: the prognostic relevance of tumour involvement within 1 mm of a resection margin. *Histopathology* 2009;55(3):277–283.
5. Oettle H, Neuhaus P, Hochhaus A, et al. Adjuvant chemotherapy with gemcitabine and long-term outcomes among patients with resected pancreatic cancer: the CONKO-001 randomized trial. *JAMA* 2013;310(14):1473–1481.
6. Oettle H, Post S, Neuhaus P, et al. Adjuvant chemotherapy with gemcitabine vs observation in patients undergoing curative-intent resection of pancreatic cancer: a randomized controlled trial. *JAMA* 2007;297(3):267–277.
7. Neoptolemos JP, Stocken DD, Friess H, et al. A randomized trial of chemoradiotherapy and chemotherapy after resection of pancreatic cancer. *N Engl J Med* 2004;350(12):1200–1210.
8. Willett CG, Lewandrowski K, Warshaw AL, et al. Resection margins in carcinoma of the head of the pancreas. Implications for radiation therapy. *Ann Surg* 1993;217(2):144–148.
9. Nitecki SS, Sarr MG, Colby TV, et al. Long-term survival after resection for ductal adenocarcinoma of the pancreas. Is it really improving? *Ann Surg* 1995;221(1):59–66.
10. Nishimura Y, Hosotani R, Shibamoto Y, et al. External and intraoperative radiotherapy for resectable and unresectable pancreatic cancer: analysis of survival rates and complications. *Int J Radiat Oncol Biol Phys* 1997;39(1):39–49.
11. Millikan KW, Deziel DJ, Silverstein JC, et al. Prognostic factors associated with resectable adenocarcinoma of the head of the pancreas. *Am Surg* 1999;65(7):618–623; discussion 623–624.
12. Benassai G, Mastrorilli M, Quarto G, et al. Factors influencing survival after resection for ductal adenocarcinoma of the head of the pancreas. *J Surg Oncol* 2000;73(4):212–218.
13. Bouvet M, Gamagami RA, Gilpin EA, et al. Factors influencing survival after resection for periampullary neoplasms. *Am J Surg* 2000;180(1):13–17.
14. Sohn TA, Yeo CJ, Cameron JL, et al. Resected adenocarcinoma of the pancreas-616 patients: results, outcomes, and prognostic indicators. *J Gastrointest Surg* 2000;4(6):567–579.

15. Ahmad NA, Lewis JD, Ginsberg GG, et al. Long term survival after pancreatic resection for pancreatic adenocarcinoma. *Am J Gastroenterol* 2001;96(9):2609–2615.
16. Pingpank JF, Hoffman JP, Ross EA, et al. Effect of preoperative chemoradiotherapy on surgical margin status of resected adenocarcinoma of the head of the pancreas. *J Gastrointest Surg* 2001;5(2):121–130.
17. Richter A, Niedergethmann M, Sturm JW, et al. Long-term results of partial pancreaticoduodenectomy for ductal adenocarcinoma of the pancreatic head: 25-year experience. *World J Surg* 2003;27(3):324–329.
18. Wagner M, Redaelli C, Lietz M, et al. Curative resection is the single most important factor determining outcome in patients with pancreatic adenocarcinoma. *Br J Surg* 2004;91(5):586–594.
19. Kuhlmann KF, de Castro SM, Wesseling JG, et al. Surgical treatment of pancreatic adenocarcinoma; actual survival and prognostic factors in 343 patients. *Eur J Cancer* 2004;40(4):549–558.
20. Jarufe NP, Coldham C, Mayer AD, et al. Favourable prognostic factors in a large UK experience of adenocarcinoma of the head of the pancreas and periampullary region. *Dig Surg* 2004;21(3):202–209.
21. Winter JM, Cameron JL, Campbell KA, et al. 1423 pancreaticoduodenectomies for pancreatic cancer: A single-institution experience. *J Gastrointest Surg* 2006;10(9):1199-210; discussion 1210–1211.
22. Moon HJ, An JY, Heo JS, et al. Predicting survival after surgical resection for pancreatic ductal adenocarcinoma. *Pancreas* 2006;32(1):37–43.
23. Han SS, Jang JY, Kim SW, et al. Analysis of long-term survivors after surgical resection for pancreatic cancer. *Pancreas* 2006;32(3):271–275.
24. Howard TJ, Krug JE, Yu J, et al. A margin-negative R0 resection accomplished with minimal postoperative complications is the surgeon's contribution to long-term survival in pancreatic cancer. *J Gastrointest Surg* 2006;10(10):1338–1345; discussion 1345–1346.
25. Verbeke CS, Menon KV. Redefining the R1 resection in pancreatic cancer. *Br J Surg* 2006;93(10):1232–1237.
26. Murakami Y, Uemura K, Sudo T, et al. Postoperative adjuvant chemotherapy improves survival after surgical resection for pancreatic carcinoma. *J Gastrointest Surg* 2008;12(3):534–541.
27. Schnelldorfer T, Ware AL, Sarr MG, et al. Long-term survival after pancreatoduodenectomy for pancreatic adenocarcinoma: is cure possible? *Ann Surg* 2008;247(3):456–462.
28. Fusai G, Warnaar N, Sabin CA, et al. Outcome of R1 resection in patients undergoing pancreaticoduodenectomy for pancreatic cancer. *Eur J Surg Oncol* 2008;34(12):1309–1315.
29. Westgaard A, Tafjord S, Farstad IN, et al. Resectable adenocarcinomas in the pancreatic head: the retroperitoneal resection margin is an independent prognostic factor. *BMC Cancer* 2008;8:5.
30. Kinsella TJ, Seo Y, Willis J, et al. The impact of resection margin status and postoperative CA19-9 levels on survival and patterns of recurrence after postoperative high-dose radiotherapy with 5-FU-based concurrent chemotherapy for resectable pancreatic cancer. *Am J Clin Oncol* 2008;31(5):446–453.
31. Bilimoria KY, Talamonti MS, Sener SF, et al. Effect of hospital volume on margin status after pancreaticoduodenectomy for cancer. *J Am Coll Surg* 2008;207(4):510–519.
32. Ueda M, Endo I, Nakashima M, et al. Prognostic factors after resection of pancreatic cancer. *World J Surg* 2009;33(1):104–110.
33. Van den Broeck A, Sergeant G, Ectors N, et al. Patterns of recurrence after curative resection of pancreatic ductal adenocarcinoma. *Eur J Surg Oncol* 2009;35(6):600–604.
34. Hernandez J, Mullinax J, Clark W, et al. Survival after pancreaticoduodenectomy is not improved by extending resections to achieve negative margins. *Ann Surg* 2009;250(1):76–80.
35. Chang DK, Johns AL, Merrett ND, et al. Margin clearance and outcome in resected pancreatic cancer. *J Clin Oncol* 2009;27(17):2855–2862.
36. Jamieson NB, Foulis AK, Oien KA, et al. Positive mobilization margins alone do not influence survival following pancreatico-duodenectomy for pancreatic ductal adenocarcinoma. *Ann Surg* 2010;251(6):1003–1010.
37. Fatima J, Schnelldorfer T, Joshua Barton J, et al. Pancreatoduodenectomy for ductal adenocarcinoma: implications of positive margin on survival. *Arch Surg* 2010;145(2):167–172.
38. Hartwig W, Hackert T, Hinz U, et al. Pancreatic cancer surgery in the new millennium: better prediction of outcome. *Ann Surg* 2011;254(2):311–319.
39. Gnerlich JL, Luka SR, Deshpande AD, et al. Microscopic margins and patterns of treatment failure in resected pancreatic adenocarcinoma. *Arch Surg* 2012;147(8):753–760.
40. Sugiura T, Uesaka K, Mihara K, et al. Margin status, recurrence pattern, and prognosis after resection of pancreatic cancer. *Surgery* 2013;154(5):1078–1086.

41. Tummala P, Howard T, Agarwal B. Dramatic survival benefit related to R0 resection of pancreatic adenocarcinoma in patients with tumor </=25 mm in size and </=1 involved lymph nodes. *Clin Transl Gastroenterol* 2013;4:e33.

42. Jamieson NB, Chan NI, Foulis AK, et al. The prognostic influence of resection margin clearance following pancreaticoduodenectomy for pancreatic ductal adenocarcinoma. *J Gastrointest Surg* 2013;17(3):511–521.

43. Kimbrough CW, St Hill CR, Martin RC, et al. Tumor-positive resection margins reflect an aggressive tumor biology in pancreatic cancer. *J Surg Oncol* 2013;107(6):602–607.

44. Klinkenbijl JH, Jeekel J, Sahmoud T, et al. Adjuvant radiotherapy and 5-fluorouracil after curative resection of cancer of the pancreas and periampullary region: phase III trial of the EORTC gastrointestinal tract cancer cooperative group. *Ann Surg* 1999;230(6):776–782; discussion 782–784.

45. Regine WF, Winter KA, Abrams RA, et al. Fluorouracil vs gemcitabine chemotherapy before and after fluorouracil-based chemoradiation following resection of pancreatic adenocarcinoma: a randomized controlled trial. *JAMA* 2008;299(9):1019–1026.

46. Delpero JR, Bachellier P, Regenet N, et al. Pancreaticoduodenectomy for pancreatic ductal adenocarcinoma: a French multicentre prospective evaluation of resection margins in 150 evaluable specimens. *HPB (Oxford)* 2014;16(1):20–33.

Pancreatoduodenectomy: Key Question 2

Are the perioperative and oncologic outcomes associated with minimally invasive pancreatoduodenectomy for resectable adenocarcinoma of the pancreas equivalent to those associated with an open operation?

INTRODUCTION

Interest in minimally invasive pancreatoduodenectomy (PD), despite its complexity and need for highly specialized training and skills, has continued to grow since its first description by Gagner and Pomp in 1994.[1] However, many surgeons have been reluctant to use the technique in the setting of malignancy, especially pancreatic adenocarcinoma, because few data about the short- and long-term oncologic outcomes of the procedure in this setting have been published. Questions regarding important oncologic metrics such as adequacy of resection (as indicated by lymph node yield and margin-negative resection rates) and recurrence-free and overall survival must be answered to determine the clinical equipoise of minimally invasive PD and traditional open PD. Furthermore, in today's health care environment, the costs of the minimally invasive approach and its value relative to open PD must be clearly established before the procedure will be supported by hospitals and reimbursed by payers. Therefore, a careful, critical evaluation of minimally invasive PD for patients with pancreatic adenocarcinoma, for whom postoperative recovery is frequently complicated and cure is exceedingly rare, is warranted.

METHODOLOGY

The MEDLINE, Cochrane CENTRAL Register of Controlled Trials, EMBASE, and Ovid databases were searched to retrieve studies published between January 1990 and March 2013 that investigated the use of minimally invasive PD for adenocarcinoma. The MeSH search terms used included "laparoscopy," "pancreaticoduodenectomy," and "pancreatic neoplasm." These terms and combinations of them, as well the terms "pancreas," "adenocarcinoma," "pancreatectomy," "Whipple," "robotic," and "minimally invasive surgery," were used in text word searches. The "related articles" function was utilized to broaden the search. The reference lists of selected articles were also examined to identify relevant studies that were not discovered during the initial database searches. Articles were selected for final review if they reported at least 10 cases of minimally invasive PD for pancreatic adenocarcinoma. Each reviewed article was given a final grade of recommendation using the Grades of Recommendation, Assessment, Development, and Evaluation system.

A flow chart illustrating the literature review is given in Figure 14-9. The initial search yielded 88 articles published between January 1990 and March 2013. Of these, 62 were excluded because they were not relevant based on a detailed review of the title and abstract. Of the remaining 26 abstracts, 8 were excluded because they did

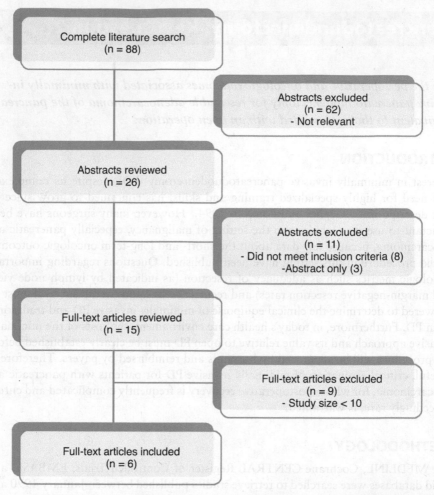

FIGURE 14-8 CONSORT diagram.

not pertain specifically to PD for resectable adenocarcinoma of the head or uncinate of the pancreas and 3 were excluded because they were abstracts that were presented at meetings only and yielded no subsequent manuscript. A total of 15 articles were reviewed in detail; of these, 9 were excluded because they reported on fewer than 10 patients with histologically proven adenocarcinoma. Thus, only 6 studies were identified and reviewed in detail.[2-7]

FINDINGS

The findings of the six studies reviewed in detail are summarized in Table 14-4. Three of the identified studies investigated robot-assisted laparoscopic PD, and three investigated totally laparoscopic PD. All six of these studies described initial experiences

TABLE 14-4 Six Studies Meeting All Inclusion Criteria

Author, Year	Procedure Type(s)	Grade	No. of Patients	Operative Time, Minutes	Blood Loss, mL	LOS, Days	Margin Positivity Rate	No. of Lymph Nodes	Recurrence/Survival
Kendrick and Cusati, 2010[4]	LPD	D	31	Median (range): 368 (258–608)	Median (range): 240 (30–1200)	Median (range): 7 (4–69)	11%	Median (range): 15 (6–31)	Of the 45 patients with malignancy, hepatic or pulmonary recurrence was identified in 7 (16%) within a mean time of 7.4 months; 6 of these patients died of progressive malignancy a mean time of 9 months (range, 3–14 months) after resection. No port site recurrences were identified in any patient during the observation period.
Guilianotti et al, 2010[3]	RALPD	D	19	Mean (range): 421 (240–660)	Mean (range): 394 (80–1500)	Mean (range): 22 (5–85)	0% (Italy); 21% (USA)	Mean (range): 21 (5–37) (Italy), 14 (12–45) (USA)	Two patients died in the postoperative period. Five patients died of recurrence 20, 11, 11, 9, and 7 months, respectively, after surgery. Three patients were alive with recurrences (1 each with pulmonary, local and hepatic, and local recurrence) 12, 11, and 11 months, respectively, after surgery. Nine patients were alive with no recurrence at a mean follow-up time of 16.8 months (range, 8–47 months).

(continued)

237

TABLE 14-4 Six Studies Meeting All Inclusion Criteria (continued)

Author, Year	Procedure Type(s)	Grade	No. of Patients	Operative Time, Minutes	Blood Loss, mL	LOS, Days	Margin Positivity Rate	No. of Lymph Nodes	Recurrence/Survival
Palanivelu et al, 2009[2]	LPD	D	23	Mean (range): 357 (270–650)	Mean (range): 74 (range 35–410)	Mean (range): 8.2 (6–42)	2.6%	Mean (range): 14 (8–22)	NA
Buchs et al, 2011[5]	RALPD, OPD	D	22 (RALPD), 12 (OPD)	Mean ± SD (range): 444 ± 93.5 (240–720) (RALPD), 559 ± 135 (320–850) (OPD), P <.001	Mean ± SD (range): 387 ± 334 (50–1500) (RALPD), /827 ±439 (200–2500) (OPD), P = .0001	Mean ± SD (range): 13 ± 7.5 (5–40) (RALPD), 14.6 ± 9.5 (6–47), P = .4	9.1% (RALPD), 18.5% (OPD), P = .45	Mean ± SD (range): 16.8 ± 10 (2–45) (RALPD), 11 ± 6.3 (2–26) (OPD), P = .02	NA
Asbun and Stauffer, 2012[6]	LPD, OPD	D	22 (TLPD), 100 (OPD)	Mean ± SD: 541 ± 88 (TLPD), 401 ± 108 (OPD), P <.001	Mean ± SD: 195 ± 136 (TLPD), 1032 ± 1151 (OPD), P <.001	Mean ± SD: 8 ± 3.2 (TLPD), 12.4 ± 8.5 (OPD), P <.001	5.1% (TLPD), 17% (OPD)	Mean ± SD: 23.44 ± 10.1 (TLPD), 16.84 ± 10.6 (OPD), P <.001	There was no difference in mean time from surgery to the initiation of chemotherapy between the 2 groups. There were no port site tumor implants or metastases in the LPD group.
Chalikonda et al, 2012[7]	RALPD, OPD	D	14 (RALPD), 14 (OPD)	Mean (range): 476 (363–727) (RALPD), 366.48 (213–602), P <.005	Mean (range): 485 (50–3500) (RALPD), 775 (100–5000) (OPD, P = .13	Mean: 9.79 (RALPD), 13.26 (OPD), P = .043	0% (RALPD), 13% (OPD), P = .02	Mean (range): 13.2 (1–37) (RALPD), 11.76 (1–34) (OPD), P = .25	NA

All studies were retrospective. Metrics provided may reflect those of the entire group studied and do not necessarily reflect those of pancreatic cancer patients alone.
LOS, length of stay; LPD, laparoscopic pancreatoduodenectomy; mL, milliliters; NA, not applicable; No., number; OPD, open pancreatoduodenectomy; RALPD, robotic-assisted laparoscopic pancreatoduodenectomy; TLPD, total laparoscopic pancreaticoduodenectomy.

with minimally invasive PD for a variety of benign or malignant indications (e.g., intraductal papillary mucinous neoplasms, neuroendocrine tumors, periampullary adenocarcinomas, ductal adenocarcinomas). None of the studies investigated minimally invasive PD for pancreatic adenocarcinoma exclusively, and thus the results did not necessarily reflect those specific to this malignancy. Three studies compared outcomes of patients undergoing minimally invasive PD or open PD. None evaluated cost as an outcome metric.

The mean number of patients with pancreatic adenocarcinoma was 22 (range, 14 to 31 patients). The studies' mean overall operative time for minimally invasive PD was 435 minutes (range, 357 to 541 minutes). The mean operative blood loss volume for minimally invasive PD was 296 mL (range, 35 to 1500 mL). The mean margin positivity rate of patients undergoing minimally invasive PD was 8% (range, 0% to 21%). The mean and median numbers of lymph nodes harvested in the minimally invasive PD cohort ranged from 13.2 to 23.4.

Together, the six studies' findings suggest that minimally invasive PD is favorable in terms of perioperative aspects such as operative time, blood loss, and length of hospital stay with the caveat that many of the data in these studies reflect metrics associated with multiple different pathologic diagnoses. Of the three studies that compared operative time for patients undergoing open pancreatoduodenectomy (OPD) with that for patients undergoing minimally invasive PD, two reported a longer time with minimally invasive PD, and one reported a longer time with OPD. In all three studies that compared minimally invasive PD and OPD, patients undergoing minimally invasive PD had less blood loss than those undergoing OPD did. In two of the three comparative studies, length of hospital stay for the minimally invasive PD group was shorter than that for the OPD group. In the one study that evaluated it, the mean time from surgery to the initiation of chemotherapy in the minimally invasive PD group (58.6 ± 17.1 days) did not differ significantly from that of the OPD group (64.1 ± 29.2 days).

The reviewed studies' findings seem to suggest that short-term surrogate metrics of oncologic outcomes, including margin positivity rate and lymph node yield, for patients undergoing minimally invasive PD also compare favorably with those patients undergoing open PD. Of the three studies that compared the margin positivity rates of patients undergoing OPD and patients undergoing minimally invasive PD, two reported no statistically significant difference in margin positivity rates between the two groups. However, Chalikonda et al[7] reported that the margin positivity rate of a cohort of 14 patients undergoing minimally invasive PD (0%) was significantly lower than that of a cohort of 14 patients undergoing OPD (13%; $P = .02$). Of the three studies that compared OPD and minimally invasive PD, two reported that minimally invasive PD yielded more lymph nodes than OPD did (16.8 nodes versus 11 nodes and 23.4 nodes versus 16.8 nodes, respectively). The third study did not show any difference in the number of nodes harvested between the two groups.

The reviewed studies offered a paucity of data regarding recurrence and survival following PD for adenocarcinoma using either open or minimally invasive approaches.

Of the six studies reviewed, only two provided some information on short-term over-all and recurrence-free survival following minimally invasive PD. (Of note, these studies both reported no port site recurrences.) In one study, Kendrick and Cusati[4] described recurrence and survival in 45 patients who underwent PD for adenocarcinoma (31 patients) or other neoplasm (14 patients). Among these 45 patients, distant hepatic or pulmonary recurrence was identified in 7 (16%) within a mean time of 7.4 months; 6 of these patients died of progressive malignancy at a mean time of 9 months (range, 3 to 14 months) after resection. In the other study, Giulianotti et al[3] described recurrence and survival in 19 patients who underwent PD for pancreatic adenocarcinoma. Of these patients, 2 died in the immediate postoperative period, and 5 patients died of recurrence at 20, 11, 11, 9, and 7 months, respectively, after surgery. At the time of the study's publication, 3 patients were alive with either local, distant, or combined recurrences at 12, 11, and 11 months, respectively, after surgery, and 9 patients were alive with no recurrence at mean follow-up time of 16.8 months (range, 8 to 47 months).

CONCLUSION

Several centers have described their initial experiences with minimally invasive PD, but there are still extraordinarily few data regarding the procedure's oncologic results in the setting of pancreatic adenocarcinoma. At best, it appears that minimally invasive PD performed by skilled surgeons is feasible in the setting of pancreatic adenocarcinoma and offers the typical benefits of a minimally invasive approach in terms of hospital stay and operative blood loss. However, minimally invasive PD has no obvious advantage over OPD with regard to short-term surrogates of oncologic metrics such as number of lymph nodes harvested and margin positivity rate. Studies comparing minimally invasive PD to OPD that specifically assess overall and recurrence-free survival, as well as the costs and health care value associated with these procedures, are clearly needed before any meaningful conclusions about the use of one approach versus the other can be made.

Given the relative infrequency of resectable pancreatic ductal adenocarcinoma in general, the limited number of centers performing minimally invasive pancreatic resections, and the lack of regionalization of many patients with resectable pancreatic ductal adenocarcinoma to specialized centers, randomized trials comparing minimally invasive with open PD are exceedingly unlikely. It may therefore be prudent to establish a formal registry for vital oncologic outcomes information from various centers at which minimally invasive PD is performed. Such a registry may provide the means to obtain needed insight and data for subsequent recommendations regarding the use of minimally invasive PD.

In summary, current evidence suggests that the performance of pancreatoduodenectomy using a minimally invasive approach for well-selected patients with resectable adenocarcinoma of the head or uncinate of the pancreas by experienced surgeons is feasible and safe. Outcomes should be carefully monitored and recorded in a prospective registry.

REFERENCES

1. Gagner M, Pomp A. Laparoscopic pylorus-preserving pancreatoduodenectomy. *Surg Endosc* 1994;8(5):408–410.
2. Palanivelu C, Rajan PS, Rangarajan M, et al. Evolution in techniques of laparoscopic pancreaticoduodenectomy: a decade long experience from a tertiary center. *J Hepatobiliary Pancreat Surg* 2009;16(6):731–740.
3. Giulianotti PC, Sbrana F, Bianco FM, et al. Robot-assisted laparoscopic pancreatic surgery: single-surgeon experience. *Surg Endosc* 2010;24(7):1646–1657.
4. Kendrick ML, Cusati D. Total laparoscopic pancreaticoduodenectomy: feasibility and outcome in an early experience. *Arch Surg* 2010;145(1):19–23.
5. Buchs NC, Addeo P, Bianco FM, et al. Robotic versus open pancreaticoduodenectomy: a comparative study at a single institution. *World J Surg* 2011;35(12):2739–2746.
6. Asbun HJ, Stauffer JA. Laparoscopic vs open pancreaticoduodenectomy: overall outcomes and severity of complications using the Accordion Severity Grading System. *J Am Coll Surg* 2012;215(6):810–819.
7. Chalikonda S, Aguilar-Saavedra JR, Walsh RM. Laparoscopic robotic-assisted pancreaticoduodenectomy: a case-matched comparison with open resection. *Surg Endosc* 2012;26(9):2397–2402.

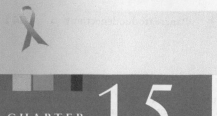

CHAPTER 15

Distal Pancreatectomy

CRITICAL ELEMENTS

- Proximal Parenchymal Transection and Retroperitoneal Dissection
- Radical Lymphadenectomy
- Resection of Adjacent Organs, Superior Mesenteric Vein/Portal Vein, and/or Celiac Axis

1. PROXIMAL PARENCHYMAL TRANSECTION AND RETROPERITONEAL DISSECTION

Recommendation: The pancreatic parenchyma should be transected proximal to all gross disease within normal-appearing gland. Confirmation of a margin-negative resection by intraoperative analysis of the pancreatic neck margin should be considered but is not obligatory, particularly if re-resection is likely to result in the sacrifice of a significant amount of normal pancreatic parenchyma. The posterior plane of the dissection should be carried deep relative to gross tumor and include a rim of normal tissue between the tumor and posterior dissection surface.

Type of Data: Primarily retrospective; two small single-institution prospective.

Strength of Recommendation: Weak.

Rationale

Most patients with tumors of the body or tail of the pancreas are not candidates for potentially curative surgery owing to the presence of either locally advanced or metastatic disease at the time of their initial presentation.[1] Among patients who do undergo resection with curative intent, the 5-year overall survival rates range from 6% to 30% in small, single-institution series.[2] A recent multicenter analysis of patients undergoing left pancreatectomy reported a median survival duration of 16 months and found that positive resection margins were independently associated with poorer survival.[3]

242

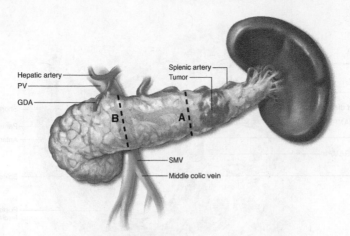

FIGURE 15-1 The pancreatic parenchyma should be divided proximal to the tumor with the goal of achieving a margin-negative resection (*line A*). A more radical parenchymal resection with division of the pancreas at the neck of the gland (*line B*) is unnecessary when the primary tumor is in the distal body or tail, and it may increase the risk for postoperative exocrine and/or endocrine insufficiency.

Classic distal pancreatectomy is characterized by the development of a posterior dissection plane between the pancreas and anterior renal fascia and parenchymal transection just proximal to the cancer (Figs. 15-1 and 15-2). The oncologic integrity of this approach has recently been questioned; of particular concern is the perceived inability of the operation to optimize rates of margin-negative resection given its limited proximal and posterior anatomic scope. The radical antegrade modular pancreaticosplenectomy (RAMPS) procedure, which was developed specifically to address this concern, epitomizes a more exhaustive local resection. In this operation, the pancreatic parenchyma is transected proximally at the neck of the gland (see Fig. 15-1), and the posterior dissection is performed in one of two planes, both of which lie deep to the anterior renal fascia, regardless of the posterior extent of the primary cancer.[4] If a rim of normal pancreas lies posterior to the tumor, a superficial dissection just deep to the fascia on the surface of the left adrenal gland is performed (see Fig. 15-2). If the posterior aspect of the tumor contacts or breaks through the posterior capsule of the gland, an even deeper plane that includes the adrenal gland and Gerota fascia of the left kidney is dissected. In addition to facilitating the soft tissue clearance needed to maximize both R0 rates and nodal clearance, the proximal transection plane with proximal ligation of the splenic vessels has been suggested to reduce the risk for splenic vein thrombosis associated with more distal ligation of the vein.[5,6]

In a recent long-term follow-up study of 47 patients who underwent RAMPS at a single institution, the R0 rate was 81%, and the 5-year overall survival rate was 35.5%; other centers have reported similar outcomes.[2,7] Although these numbers are favorable, they are difficult to interpret, particularly because the oncologic status of the tangential margins (i.e., the anterior and posterior surfaces) has been

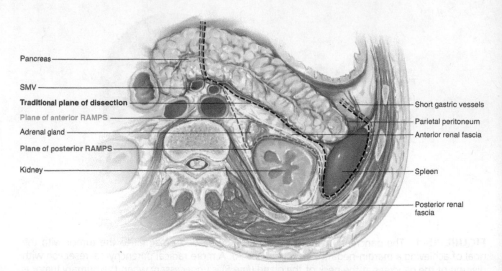

Pancreas

SMV

Traditional plane of dissection

Plane of anterior RAMPS

Adrenal gland

Plane of posterior RAMPS

Kidney

Short gastric vessels

Parietal peritoneum

Anterior renal fascia

Spleen

Posterior renal fascia

FIGURE 15-2 Several deep dissection planes may be used to elevate the pancreas from the underlying retroperitoneum. The standard approach utilizes a plane, determined intraoperatively, carried deep to all gross disease. The radical antegrade modular pancreatosplenectomy procedure utilizes anterior and posterior planes prospectively determined by analysis of the relationship of the tumor to the pancreatic capsule on preoperative imaging; existing data does not clearly support the use of these deep planes unless required to obtain a negative margin.

rarely reported in other series of distal pancreatectomy.[2] Two small studies comparing RAMPS to conventional distal pancreatectomy reported no difference in actuarial survival and mixed results with regards to achieving negative tangential and retroperitoneal margins.[8,9] However, these studies were retrospective and underpowered, and further work is clearly needed to make any substantial conclusions.

The potential disadvantages associated with more radical soft tissue clearance must also be considered. RAMPS has been associated with a severe complication rate of 29%[2]; however, the extent to which these complications result from the more proximal parenchymal transection or deeper posterior dissection associated with the operation, rather than the more radical lymphadenectomy, is unclear. Furthermore, the risk for endocrine insufficiency, in particular, should be carefully considered prior to the resection of normal, functioning pancreatic parenchyma.[10]

Given the unclear advantages associated with uniform transection of the pancreas at the neck and a deep posterior dissection, the routine use of these techniques cannot be advocated at present. Instead, the pancreas should be divided proximal to the site of disease, and the posterior dissection should be carried out deep to the tumor, with a rim of grossly uninvolved soft tissue included both proximally and posteriorly. Although no data support the routine intraoperative evaluation of either the pancreatic neck margin or posterior surface, subjecting both to frozen section analysis would seem reasonable if there is additional soft tissue that could be re-resected if positive margins are found.

2. RADICAL LYMPHADENECTOMY

Recommendation: Lymphadenectomy performed as part of distal pancreatectomy for cancer should routinely include the nodal basins along the splenic artery, at the supra- and infrapancreatic border, and at the splenic hilum.

Type of Data: Primarily retrospective, low-level evidence.

Strength of Recommendation: Weak.

Rationale

Adenocarcinomas of the pancreatic body and tail frequently metastasize to regional lymph nodes. In cases of resectable adenocarcinomas of the body and tail, positive lymph nodes are found in 47% to 80% of resected specimens.[11] Lymphatic spread appears to occur quite early, as reflected by the presence of lymph node metastases in more than 50% of patients with small cancers (<2 cm).[12,13] Positive lymph nodes are associated with poor prognosis.[14] Although a direct effect of lymphadenectomy on survival has not been established, resection of the regional lymph nodes should be performed for staging, if not for therapeutic purposes, as part of potentially curative resections of the pancreatic body or tail.[15]

Lymphatic drainage from cancers in the distal pancreas initially travels to a superficial ring composed of four groups of named nodes—the splenic, gastrosplenic, suprapancreatic, and infrapancreatic nodes—and then to a deeper group of nodes that includes the preaortic nodes, lateral aortic nodes, and interaortocaval nodes.[16,17] In a recent study of 85 patients who underwent radical pancreatectomy with routine dissection of lymph nodes along the common hepatic artery, splenic artery, inferior edge of the pancreas, and splenic hilum and selective dissection of aortocaval nodes, metastases were identified in 5 of 60 (8.3%) common hepatic artery nodes, 19 of 70 (27%) splenic artery nodes, 5 of 31 (16%) nodes along the inferior edge of the pancreas, and 2 of 62 (3%) hilar nodes.[14] Positive nodes were also found along the SMA (9 of 31 nodes, 29%) and celiac trunk (6 of 17 nodes, 35%). In another recent investigation of 1,461 lymph nodes resected from 50 patients at distal pancreatectomy, lymph nodes attached to the pancreas accounted for 78% of positive lymph nodes, and positive extrapancreatic lymph nodes were found in only 6.5% of patients in whom no positive lymph nodes were attached to the pancreas.[18]

Despite this general understanding of the anatomy of the lymphatics associated with the pancreatic body and tail, few data are available for guiding decisions regarding the extent of lymphadenectomy at the time of distal pancreatectomy.[15,19,20] According to the American Joint Committee on Cancer, standard lymphadenectomy for cancers in the body and tail of the pancreas should routinely include lymph nodes along the common hepatic artery, celiac axis (CA), splenic artery, and splenic hilum.[21] In practice, however, many surgeons perform a more limited lymphadenectomy that includes nodes above and below the body and tail of the pancreas but not nodes at the common hepatic artery or CA. Because no studies have compared survival or quality of life outcomes following more limited or extended resections, the benefits and costs associated with each extent of lymphatic resection is unclear. Given available data, however, it would seem reasonable to remove at least the nodes along the upper and lower border of the pancreas, the nodes at the splenic hilum, and those along the splenic vessels (see Fig. 14-4).

Technical Aspects

During lymphatic dissection for distal pancreatectomy, the draining lymphatics along the course of the major vasculature must be securely ligated. This can be accomplished using a variety of techniques. For the ligation of lymphatics along the leftmost border of the SMA and the CA, clips and sutures should be used to help decrease the incidence of postoperative chyle leaks. In general, the lymphatic basins are most readily dissected en bloc as part of the pancreatectomy, but this is not an essential requirement; if necessary, nodal basins along the celiac and SMA can be dissected separately.

Lateral Portion of the Dissection

Splenectomy to harvest lymph nodes in the splenic and gastrosplenic basins is mandatory for cases of pancreatic adenocarcinoma of the pancreatic body or tail. Optimal harvest of the gastrosplenic nodes should be accomplished by dissecting the short gastric vessels in close proximity to the stomach, thereby leaving the maximum amount of fibrofatty tissue from the gastrosplenic ligament with the specimen.

Superior Portion of the Dissection

The suprapancreatic nodes run along the course of the splenic artery, so dissection directly along the course of the artery should not be conducted. Rather, the retroperitoneal fat along the cephalad aspect of the pancreatic tail and splenic artery should be resected en bloc with the tumor.

Inferior Portion of the Dissection

Ensuring inclusion of the infrapancreatic nodes in the specimen requires that dissection along the caudal aspect of the pancreatic body similarly not proceed directly on the substance of the gland itself. Rather, dissection should include some of the retroperitoneal fat in this location. Because the mesocolic nodes lie within the leaflets of the transverse mesocolon at its junction with the pancreas, the mesocolon should be separated off the gland in such a way as to include the most posterior of its attachments with the specimen.[22]

Medial Portion of the Dissection

As discussed, the role of resecting the nodes around the hepatic artery, celiac trunk, and SMA is unclear. When performed, lymphadenectomy of these basins is usually facilitated by identifying the proper hepatic artery and following it proximally towards the origin of the gastroduodenal artery. Ligation of the right gastric artery may be performed to facilitate the lymphadenectomy and to better visualize the anterior surface of the portal vein at the cephalad border of the pancreatic neck. The nodes along the hepatic artery, the left border of the portal vein, and the right crus are swept medially with the specimen until the origin of the splenic artery is identified. Once the splenic artery has been ligated and the celiac nodes have been dissected, the dissection continues posteriorly in a sagittal plane until the SMA is encountered.[23] The proximal SMA can first be identified in the root of the mesentery just as it crosses the left renal vein.

3. RESECTION OF ADJACENT ORGANS, SUPERIOR MESENTERIC VEIN/PORTAL VEIN, AND/OR CELIAC AXIS

Recommendation: Extended operations that involve the resection of adjacent organs, a segment of the superior mesenteric vein (SMV)/portal vein (PV), or even the celiac axis (CA) concomitantly with distal pancreatectomy are occasionally justified in highly selected patients in whom a margin-negative resection is anticipated.

Type of Data: Primarily retrospective, low-level evidence.

Strength of Recommendation: Weak.

Rationale

Because they do not cause symptoms until late in the disease course, tumors in the body and tail of the pancreas tend to be more advanced at presentation than tumors in the head of the pancreas. Nonetheless, the primary goal of potentially curative surgery for distal pancreas cancers is identical to that for pancreatic head cancers: complete extirpation of all disease to microscopically negative margins. Owing to the unique anatomic relationships of the pancreatic body and tail, resection to negative margins may require en bloc resection of the SMV/PV (Fig. 15-3A,B), adjacent organs, or even the CA in addition to the spleen.

Historically, extended operations for distal pancreatic cancers were considered uniformly inappropriate because the survival of patients with distal pancreatic cancer was so poor. However, recent series have demonstrated that extended operations may yield R0 resection and may be associated with rates of morbidity and long-term mortality that are higher than those associated with standard operations but still acceptable in a relatively small group of highly selected patients.[1,24–27] In a series of 513 patients who presented to Memorial Sloan Kettering Cancer Center for treatment of an adenocarcinoma of the pancreatic body or tail between 1983 and 2000, the 5-year overall survival rate of patients who underwent extended distal pancreatectomy (22%) was similar to that of patients who underwent standard distal pancreatectomy (8%) and superior to that of patients who received palliative therapy. However, only 57 (11%) patients underwent resection, and of these patients, only 22 underwent extended operations.[1] The infrequency with which extended operations were conducted even in this high-volume center notwithstanding, one can expect the number of patients who may reasonably be considered for these procedures to increase as novel systemic therapies increasingly prolong the survival of patients with localized pancreatic ductal adenocarcinoma (PDAC) and as preoperative therapy is increasingly used to select patients with biologically favorable tumors for increasingly aggressive operations. Nevertheless, given their technical challenges, extended operations of the distal pancreas, particularly those that require vascular resection, should be performed only at high-volume treatment centers by surgeons skilled in the techniques necessary for the procedures.

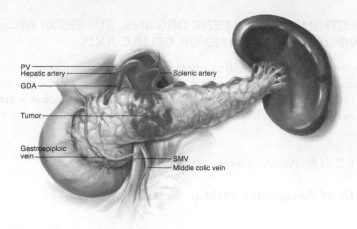

PV
Hepatic artery
GDA
Splenic artery
Tumor
Gastroepiploic vein
SMV
Middle colic vein

A

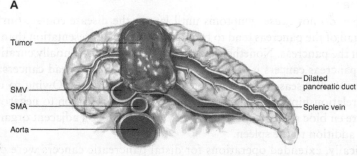

Tumor
Dilated pancreatic duct
SMV
SMA
Splenic vein
Aorta

B

FIGURE 15-3 Tumors of the proximal body of the pancreas may infiltrate proximally into the pancreatic neck to involve the venous confluence. **A:** Coronal view and **(B)** axial view.

Technical Aspects

Superior Mesenteric Vein/Portal Vein Resection

In most cases, involvement of the SMV/PV confluence is evident from the findings of preoperative imaging studies. In some instances, venous involvement is evident by the surgeon's inability to create a retropancreatic tunnel over the SMV/PV. Even if a tunnel is created, however, there may still be vein involvement at the left lateral aspect of the SMV/PV that will not be apparent until the neck of the pancreas is transected. If tumor involvement of the splenic vein extending to or beyond the vein's confluence with the SMV/PV is present, a tangential or segmental resection of the involved portion of the SMV/PV is advised if a complete macroscopically negative resection is otherwise expected (Fig. 15-4A–C).

The remainder of the specimen is mobilized by dividing the lateral attachments of the spleen, the attachments of the body and/or tail of the pancreas, and any adjacent organs that may be involved. Such division may require the ligation of the inferior mesenteric vein if it inserts into the splenic vein. The specimen can then be elevated and retracted to the right to expose the SMA. The anterior and left lateral aspects of the SMA should be skeletonized and completely separated from the specimen. After this separation is complete, the specimen is entirely free except for the attachment at the vein.

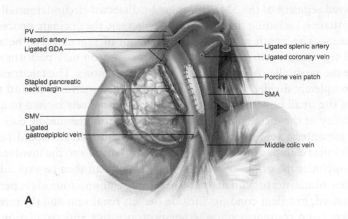

A

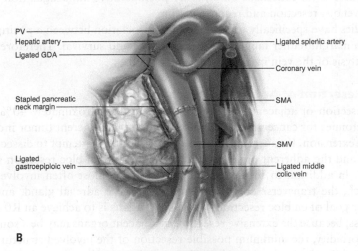

B

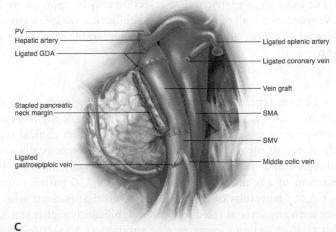

C

FIGURE 15-4 Reconstruction of the portal vein or superior mesenteric vein may be accomplished using a patch venoplasty **(A)**, primary end-to-end reconstruction **(B)**, or interposition graft **(C)**.

The involved segment of the SMV/PV must be dissected circumferentially from the surrounding tissues, including the head of the pancreas, the uncinate process, and the retroperitoneum. The length of the involved segment of vein can then be assessed. If the involved segment of vein is short (<3 cm), the surgeon may perform maneuvers to maximize the possibility of a primary venous anastomosis. The falciform ligament should be completely divided to free the liver from the anterior wall and the peritoneal lining of the small bowel mesentery should be transversely incised to allow more upward mobility of the distal end of the vein. In addition, the middle colic vein (and the inferior mesenteric vein, if it inserts directly into the SMV) should be ligated if necessary. Vascular clamps are placed proximally and distally to the involved segment, which often includes the origin of the SV; the segment can then be excised. Systemic heparin is then administered, and an end-to-end vascular anastomosis is performed. If a graft is required, excellent conduits include the left renal vein and the internal jugular vein. There is no consensus on whether postoperative anticoagulation is needed following venous resection and reconstruction.

No studies have specifically investigated the association between a positive venous transection margin (either tangential or segmental) and survival. Therefore, intraoperative analysis of the vein margins is not advocated.

En Bloc Resection of Adjacent Organs

En bloc resection of adjacent organs is performed in approximately 40% of distal pancreatectomies for cancer.[1,25] One should assume that adherent tumor indicates direct tumor extension. If adherent tumor is encountered, no attempt to dissect between the tumor and the adherent organ should be made, and en bloc resection should be performed. In addition to the spleen, adjacent organs most often involved include the stomach, the transverse colon (mesentery), the left adrenal gland, and the left kidney. The goal of en bloc resection of adjacent organs is to achieve an R0 resection. Nonetheless, because the extensive resection of adjacent organs may be a source of additional morbidity, the minimum possible resection of the involved structures should be performed. For example, a gastric wedge resection may be appropriate if tumor focally involves the posterior wall of the stomach. Similarly, a wedge or partial resection of involved adrenal gland or kidney, if feasible, is preferable to total adrenalectomy or nephrectomy.

Celiac Axis Resection

No fewer than 12 case reports and small series of CA resection at the time of distal pancreatectomy were published in 2013 alone. The size of the body of literature related to this procedure is disproportionately larger than its clinical relevance can possibly justify. A recent meta-analysis of 26 studies that specifically evaluated the role of arterial resection at pancreatectomy reported that only 366 of 2,479 patients underwent resection of any mesenteric artery and only 130 patients underwent resection of the CA.[28] The results of that study showed that patients who underwent pancreatectomy with any arterial resection had a significantly higher rate of operative mortality (odds ratio, 5.04) and lower rate of survival at 3 years (odds ratio, 0.39) than did patients who underwent standard pancreatectomy.

In general, two technical principles should be considered in planning and performing CA resection to achieve an R0 resection. First, there must be a plan for arterial perfusion of the liver following division of the CA. Because the division of the CA disrupts blood flow through the proper hepatic artery, the gastroduodenal artery must be preserved for adequate liver perfusion unless a replaced right hepatic artery is present. Second, aborting the resection should be seriously considered if the cancer involves both the SMV/PV and the CA, as combined arterial and venous invasion indicates biologically aggressive disease and combined vascular resection significantly increases the risks of hepatic insufficiency and perioperative mortality.[26,29]

REFERENCES

1. Shoup M, Conlon KC, Klimstra D, et al. Is extended resection for adenocarcinoma of the body or tail of the pancreas justified? *J Gastrointest Surg* 2003;7(8):946–952; discussion 952.
2. Mitchem JB, Hamilton N, Gao F, et al. Long-term results of resection of adenocarcinoma of the body and tail of the pancreas using radical antegrade modular pancreatosplenectomy procedure. *J Am Coll Surg* 2012;214(1):46–52.
3. Kooby DA, Hawkins WG, Schmidt CM, et al. A multicenter analysis of distal pancreatectomy for adenocarcinoma: is laparoscopic resection appropriate? *J Am Coll Surg* 2010;210(5):779–785, 786–787.
4. Strasberg SM, Linehan DC, Hawkins WG. Radical antegrade modular pancreatosplenectomy procedure for adenocarcinoma of the body and tail of the pancreas: ability to obtain negative tangential margins. *J Am Coll Surg* 2007;204(2):244–249.
5. Kang CM, Chung YE, Jung MJ, et al. Splenic vein thrombosis and pancreatic fistula after minimally invasive distal pancreatectomy. *Br J Surg* 2014;101(2):114–119.
6. Stamou KM, Toutouzas KG, Kekis PB, et al. Prospective study of the incidence and risk factors of postsplenectomy thrombosis of the portal, mesenteric, and splenic veins. *Arch Surg* 2006;141(7):663–669.
7. Chang YR, Han S-S, Park S-J, et al. Surgical outcome of pancreatic cancer using radical antegrade modular pancreatosplenectomy procedure. *World J Gastroenterol* 2012;18(39):5595–5600.
8. Latorre M, Ziparo V, Nigri G, et al. Standard retrograde pancreatosplenectomy versus radical antegrade modular pancreatosplenectomy for body and tail pancreatic adenocarcinoma. *Am Surg* 2013;79(11):1154–1158.
9. Park HJ, You DD, Choi DW, et al. Role of radical antegrade modular pancreatosplenectomy for adenocarcinoma of the body and tail of the pancreas. *World J Surg* 2014;38(1):186–193.
10. DiNorcia J, Ahmed L, Lee MK, et al. Better preservation of endocrine function after central versus distal pancreatectomy for mid-gland lesions. *Surgery* 2010;148(6):1247–1254; discussion 1254–1256.
11. Sun W, Leong CN, Zhang Z, et al. Proposing the lymphatic target volume for elective radiation therapy for pancreatic cancer: a pooled analysis of clinical evidence. *Radiat Oncol* 2010;5:28.
12. Franko J, Hugec V, Lopes TL, et al. Survival among pancreaticoduodenectomy patients treated for pancreatic head cancer <1 or 2 cm. *Ann Surg Oncol* 2013;20(2):357–361.
13. Hermanek P. Pathology and biology of pancreatic ductal adenocarcinoma. *Langenbecks Arch Surg* 1998;383(2):116–120.
14. Sahin TT, Fujii T, Kanda M, et al. Prognostic implications of lymph node metastases in carcinoma of the body and tail of the pancreas. *Pancreas* 2011;40(7):1029–1033.
15. Pavlidis TE, Pavlidis ET, Sakantamis AK. Current opinion on lymphadenectomy in pancreatic cancer surgery. *Hepatobiliary Pancreat Dis Int* 2011;10(1):21–25.
16. Deki H, Sato T. An anatomic study of the peripancreatic lymphatics. *Surg Radiol Anat* 1988;10(2):121–135.
17. Nagakawa T, Kobayashi H, Ueno K, et al. The pattern of lymph node involvement in carcinoma of the head of the pancreas. A histologic study of the surgical findings in patients undergoing extensive nodal dissections. *Int J Pancreatol* 1993;13(1):15–22.
18. Fujita T, Nakagohri T, Gotohda N, et al. Evaluation of the prognostic factors and significance of lymph node status in invasive ductal carcinoma of the body or tail of the pancreas. *Pancreas* 2010;39(1):e48–e54.
19. Farnell MB, Aranha GV, Nimura Y, et al. The role of extended lymphadenectomy for adenocarcinoma of the head of the pancreas: strength of the evidence. *J Gastrointest Surg* 2008;12(4):651–656.

20. Michalski CW, Kleeff J, Wente MN, et al. Systematic review and meta-analysis of standard and extended lymphadenectomy in pancreaticoduodenectomy for pancreatic cancer. *Br J Surg* 2007;94(3):265–273.

21. Edge SB, Byrd DR, Compton CC, et al, eds; American Joint Committee on Cancer. *AJCC Cancer Staging Manual*. 7th ed. New York, NY: Springer; 2010.

22. Rosso E, Langella S, Addeo P, et al. A safe technique for radical antegrade modular pancreato-splenectomy with venous resection for pancreatic cancer. *J Am Coll Surg* 2013;217(5):e35–e39.

23. Strasberg SM, Drebin JA, Linehan D. Radical antegrade modular pancreatosplenectomy. *Surgery* 2003;133(5):521–527.

24. Baumgartner JM, Krasinskas A, Daouadi M, et al. Distal pancreatectomy with en bloc celiac axis resection for locally advanced pancreatic adenocarcinoma following neoadjuvant therapy. *J Gastrointest Surg* 2012;16(6):1152–1159.

25. Christein JD, Kendrick ML, Iqbal CW, et al. Distal pancreatectomy for resectable adenocarcinoma of the body and tail of the pancreas. *J Gastrointest Surg* 2005;9(7):922–927.

26. Okada K, Kawai M, Tani M, et al. Surgical strategy for patients with pancreatic body/tail carcinoma: who should undergo distal pancreatectomy with en-bloc celiac axis resection? *Surgery* 2013;153(3):365–372.

27. Hirano S, Kondo S, Hara T, et al. Distal pancreatectomy with en bloc celiac axis resection for locally advanced pancreatic body cancer: long-term results. *Ann Surg* 2007;246(1):46–51.

28. Mollberg N, Rahbari NN, Koch M, et al. Arterial resection during pancreatectomy for pancreatic cancer: a systematic review and meta-analysis. *Ann Surg* 2011;254(6):882–893.

29. Nakao A, Takeda S, Inoue S, et al. Indications and techniques of extended resection for pancreatic cancer. *World J Surg* 2006;30(6):976-982; discussion 983–984.

Distal Pancreatectomy: Key Question 1

For patients with adenocarcinoma of the pancreatic body or tail, does radical antegrade modular pancreatosplenectomy (RAMPS) or standard distal pancreatectomy and splenectomy offer better overall survival?

INTRODUCTION

Historically, distal pancreatectomy for invasive ductal adenocarcinoma in the body and tail of the pancreas has been associated with poor lymph node retrieval, a high rate of positive margins, and dismal overall survival. In an early series from the Mayo Clinic of 26 patients undergoing standard distal pancreatectomy and splenectomy, the median overall survival duration was only 10 months, and the 5-year overall survival rate was only 8%.[1] A more recent study from the Mayo Clinic showed persistently poor outcomes, with 5-year overall survival of 9.6% after distal pancreatectomy and splenectomy, including resection of adjacent organs in 39% of the patients.[2]

Standard distal pancreatectomy and splenectomy is routinely performed in a left-to-right retrograde fashion and involves mobilization of the spleen and tail of the pancreas followed by vascular control and division of the pancreas. This approach has been suggested to result in an inadequate lymph node yield, poor visualization of the posterior dissection plane, and late vascular control. A novel approach to resecting adenocarcinoma in the body and tail of the pancreas, RAMPS, was introduced by Strasberg et al[3] in 2003. The primary goal of RAMPS is to maximize local control and overall survival following the resection of adenocarcinomas of the body or tail of the pancreas by optimizing lymphadenectomy and clearing the tumor to negative tangential margins. In contrast to standard distal pancreatectomy and splenectomy, RAMPS is performed in a right-to-left antegrade fashion and involves early parenchymal transection at the neck of the pancreas and control of the splenic vessels; dissection of the lymph nodes and perineural plexus around the celiac axis and superior mesenteric artery; and retroperitoneal dissection under direct visualization. Based on preoperative imaging findings, the posterior extent of resection can be adjusted to proceed anterior to the left adrenal gland and Gerota's fascia (anterior RAMPS) or posterior to the adrenal gland and Gerota's fascia (posterior RAMPS).

Single-institution retrospective series have reported that, compared with standard distal pancreatectomy, RAMPS is associated with higher rates of negative surgical margins and lymph node yield. However, whether RAMPS or standard distal pancreatectomy results in better local control and/or overall survival remains unknown.

METHODOLOGY

In January 2014, we performed an organized search of PubMed for articles published from January 1990 through January 2014. MeSH terms used for the search were "pancreatic cancer" and "pancreatectomy," and additional search terms were "distal pancreatectomy" and "antegrade modular pancreatosplenectomy"; the final PubMed query was "(("pancreatic neoplasms/surgery"[Majr]) AND "pancreatectomy"[Mesh] AND (distal pancreatectomy [text] OR radical antegrade modular pancreatosplenectomy [text])". Directed searches of the references embedded in the primary articles were also performed. The Grades of Recommendation, Assessment, Development, and Evaluation system was used to assign a grade to each article's level of evidence.[4]

Our initial search yielded 411 unique English language articles, whose abstracts and titles were reviewed by two reviewers. Of these 411 articles, 379 were excluded because they were case reports or were not about pancreatic adenocarcinoma. Of the remaining 32 articles, 12 were excluded because they focused on vascular resection and did not address the clinical question of interest. An additional 13 articles were excluded because they were review articles or because they focused on adjacent organ resection, included patients with metastatic disease, described the technique only, or had inadequate follow-up data (Fig. 15-5). The final 7 manuscripts were reviewed by both reviewers who assigned each article a grade of evidence (Table 15-1).

FINDINGS

Lymph Node Yield

Single-institution retrospective studies have reported that RAMPS yields median lymph node counts of 14 and higher, with a wide range of lymph node counts of between 1 and 60. In the two retrospective studies comparing RAMPS to standard distal pancreatectomy, RAMPS was associated with a significantly higher number of retrieved lymph nodes.[5,6] Although the early division of the neck of the pancreas in RAMPS affords better visualization and dissection of lymph nodes around the celiac axis and superior mesenteric artery, there is no direct evidence that removing these lymph nodes provides a survival benefit. It has been suggested that higher lymph node yield in surgery for pancreatic cancer is associated with improved survival[7]; an inadequate number of evaluated lymph nodes may result in understaging of the cancer or may represent a surrogate marker of poor surgical technique overall. However, other data suggest that patients with pancreatic body or tail tumors involving the lymph nodes along the celiac and superior mesenteric arteries have a dismal prognosis regardless of whether these nodes are removed and that increasing the extent of lymphadenectomy at the time of cancer resection does not improve survival.[8,9]

MARGIN STATUS

Adenocarcinomas in the body and tail of the pancreas frequently infiltrate the retroperitoneal tissues. In a standard distal pancreatectomy and splenectomy, this retroperitoneal plane is approached in a retrograde manner, with blunt dissection posterior to the spleen and pancreas and poor visualization of the retroperitoneal tissue planes.[10] Blunt division of the posterior tissue planes without visualization theoretically contributes to the high positive margin rate with standard distal pancreatectomy and splenectomy. In contrast, RAMPS proceeds in an antegrade manner, with sharp dissection of the retroperitoneal dissection plane under direct vision. The decision to perform anterior or posterior RAMPS is made preoperatively and is based on triphasic computed

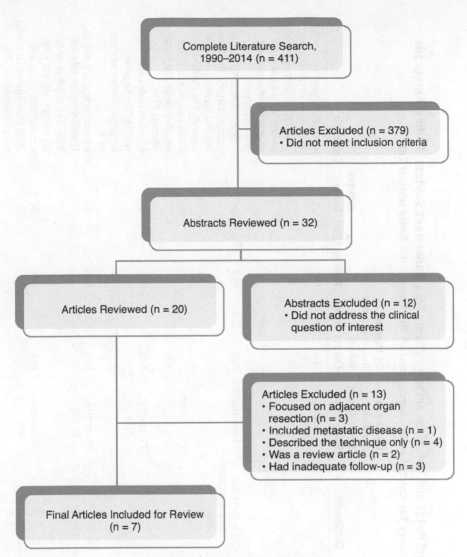

FIGURE 15-5 CONSORT diagram.

tomography findings. The dissection plane for anterior RAMPS is established by identifying the left adrenal vein and lifting the specimen off this vein until the surface of the left adrenal gland is exposed. In conventional distal pancreatectomy, this plane is difficult to dissect because there is no indicator of the left border of the adrenal gland. In posterior RAMPS, the left adrenal vein is divided, and dissection proceeds under direct visualization posterior to the adrenal gland and behind Gerota's fascia.

Retrospective studies have shown that RAMPS results in negative tangential margin rates of 75% to 95%. The rate of positive pancreatic neck margins among patients who undergo RAMPS is significant; Mitchem et al reported a rate of 8.5%.[11]

TABLE 15-1 Overall Survival Rates and Durations among Patients Who Underwent Subtotal Radical Antegrade Modular Pancreatosplenectomy for Ductal Adenocarcinoma of the Pancreatic Body and/or Tail

Author, Year	No. of Patients	Outcome(s)	OS Median Duration, 5-Year Rate in Study Group	OS Median Duration, 5-Year Rate in Control Group	Relative Effect	Evidence Grade	Comments
Shimada et al, 2006[8]	88 (including 12 undergoing Appleby procedure)	OS	22 months, 19%	N/A	N/A	2C	The negative margin rate was 75%. 61% of patients received routine IORT. Surgery included routine left adrenal gland resection and para-aortic node dissection.
Fernandez-Cruz et al, 2007[14]	13	OS, lymph node harvest, resection margin	14 months, N/A	N/A	N/A	2C	Ten patients underwent laparoscopic surgery. The SMA was not skeletonized in 10 patients. The mean node count was 14.5 ± 3. The negative tangential margin rate was 77%.
Strasberg et al, 2007[15]	23	OS	21 months, 26%	N/A	N/A	2C	The median node count was 15. The negative tangential margin rate was 91%.
Mitchem et al, 2012[11]	47	OS	26 months, 35.5%	N/A	N/A	2C	The mean node count was 18. The R0 resection rate was 81%. The negative tangential margin rate was 89%.
Chang et al, 2012[16]	24 (including 3 undergoing total pancreatectomy)	OS	18.2 months, N/A	N/A	N/A	2C	The mean node count was 20.9. The negative tangential margin rate was 91.7%.

Study	Patients			Outcomes		Level of Evidence	Results
Latorre et al, 2013[5]	8 RAMPS, 17 standard	14 months, 26%	17 months, 29%	OS, resection margin	N/A	2C	All patients in the RAMPS group underwent anterior RAMPS. The mean node counts in the RAMPS and standard surgery groups were 20.7 and 16.2, respectively. Both the RAMPS and standard groups had an R0 resection rate of 88%.
Park et al, 2014[6]	38 RAMPS, 54 standard	24.6 months, 40.1%	15.5 months, 12%	OS, lymph node harvest	Univariate HR, 2.201; 95% CI, 1.142–3.574	2C	Multivariate analysis revealed adjuvant chemoRT and resection margins, but not operative approach, to be predictors of OS. The median node counts in the RAMPS and standard groups were 14 and 9, respectively. The R0 resection rates in the RAMPS and standard groups were 89% and 85%, respectively.

CI, confidence interval; HR, hazard ratio; IORT, intraoperative radiation therapy; OS, overall survival; RAMPS, radical antegrade modular pancreatosplenectomy; RT, radiation therapy; SMA, superior mesenteric artery.

In patients undergoing standard distal pancreatectomy and splenectomy, microscopic positive margin rates as high as 62% have been published.[12] The margin clearance rates that different studies have reported for RAMPS and standard distal pancreatectomy are difficult to compare because the techniques used to evaluate and report the status of the margins are not standardized.[13] Furthermore, the two retrospective studies that have compared RAMPS to standard distal pancreatectomy found that operative approach did not affect rates of overall R0 resection.[5,6]

SURVIVAL

Survival data are limited to single-institution retrospective studies, and only two of these studies have compared the survival associated with RAMPS to that associated with standard distal pancreatectomy.[5,6] Park et al[6] compared survival outcomes in 38 and 54 patients who underwent RAMPS or standard distal pancreatectomy, respectively. Univariate but not multivariate analysis revealed that standard distal pancreatectomy was associated with worse overall survival; multivariate analysis showed that adjuvant chemoradiation and R0 resection were the sole independent predictors of survival. In this study, the fact that a higher proportion of patients undergoing RAMPS received adjuvant chemoradiation may have accounted for univariate analysis showing better survival associated with RAMPS. Latorre et al[5] reported overall survival rates for 8 patients who underwent RAMPS and 17 patients who underwent standard distal pancreatectomy that were similar to those reported by Park et al.[6] Although RAMPS was associated with a higher number of harvested lymph nodes and a higher rate of negative tangential margins, these factors did not result in improved overall survival.

CONCLUSION

Since its introduction, RAMPS has been embraced by many surgeons not only because of its theoretical oncologic benefits but also because of its emphasis on early vascular control and direct visualization of dissection planes. RAMPS is associated with a higher lymph node yield than standard distal pancreatectomy is. However, small, single-institution retrospective studies have not found this benefit to translate into an improvement in overall survival. A randomized controlled trial comparing RAMPS to standard distal pancreatectomy is not feasible because it would require the enrollment of more than 550 patients to detect a significant difference.[11]

In summary, available data do not support the routine use of RAMPS for adenocarcinomas in the head or neck of the pancreas.

REFERENCES

1. Dalton RR, Sarr MG, van Heerden JA, et al. Carcinoma of the body and tail of the pancreas: is curative resection justified? *Surgery* 1992;111:489–494.
2. Christein JD, Kendrick ML, Iqbal CW, et al. Distal pancreatectomy for resectable adenocarcinoma of the body and tail of the pancreas. *J Gastrointest Surg* 2005;9:922–927.
3. Strasberg SM, Drebin JA, Linehan D. Radical antegrade modular pancreatosplenectomy. *Surgery* 2003;133:521–527.
4. Atkins D, Best D, Briss PA, et al. Grading quality of evidence and strength of recommendations. *BMJ* 2004;328:1490.

5. Latorre M, Ziparo V, Nigri G, et al. Standard retrograde pancreatosplenectomy versus radical antegrade modular pancreatosplenectomy for body and tail pancreatic adenocarcinoma. *Am Surg* 2013;79:1154–1158.
6. Park HJ, You DD, Choi DW, et al. Role of radical antegrade modular pancreatosplenectomy for adenocarcinoma of the body and tail of the pancreas. *World J Surg* 2014;38:186–193.
7. Schwarz RE, Smith DD. Extent of lymph node retrieval and pancreatic cancer survival: information from a large US population database. *Ann Surg Oncol* 2006;13:1189–1200.
8. Shimada K, Sakamoto Y, Sano T, et al. Prognostic factors after distal pancreatectomy with extended lymphadenectomy for invasive pancreatic adenocarcinoma of the body and tail. *Surgery* 2006;139:288–295.
9. Hsu CC, Herman JM, Corsini MM, et al. Adjuvant chemoradiation for pancreatic adenocarcinoma: the Johns Hopkins Hospital–Mayo Clinic collaborative study. *Ann Surg Oncol* 2010;17:981–990.
10. Lowy AM, Leach SD, Philip PA. *Pancreatic Cancer.* New York: Springer Science + Business Media; 2008.
11. Mitchem JB, Hamilton N, Gao F, et al. Long-term results of resection of adenocarcinoma of the body and tail of the pancreas using radical antegrade modular pancreatosplenectomy procedure. *J Am Coll Surg* 2012;214:46–52.
12. Sasson AR, Hoffman JP, Ross EA, et al. En bloc resection for locally advanced cancer of the pancreas: is it worthwhile? *J Gastrointest Surg* 2002;6:147–157; discussion 57–58.
13. Katz MH, Merchant NB, Brower S, et al. Standardization of surgical and pathologic variables is needed in multicenter trials of adjuvant therapy for pancreatic cancer: results from the ACOSOG Z5031 trial. *Ann Surg Oncol* 2011;18:337–344.
14. Fernandez-Cruz L, Cosa R, Blanco L, et al. Curative laparoscopic resection for pancreatic neoplasms: a critical analysis from a single institution. *J Gastrointest Surg* 2007;11:1607–1621; discussion 21–22.
15. Strasberg SM, Linehan DC, Hawkins WG. Radical antegrade modular pancreatosplenectomy procedure for adenocarcinoma of the body and tail of the pancreas: ability to obtain negative tangential margins. *J Am Coll Surg* 2007;204:244–249.
16. Chang YR, Han SS, Park SJ, et al. Surgical outcome of pancreatic cancer using radical antegrade modular pancreatosplenectomy procedure. *World J Gastroenterol* 2012;18:5595–5600.

Distal Pancreatectomy: Key Question 2

Are the perioperative and oncologic outcomes associated with minimally invasive distal pancreatectomy for resectable adenocarcinoma of the pancreas equivalent to those associated with an open operation?

INTRODUCTION

The use of minimally invasive distal pancreatectomy (DP) has become increasingly common because it requires only moderate dissection and no formal reconstruction. Although minimally invasive DP has been found to be both feasible and safe generally, more than 90% of the cases described in the literature were performed for either benign or cystic disease, and few studies have assessed outcomes using the technique in the setting of pancreatic adenocarcinoma. Therefore, a careful and critical evaluation of the use of minimally invasive DP for patients with PDAC, for whom postoperative recovery is frequently complicated and cure is exceedingly rare, is warranted.

METHODOLOGY

The MEDLINE, Cochrane CENTRAL Register of Controlled Trials, EMBASE, and Ovid databases were searched to retrieve studies published between January 1990 and March 2013 that investigated the use of minimally invasive DP for adenocarcinoma. The MeSH search terms used included "laparoscopy," "pancreatectomy," and "pancreatic neoplasm." These terms and combinations of them, as well the terms "pancreas," "adenocarcinoma," "distal pancreatectomy," "robotic," and "minimally invasive surgery," were used in text word searches. The "related articles" function was utilized to broaden the search. The reference lists of selected articles were also examined to identify relevant studies not discovered during the database searches. Articles were selected for final review if they reported at least 10 cases of minimally invasive DP for pancreatic adenocarcinoma. Each reviewed article was given a final grade of recommendation using the Grades of Recommendation, Assessment, Development, and Evaluation system.

A flow chart illustrating the literature review is given in Figure 15-6. The initial search yielded 60 articles published between January 1990 and March 2013. Of these, 17 were excluded because they were not relevant based on a review of the title and abstract. Of the remaining 43 abstracts, 20 were excluded because they did not pertain to DP for resectable adenocarcinoma of the body or tail of the pancreas, and three were excluded because they were abstracts that were presented at meetings and yielded no subsequent manuscript. A total of 20 articles were reviewed in detail; of these, 14 were excluded because they did not meet the inclusion criteria after further review (two articles), reported on a duplicate patient cohort (one article), or reported on fewer than 10 patients with histologically proven adenocarcinoma (11 articles). Thus, only six studies were identified and reviewed in detail.[1-6]

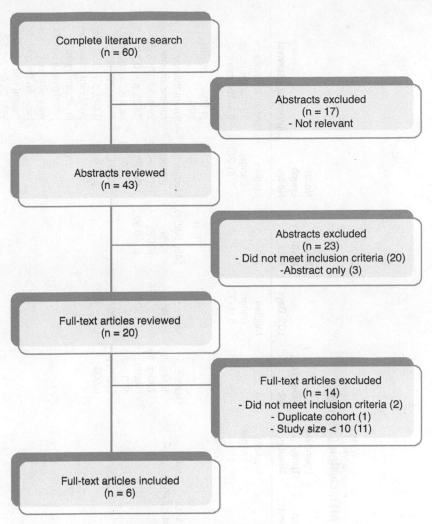

FIGURE 15-6 CONSORT diagram.

FINDINGS

The findings of the six studies reviewed in detail are summarized in Table 15-2. Of these six studies, five were single-center reviews, and one was a multicenter review. Only two of the studies specifically examined the use of minimally invasive DP in the setting of adenocarcinoma.[1,5] Both of these, one of which was the multicenter review, compared outcomes in adenocarcinoma patients undergoing minimally invasive DP or open DP. Of the other four studies, two included subgroup analyses of adenocarcinoma patients, and two combined data from patients with all histologic indications in their analyses. Thus, four studies provided specific data about the use of minimally invasive DP in the setting of adenocarcinoma.

TABLE 15-2   Six Studies Meeting All Inclusion Criteria

Author, Year	Procedure Type(s)	Grade	No. of Patients	Operative Time, Minutes	Blood Loss, mL	LOS, Days	Margin Positivity Rate	No. of Lymph Nodes	Recurrence/Survival
Marangos et al, 2012[4]	LDP	D	21	Median (range): 159 (73–313)	NA	Median (range): 5 (1–30)	7%	Median (range): 5 (0–26)	Median survival time, 19 months (range, 0.5–108 months); 3-year survival rate of PDAC patients, 30%.
Magge et al, 2013[5]	MIDP (adeno), ODP	C	28 (MIDP), 34 (ODP)	NA	Mean ± SEM: 290 ± 60 (MIDP), 570 ± 80 (ODP), p = 0.006	Mean ± SEM: 6 ± 2.75 (MIDP), 8 ± 3 (ODP), p = 0.03	14% (MIDP), 12% (ODP), p >0.99	Median (range): 11 (8–20) (MIDP), 12 (6–19) (ODP), p = 0.75	Adjuvant therapy completion rate, 89% (MIDP), 85% (ODP), p = 0.72; local recurrence rate, 7% (MIDP), 3% (ODP), p = 0.59. No significant differences in propensity-adjusted overall survival were observed between the cohorts (hazard ratio, 1.11; 95% CI, 0.47–2.62; p = 0.80).

Study		Groups	No. of Patients	Operative Time	EBL	Length of Stay	Complications		Survival
Song et al, 2011[3]	D	LDP (RAMPS)	24	Median (range): 225 (95–360)	NA	Median (range): 9.5 (5–22)	8%	Mean ± SEM: 10.3 ± 8.6	2-year overall survival rate, 85.2%.
Kooby et al, 2010[3]	B	LDP (adeno), ODP	23 (LDP), 189 (ODP)	Mean ± SD: 238.4 ± 68.1 (LDP), 230.4 ± 80.4 (ODP), p = 0.65	Mean ± SD: 422 ± 473 (LDP), 790 ± 828 (ODP), p = 0.04	Mean ± SD: 7.4 ± 3.4 (LDP), 10.7 ± 6.3 (ODP), p = 0.03	26% (LDP), 27% (ODP), p = 0.98	Mean ± SD: 13.8 ± 8.5 (LDP), 12.5 ± 8.4 (ODP), p = 0.47	Median follow-up time, 10 months; median survival time, 16 months for both LDP and ODP, p = 0.71. Resection method was not associated with survival.
Jayaraman et al, 2010[6]	D	LDP, ODP	17 (LDP), 236 (ODP)	Median: 193 (LDP), 164 (ODP), p <0.001	Median: 150 (LDP), 350 (ODP), p <0.001	Median: 5 (LDP), 7 (ODP), p <0.001	3% (LDP), 4% (ODP), p = 0.76	Median: 6 (LDP), 7 (ODP), p = 0.53	NA
Fernandez-Cruz et al, 2007[2]	D	LDP	13	Mean ± SD (range): 310 ± 20 (280–330)	Mean ± SD (range): 720 ± 450 (300–1300)	Mean (range): 8 (7–11)	13%	Mean ± SD (range): 14.5 ± 3 (6–20)	Median survival time, 14 months

Note: All studies were retrospective. The study by Kooby et al at involved multiple institutions.

Abbreviations: CI, confidence interval; LDP, laparoscopic distal pancreatectomy; LOS, length of stay; MIDP, minimally invasive distal pancreatectomy; NA, not applicable; ODP, open distal pancreatectomy; PDAC, pancreatic ductal adenocarcinoma; SD, standard deviation; SEM, standard error of the mean.

NB: Metrics provided may reflect those of the entire group studied, and do not necessarily reflect those of pancreatic cancer patients alone.

The mean number of pancreatic adenocarcinoma patients in the six studies was 21 (range, 13 to 28 patients). The studies' mean operative time for minimally invasive DP was 225 minutes (range, 159 to 310 minutes). The mean operative blood loss volume for minimally invasive DP was 430 mL (range, 150 to 1300 mL). The mean margin positivity rate of patients undergoing LDP was 11.8% (range, 3% to 26%). The mean and median numbers of lymph nodes harvested using minimally invasive DP ranged from 6 to 14.5.

Together, the six studies' findings suggest that minimally invasive DP is favorable to ODP in terms of perioperative aspects including operative time, blood loss, and length of hospital stay for a variety of diagnoses. The one study that compared minimally invasive DP and ODP for adenocarcinoma revealed no significant difference in operative time between the two approaches. Two studies showed that patients undergoing minimally invasive DP had significantly less blood loss than those undergoing ODP. Three studies reported that patients undergoing minimally invasive DP for all indications had an overall shorter length of hospital stay than those undergoing ODP, and two studies comparing outcomes in adenocarcinoma patients specifically reported that the length of hospital stay for patients undergoing minimally invasive DP was significantly shorter than that for patients undergoing ODP. In the one comparative study that evaluated it, adjuvant therapy completion rates of patients undergoing minimally invasive DP (89%) or ODP (85%) did not differ significantly.

The reviewed studies' findings suggest that short-term surrogate metrics of oncologic outcomes, including margin positivity rate and lymph node yield, do not differ between minimally invasive DP and ODP. Neither of the two studies that compared the margin positivity rates of patients undergoing ODP to those of patients undergoing minimally invasive DP revealed a significant difference between the groups. Furthermore, the two studies that compared the outcomes of patients who underwent minimally invasive DP or ODP for adenocarcinoma did not demonstrate a significant difference in the number of lymph nodes harvested between the minimally invasive DP and ODP groups.

Overall, the six studies provide some evidence suggesting that minimally invasive DP and ODP result in equivalent survival. Five studies reported at least some survival information for patients undergoing minimally invasive DP for adenocarcinoma. Two of these studies compared survival outcomes of patients undergoing minimally invasive DP to those of patients undergoing ODP. In one comparative study, which had a median follow-up time of 10 months, Kooby et al reported that patients undergoing minimally invasive DP or ODP both had a median overall survival duration of 16 months ($p = 0.71$). A multivariate analysis in this study that included all 212 patients undergoing minimally invasive DP or ODP revealed that resection method did not significantly affect survival. In the other comparative study, Magge et al found no difference in overall propensity score-adjusted survival between the minimally invasive DP and ODP cohorts (hazard ratio, 1.11; 95% confidence interval, 0.47 to 2.62; $p = 0.80$). In this study, the rates of local recurrence as the sole evidence of progression for patients undergoing minimally invasive DP (7%; 2 of 28 patients) and patients undergoing ODP (3%; 1 of 34 patients) did not differ significantly ($p = 0.59$).

Three studies described survival outcomes for only patients undergoing minimally invasive DP. Marangos et al reported that the median survival duration following minimally invasive DP for adenocarcinoma was 19 months (range, 0.5 to 108 months). In the study by Song et al, the 1- and 2-year overall survival rates were both 85.2%; three of the patients in the study developed distant and regional recurrences and died. Fernandez-Cruz et al reported a median survival time of 14 months. In this study, three patients developed distant and local recurrences and died within 1 year.

CONCLUSION

Although multiple centers have described their experiences with minimally invasive DP, there is only limited evidence regarding the oncologic results of this procedure in the setting of pancreatic adenocarcinoma. At best, minimally invasive DP is feasible in the setting of pancreatic adenocarcinoma and offers the typical benefits of a minimally invasive approach in terms of hospital stay and operative blood loss. However, the approach has no obvious advantage over ODP with regard to short-term surrogates of oncologic metrics, such as the number of lymph nodes harvested and margin positivity rate. Limited retrospective comparative data, at least those from studies with follow-up times of less than 1 year, indicate no difference in overall survival between patients undergoing minimally invasive DP or ODP. To date, the multicenter study by Kooby et al is the best example of the additional studies that compare minimally invasive DP and ODP and specifically assess medium- and long-term overall and recurrence-free survival that are needed before stronger conclusions about the use of minimally invasive DP or ODP in this population can be made. As surgeons' comfort and experience with minimally invasive DP increases, a formal randomized trial specifically assessing outcomes in adenocarcinoma patients following minimally invasive DP or ODP may become feasible.

Current evidence suggests distal pancreatectomy using a minimally invasive approach among patients with resectable adenocarcinoma of the body/tail of the pancreas is feasible, safe, and associated with favorable short-term perioperative outcomes and surrogates for oncologic outcomes.

REFERENCES

1. Kooby DA, Hawkins WG, Schmidt CM. A multicenter analysis of distal pancreatectomy for adenocarcinoma: is laparoscopic resection appropriate? *J Am Coll Surg* 2010;210(5):779–785, 786–787.
2. Fernandez-Cruz L, Cosa R, Blanco L, et al. Curative laparoscopic resection for pancreatic neoplasms: a critical analysis from a single institution. *J Gastrointest Surg* 2007;11(12):1607–1621; discussion 1621–1622.
3. Song KB, Kim SC, Park JB, et al. Single-center experience of laparoscopic left pancreatic resection in 359 consecutive patients: changing the surgical paradigm of left pancreatic resection. *Surg Endosc* 2011;25(10):3364–3372.
4. Marangos IP, Buanes T, Røsok BI, et al. Laparoscopic resection of exocrine carcinoma in central and distal pancreas results in a high rate of radical resections and long postoperative survival. *Surgery* 2012;151(5):717–723.
5. Magge D, Gooding W, Choudry H, et al. Comparative effectiveness of minimally invasive and open distal pancreatectomy for ductal adenocarcinoma. *JAMA Surg* 2013;148(6):525–531.
6. Jayaraman S, Gnonen M, Brennan M, et al. Laparoscopic distal pancreatectomy: evolution of a technique at a single institution. *J Am Coll Surg* 2010;211(4):503–509.

Over the decades of my career, resection for pancreatic cancer has evolved from an operation performed with high morbidity and mortality with few if any "cures" to an operation that is now performed commonly for benign, premalignant, low-grade malignant, and even locally advanced cancers with acceptable short-term results and even some optimism toward improving long-term survival. These latter improvements are due not so much to the technical advances in surgery but rather to better and more effective neoadjuvant and adjuvant therapies.

Much of this progress in surgical outcomes has been due to the centralization of this surgery in centers of excellence with surgeons and perioperative teams with significant experience. However, there are still many unresolved questions directly related to operative management of pancreatic cancer. Although single- or even multi-institutional randomized controlled trials or other published reports are available, important surgical decision making is still based on surgical preference or non–evidence-based literature. In this series of chapters, the authors have tackled a number of important questions related to the extent of operative staging, technique, and outcomes of both pancreaticoduodenectomy and distal pancreatectomy—with or without vascular resection—and even minimally invasive resection for pancreatic cancer. In each chapter, the authors have presented a series of recommendations, evaluated the available data (often using CONSORT techniques), and offered their recommendations, commenting on the strength of the evidence. The authors have both nicely illustrated the technical descriptions and provided a comprehensive list of the valuable literature used in their analysis. Thus, the end result is an excellent summary with solid recommendations that will be valuable to the practicing surgical oncologist or pancreatic surgeon.

The limitation of this, as in any similar publication, is the continued evolution and progress in many of these areas. Specifically, newer, more aggressive neoadjuvant techniques are changing the management of borderline resectable and locally advanced cancers.[1] Furthermore, the field of minimally invasive pancreatectomy continues to rapidly evolve with the largest series yet published of standard, laparoscopic, and robotic pancreaticoduodenectomy appearing in the recent literature,[2,3] providing further supporting evidence to the authors' recommendations. Certainly, these chapters will serve as a good foundation as new literature on such techniques is collected.

In conclusion, these excellent chapters define critical techniques in the surgical management of pancreatic cancer. Combined with the other very well written series of chapters on other cancers, this publication will set a high standard for defining the optimal techniques of surgical management for these important cancers. This series will be a valuable addition to the library of any surgeon who treats cancer in the current era of evidence-based medicine.

Keith D. Lillemoe, MD
Chief of Surgery
Massachusetts General Hospital
W. Gerald Austen Professor of Surgery
Harvard Medical School
Boston, Massachusetts

REFERENCES

1. Ferrone CR, Marchegiani G, Hong TS, et al. Radiological and surgical implications of neoadjuvant treatment with FOLFIRINOX for locally advanced and borderline resectable pancreatic cancer. *Ann Surg* 2015;261:12–17.
2. Zureikat AH, Moser AJ, Boone BA, et al. 250 robotic pancreatic resections: safety and feasibility. *Ann Surg* 2013;258:554–559.
3. Croome KP, Farnell MB, Que FG, et al. Total laparoscopic pancreaticoduodenectomy for pancreatic ductal adenocarcinoma: oncologic advantages over open approaches? *Ann Surg* 2014;260:633–640.

Operative Standards for Cancer Surgery provides a complete outline of the pre-operative staging and intraoperative management of patients with pancreatic cancer. This manual provides a foundation of knowledge which should accompany all surgeons in the outpatient clinic, the operating room, and perhaps most importantly, one's weekly multidisciplinary conference. An institution's multidisciplinary working group should achieve consensus on how patients are staged and optimal stage-specific management (on and off of a clinical trial). Institutional consensus on staging and stage-specific therapy is necessary to achieve the best possible patient outcome. Such consensus is not achieved without some controversy and oftentimes vigorous debate. *Operative Standards for Cancer Surgery* provides information necessary to appropriately frame the most common controversies in the management of patients with pancreatic cancer. As a further aid to the surgeon, I will comment on a few of those issues in the paragraphs below.

Two of the most frequently debated topics with regard to intraoperative management include the use of laparoscopy and the role for intraoperative evaluation of local tumor resectability. At our institution, we utilize staging laparoscopy as an extension of the "time out" procedure—performed at the time of planned definitive pancreatic resection. In general, laparoscopy is not performed as a separate staging procedure but is performed before the abdomen is opened for definitive resection in virtually all patients. Laparoscopy as an extension of the time out procedure allows abdominal exploration (laparoscopically) to be performed in all patients, allows the application of uniform staging to all patients by carefully evaluating the surface of the liver and all peritoneal surfaces, and clearly provides a level of abdominal exploration which would not occur if it was attempted after opening the abdomen (through, for example, a standard upper midline incision is usually employed). Historically, the use of laparoscopy was somewhat controversial, but that was largely in an era when laparoscopic equipment was not available in every operating room and therefore the debate over which patients should undergo laparoscopy was more compelling. In the current era of wide availability of laparoscopic equipment in virtually every operating room, simply placing a scope in the supraumbilical location prior to opening the abdomen, in all patients, is hard to argue with; such uniform staging is also critically important to the conduct of clinical trials. In contrast to laparoscopy, which evaluates the peritoneal cavity for subcentimeter peritoneal, mesenteric, and surface liver metastases (which are not well seen on preoperative imaging), the assessment of local tumor resectability is more accurately defined on preoperative imaging than intraoperative assessment. Prior to the advent of high-quality cross-sectional imaging with computed tomography or magnetic resonance imaging, surgeons would oftentimes evaluate local tumor resectability (with regard to tumors of the pancreatic head and uncinate process) by Kocherizing the duodenum and manually palpating the relationship of the tumor to the superior mesenteric artery (SMA). This is a grossly inaccurate method of assessing tumor–artery abutment or encasement. An equally inaccurate method of assessing a tumor vessel relationship is to develop the plane of dissection anterior to the SMV–portal vein confluence

268

and posterior to the pancreatic neck. If this plane was successfully developed, surgeons historically were reassured that (later in the operation) after pancreatic, gastric, and biliary transection, the tumor could be successfully separated from the SMV–portal vein confluence. The fallacy of this assumption was that tumors which were inseparable from the posterior or posterolateral aspect of the SMV or portal vein were not detected until the surgeon had already committed to resection. Contemporary cross-sectional imaging can alert the surgeon to the need for venous resection preoperatively, and the preoperative assessment of both arterial and venous abutment or encasement is a fundamental element of preoperative staging. In 2014, there is little role for intraoperative assessment of local tumor resectability; in the vast majority of patients, the surgeon should not be surprised by any aspect of local tumor anatomy, as this should have been apparent on preoperative evaluation. Again, the importance of a multidisciplinary conference in reviewing/re-reviewing such findings cannot be overstated.

The most important margin of resection during the removal of a pancreatic head or uncinate process cancer is the SMA margin. Although some may disagree, in the opinion of this reviewer, there is little excuse for not exposing the SMA at the time of pancreaticoduodenectomy. Complete exposure and visual identification of the SMA is critically important to prevent SMA injury, to individually ligate the origins of the inferior pancreaticoduodenal arterial (IPDA) branches, and to obtain an optimal oncologic margin of resection. Once the uncinate process is separated from the jejunal branch of the SMV, by dividing the small venous tributaries to the pancreas, the SMA should be identified along its anterior and right lateral borders (at the level of the uncinate process just proximal to the jejunal branch of the SMV, which typically courses posterior to the SMA). Identification of the SMA at that level is the single most important technical skill which trainees, who are learning this operation, should acquire. It is unlikely that the SMA will be inadvertently injured if it is identified and easily seen within the operative field. If there is an iatrogenic injury of the SMA and it is exposed and identified, it can be safely repaired. Further, postoperative hemorrhage, if it occurs within the first 24 hours of surgery, is virtually always due to inadequate control of the IPDAs. This can consistently be prevented by identifying the origin of the IPDAs arising from the SMA and securing them appropriately. Lastly, as systemic therapies for patients with pancreatic cancer improve, local disease control will become even more important. Removal of all tumors to include perineural extension at the level of the SMA is the most important element with respect to local disease control. All surgeons performing pancreaticoduodenectomy should be comfortable in exposing the SMA, ligating the origin of the IPDAs, and removing all soft tissue and autonomic neural tissue to the right and posterior to the SMA.

Controversy persists regarding whether or not to submit the hepatic duct transection margin and the pancreatic transection margin for frozen section analysis. It is our practice, when performing pancreaticoduodenectomy, to always send the hepatic duct and pancreatic transection margins (as en face sections of the margins) for frozen section evaluation. What we do with this information may

269

vary based on the complexity of the operation and the oncologic profile of the patient. In the vast majority of situations, we prefer to leave the operating room with no evidence of high-grade dysplasia or invasive cancer at either of these two margins. Obviously, if the patient has undergone an extensive high-risk operation associated with an unanticipated high level of blood loss or a lengthy operative time, it may not be appropriate to chase a suspected positive hepatic duct or pancreatic transection margin. Similarly, if one is in the very rare situation of having an incomplete gross resection of the primary tumor, considering re-resection of a microscopically positive hepatic or pancreatic transection margin may make little sense. However, if one is dealing with a favorable oncologic situation in an otherwise routine pancreaticoduodenectomy, we would re-resect either of these margins back to negative status. When performing distal pancreatectomy for tumors of the pancreatic body, the situation is even more complicated if a positive margin would require total pancreatectomy. Therein lies the rationale for a very detailed preoperative assessment to include a thorough discussion of this possibility with the patient and his or her family prior to operation. For relatively small tumors involving the pancreatic neck, it may be somewhat unclear as to whether the patient would be best served by an extended distal pancreatectomy or an extended Whipple procedure. In such situations, we would typically divide the pancreatic neck on the right (close to the pancreatic head) first and obtain a frozen section of that transection margin. If that margin should return negative, then either a middle segment pancreatectomy or a distal pancreatectomy would be the operation of choice. However, if that margin should return positive, then the patient would best be managed with an extended Whipple procedure. Again, an understanding of this possible intraoperative challenge prior to surgery and a thorough discussion with the patient is very important.

When managing large pancreatic body tumors with distal pancreatectomy, there is growing enthusiasm for the technique described as radical antegrade modular pancreaticosplenectomy (RAMPS). Another way to think of this operation is to review the steps involved with removal of a tumor in this location. While RAMPS emphasizes removal of all neural and soft tissue to the left of the SMA to ensure a negative margin at that location, there are other important elements involved in the removal of large tumors of the pancreatic body which may be in proximity to the celiac axis or SMA and associated with splenic vein occlusion resulting in sinistral portal hypertension. We typically begin such operations by entering the lesser sac and exposing the anterior surface of the SMV. We then completely take down the ligament of Treitz to prevent inadvertent injury of the proximal jejunum (at the ligament of Treitz) when incising the visceral peritoneum along the inferior border of the pancreas. Typically, one would enter or incise the base of the transverse colon mesentery just to the left of the middle colic vessels. In doing so, one can easily injure the proximal jejunum if the ligament of Treitz had not been taken down completely. We then widely open the lesser omentum and remove the nodal tissue anterior to the proximal common hepatic, left gastric, and splenic artery origins. The splenic artery is then encircled and ligated but not divided.

270

If access to the proximal splenic artery is viewed as impossible, one may consider preoperative splenic artery embolization. Once the splenic artery is ligated, we then take down the splenic flexure of the colon, mobilize the distal pancreas and spleen out of the left upper quadrant, and divide all of the short gastric vessels. At this point in the operation, we have now effectively eliminated all arterial inflow into the spleen. We then return to the midline and divide the pancreas anterior to the SMV–portal vein confluence, assuming that this represents an area of normal pancreas being to the right, or proximal to, the area of the primary tumor. The pancreas can be divided either with the stapling device, in which case we usually use a bioabsorbable staple line reinforcement (Gore-Tex or Seamguard pledgets), or with cautery or scalpel anticipating a suture closure. With the pancreas divided (and having ligated the splenic artery), one can then divide the splenic vein. Obviously, if the splenic vein was occluded by the tumor, division of the pancreas and the splenic vein could have occurred before mobilization of the distal pancreas and spleen to facilitate transection of the short gastric vessels. If the splenic vein is patent, then it is helpful to eliminate all arterial inflow into the spleen before the splenic vein is divided. Division of the splenic vein is made much easier by transection of the pancreas. With the pancreas divided, exposure of the junction of the splenic–SMV–portal veins is quite good and we usually divide the distal splenic vein with the endovascular stapler. With the splenic vein divided, exposure to the celiac bifurcation is greatly enhanced and the splenic artery can then be divided. Either before or after division of the splenic artery, the SMA is exposed posterior to the SMV. Similar to performing a pancreaticoduodenectomy, exposure of the SMA is critically important, prevents iatrogenic injury, and optimizes the oncologic margin as initially described in the RAMPS procedure. Frequently, the left gastric artery arises fairly proximal on the celiac artery and often courses cephalad to the pancreatic body tumor. Even in those cases where celiac resection is required, one can oftentimes remove the celiac artery distal to the origin of the left gastric artery, thereby preserving this artery. When performing a distal subtotal pancreatectomy, it is preferred, whenever possible, to preserve the left gastric artery; this preserves arterial inflow to the proximal stomach, which may prevent ischemic gastropathy and thereby preserve normal gastric emptying. In those patients who require celiac resection (Appleby procedure), preservation of the left gastric artery is important unless the celiac artery is revascularized.

I would like to congratulate the authors of *Operative Standards for Cancer Surgery* and hope that most of the procedures and recommendations will be put into practice by the many readers of this manual.

Douglas B. Evans, MD
Pancreatic Cancer Program
Department of Surgery
Medical College of Wisconsin
Milwaukee, Wisconsin

eas Synoptic Report

ative Staging

...rative Intent	Curative	Palliative	
...raoperative Staging			
Operative findings	List of noteworthy oncologic findings		
Intraoperative biopsies (if applicable)	List of extrapancreatic biopsy specimens and results of immediate histopathologic analysis		
Peritoneal cytology (if applicable)	Positive	Negative	
Final operative stage	Resectable	Locally advanced	Metastatic

Procedure Summary

Extent of Dissection and Lymphadenectomy

Plane of retroperitoneal dissection (for pancreatoduodenectomy)	Periadventitial dissection on SMA	Alternate plane of retroperitoneal dissection	
Plane of posterior dissection (for distal pancreatectomy)	Superficial to retroperitoneal fascia	Alternate plane of posterior dissection	
Site of pancreatic transection	Pancreatic neck	Alternate site of pancreatic transection	
Extent of lymphadenectomy	Standard (8a, 12a2, 12p2, 12b2, 12c, 13a, 13b, 17a, 17b, 14a, 14b for pancreatoduodenectomy; 10, 11, 18 for distal pancreatectomy)	Alternate extent of lymphadenectomy (list resected basins)	

Management of Vascular Involvement by Tumor

Portal vein	Anatomic extent of vessel involvement and precise description of surgical methods used for vascular resection and reconstruction		
Superior mesenteric vein	Anatomic extent of vessel involvement and precise description of surgical methods of vascular resection and reconstruction		
Superior mesenteric artery	Anatomic extent of vessel involvement and precise description of surgical methods of vascular resection and reconstruction		
Common hepatic artery	Anatomic extent of vessel involvement and precise description of surgical methods of vascular resection and reconstruction		
Celiac trunk	Anatomic extent of vessel involvement and precise description of surgical methods of vascular resection and reconstruction		

Intraoperative Margin Assessment

Pancreatic transection margin	Positive	Negative	Not evaluated/ applicable
Bile duct margin	Positive	Negative	Not evaluated/ applicable
Other "margin(s)" (describe)	Positive	Negative	
Final intraoperative assessment of radicality	R0	R1	R2

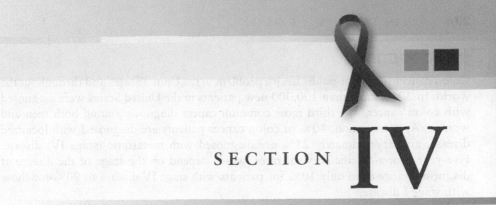

SECTION IV

COLON

INTRODUCTION

Colon cancer is a major public health problem in the United States and throughout the world. In 2013, more than 100,000 new patients in the United States were diagnosed with colon cancer,[1] the third most common cancer diagnosis among both men and women. At presentation, 40% of colon cancer patients are diagnosed with localized disease, and approximately 21% are diagnosed with metastatic (stage IV) disease. Five-year cancer-specific survival rates, which depend on the stage of the disease at diagnosis, range from only 10% for patients with stage IV disease to 90% for those with stage I disease.

Although the treatment of colon cancer patients is based on multidisciplinary principles, the primary and sometimes only necessary treatment for patients with localized disease is surgical resection. Preoperative evaluation of colon cancer patients includes a full colonoscopy; an assessment of the serum carcinoembryonic antigen level; and computed tomography of the chest, abdomen, and pelvis to characterize the extent of disease, identify the presence of distant metastases, and plan the definitive surgical resection. Although detailed description of the preoperative evaluation of colon cancer patients is beyond the scope of this document, it must be emphasized that colon cancers should be clinically staged before patients undergo elective surgical therapy. Patients with distant metastases and an asymptomatic primary tumor should be considered for primary systemic therapy. The preoperative workup should also include an assessment for synchronous cancers, as the risk for such cancers may be as high as 5% in the general population.[2]

Surgery for colon cancer includes a thorough exploration and en bloc removal of the involved segment of colon, all associated regional lymph nodes, and any involved adjacent structures. En bloc resection is the complete removal of the tumor, attached mesentery, and adherent tissues or organs as a whole. Colon cancer occurs at various sites (e.g., cecum, transverse colon, sigmoid colon), and the site of the disease determines the operation performed and has implications for reconstruction. However, the fundamental oncologic principles underlying the surgical treatment of colon cancer are the same regardless of the site of the disease. For a unique subset of patients with very early cancer arising within a polyp, endoluminal approaches, including standard polypectomy, and more advanced endoscopic mucosal resection may be adequate therapy. For patients who have tumors that are technically eligible for endoluminal treatment but have high-risk features, radical resection is indicated according to the same treatment principles of more advanced disease. In this section, therefore, we apply the discussion broadly to the oncologic surgical principles independent of the actual site of disease.

Recently, there has been renewed interest in the role of extended lymphadenectomy and standardized resection in the surgical treatment of colon cancer. Currently, the quality of surgical resection and pathologic evaluation, as determined by the number of lymph nodes assessed or the completeness of the mesenteric excision at surgery, varies significantly. Such variations in surgical technique result in disparate survival outcomes, and this highlights the importance of establishing and adhering to the surgical principles for colon cancer surgery.[3–5] Some authors have recently promoted the concept of complete mesocolic excision as one approach to surgical standardization.[6,7] Complete mesocolic excision is often described in conjunction with central vascular ligation, which shares many principles with the Japanese Society for Colorectal Cancer's approach to extended D3 lymph node dissection.[8] One important benefit of discussing these and other approaches to standardized surgery for colon cancer, independent of their potential effects on outcomes, has been a renewed interest in the oncologic principles underlying colon cancer surgery and the promotion of a common terminology for discussing these techniques.

Finally, the management of colon cancer patients who have metastatic disease continues to evolve. Advances in systemic therapy are increasing the potential for the curative treatment of selected patients with metastases to distant sites such as the liver, lung, or extraregional lymph nodes. One major question that remains is whether curative resection should be synchronous or staged, and we explore this question in greater detail in this section. Another area of recent interest is the methodology used for sentinel lymph node mapping to optimize lymph node staging by identifying aberrant nodal involvement. Although investigations of novel localizing agents and techniques continue to generate interest, this technique has no established role in colon cancer, and thus a more detailed discussion is not included here.

In this section, we provide a focused discussion of five critical oncologic elements of colon cancer surgery. Additionally, we address in detail two key questions guiding the standardized intraoperative management of colon cancer. We also identify the key components that must be included in a synoptic operative report.

REFERENCES

1. Siegel R, Ma J, Zou Z, et al. Cancer statistics. *CA Cancer J Clin* 2014;64:9–29.
2. Barillari P, Ramacciato G, De Angelis R, et al. Effect of preoperative colonoscopy on the incidence of synchronous and metachronous neoplasms. *Acta Chir Scand* 1990;156:163–166.
3. Hermanek P Jr, Wiebelt H, Riedl S, et al. Long-term results of surgical therapy of colon cancer. Results of the Colorectal Cancer Study Group [article in German]. *Chirurg* 1994;65:287–297.
4. West NP, Morris EJ, Rotimi O, et al. Pathology grading of colon cancer surgical resection and its association with survival: a retrospective observational study. *Lancet Oncol* 2008;9:857–865.
5. Bilimoria KY, Bentrem DJ, Stewart AK, et al. Lymph node evaluation as a colon cancer quality measure: a national hospital report card. *J Natl Cancer Inst* 2008;100:1310–1317.
6. Hohenberger W, Weber K, Matzel K, et al. Standardized surgery for colonic cancer: complete mesocolic excision and central ligation–technical notes and outcome. *Colorectal Dis* 2009;11: 354–364; discussion 364–365.
7. West NP, Hohenberger W, Weber K, et al. Complete mesocolic excision with central vascular ligation produces an oncologically superior specimen compared with standard surgery for carcinoma of the colon. *J Clin Oncol* 2010;28:272–278.
8. West NP, Kobayashi H, Takahashi K, et al. Understanding optimal colonic cancer surgery: comparison of Japanese D3 resection and European complete mesocolic excision with central vascular ligation. *J Clin Oncol* 2012;30:1763–1769.

Colon Resection

CRITICAL ELEMENTS

- Abdominal Exploration
- Extent of Bowel Mobilization and Resection
- Proximal Vascular Ligation and Regional Lymphadenectomy
- Multivisceral Resection
- Removal of Lymphadenopathy Beyond the Primary Distribution

1. ABDOMINAL EXPLORATION

Recommendation: A thorough exploration of the peritoneal cavity should be performed at the time of surgery, and the findings of this exploration should be recorded in the operative report.

Type of Data: Retrospective observational studies and expert consensus.

Strength of Recommendation: Strong.

Rationale

The operative management of colon cancer should begin with a thorough exploration of the abdominal cavity.[1,2] The rationale for this exploration is unassailable; appropriate treatment requires accurate staging, and unexpected findings may warrant a change in the surgical approach. Some patients' surgeries will yield unanticipated findings regardless of the type and quality of preoperative imaging performed, an eventuality supported by previous studies. For example, one study reported that the sensitivity of preoperative computed tomography (CT), magnetic resonance imaging,[3] and fluorodeoxyglucose positron emission tomography for the detection of liver metastases ranges from 74% to 81% on a per lesion basis, suggesting that a significant number of metastatic lesions may be below the limit of identification and go undetected prior to surgery.[4] Another study found that although preoperative CT could detect liver metastases in 99% of patients,

276

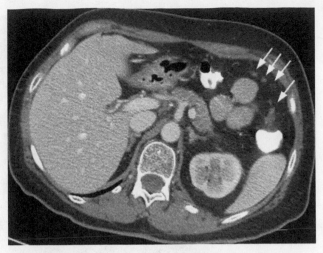

FIGURE 16-1   CT scan showing carcinomatosis (*arrows*).

it could detect locally advanced lesions in 86% of patients and peritoneal carcinomatosis in only 33% of patients[5] (Fig. 16-1). Few studies have specifically investigated the potential impact of abdominal exploration on survival or the frequency with which findings from such an exploration alter planned treatment in the era of modern preoperative staging. Given the importance that a complete evaluation has for both treatment and prognosis, however, we support existing guidelines advocating this approach.

A thorough abdominal exploration should be performed regardless of whether a minimally invasive or open operative approach is used. To the extent possible without subjecting the patient to additional risk, the surgeon should examine the liver, peritoneal surfaces, omentum, mesentery, regional and extraregional (e.g., periaortic or periportal) lymph nodes, retroperitoneum, and adnexa (if present) and document the findings of this examination (Figs. 16-2 to 16-4). The surgeon should also evaluate

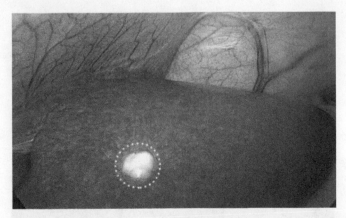

FIGURE 16-2   Intraoperative image of occult hepatic metastasis (marked by *circle*).

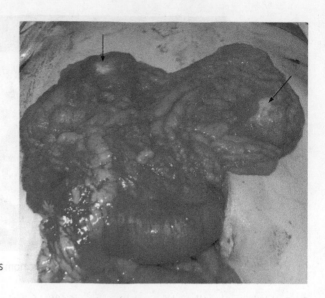

FIGURE 16-3 Carcinomatosis with omental implants (*arrows*).

primary tumor site for the presence or absence of full-thickness extension through the bowel wall and the presence of a confirmatory tattoo, if applicable (Fig. 16-5). The surgeon should also note the presence of ascites or other coexisting pathology. If it has not been completely evaluated preoperatively, the proximal colon should be examined for the presence of a synchronous cancer. The identification of unsuspected carcinomatosis during initial exploration indicates the presence of systemic disease. In an otherwise asymptomatic patient, primary tumor resection in this setting is contraindicated and the early initiation of systemic therapy should be considered. If the peritoneal disease is limited and favorable tumor biology has been demonstrated by the tumor's response to systemic therapy, subsequent resection with cytoreduction may be considered in the context of multidisciplinary treatment.

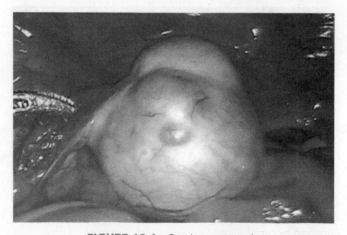

FIGURE 16-4 Ovarian metastasis.

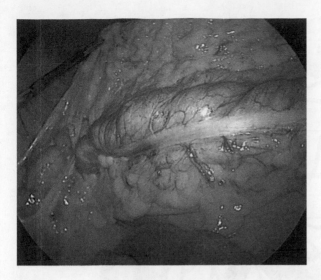

FIGURE 16-5 Tumor localized by tattoo marking.

2. EXTENT OF BOWEL MOBILIZATION AND RESECTION

Recommendation: The length of colon to be resected is determined by the primary tumor's location with respect to the colon's associated arterial supply.

Type of Data: Retrospective observational studies and expert consensus.

Strength of Recommendation: Moderate.

Rationale

The lymphatics parallel the arterial supply (Fig. 16-6). The lymphatic drainage of the right colon and proximal transverse colon courses along the branches of the superior mesenteric artery. The lymphatics of the distal transverse colon, descending colon, and sigmoid colon segments drain along the course of the inferior mesenteric artery. Lymphatic drainage is often continuous, first from the pericolonic lymph nodes, then to the intermediate lymph nodes along the right colic artery, middle colic artery, left colic artery, and sigmoid arteries and then to the central nodes at the origin of the superior or inferior mesenteric artery. In general, the extent of bowel mobilization is dictated by the colonic blood supply and whether mesenteric resection will be adequate to provide an appropriate assessment of the associated lymph nodes. The resection of carcinoma located between two drainage areas should include both lymphatic drainage pathways, which may require that a longer segment of colon be removed (Fig. 16-7A–F).

The surgical margin generally accepted to result in an R0 resection for colon cancer is 5 cm. In most circumstances, however, the margin will be greater depending on the arterial supply to the involved colon segment, emphasizing the importance of the blood supply and its impact on the lymphatic drainage rather than simple length of the colon. The surgical margin is particularly important in patients with locally advanced

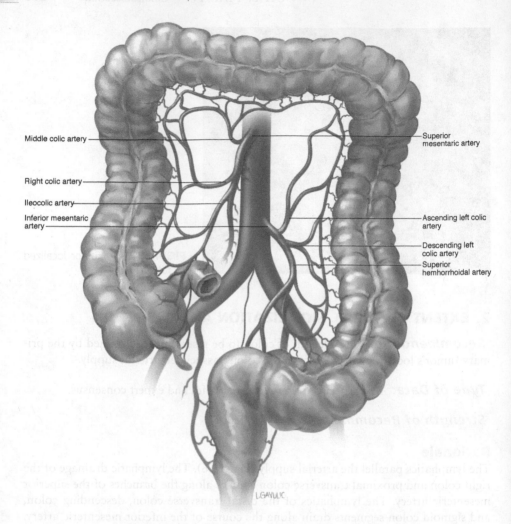

Middle colic artery

Right colic artery

Ileocolic artery

Inferior mesentaric artery

Superior mesentaric artery

Ascending left colic artery

Descending left colic artery

Superior hemhorrhoidal artery

L.GAVULIC

FIGURE 16-6   Illustration of the arterial anatomy of the colon.

lesions (T3 or T4 disease). Whereas stage I and II cancers have low recurrence rates, stage III cancers have a high risk of recurrence even if the resection margins are at least 5 cm.[6] An oncologic advantage of extended resection (e.g., resection of the terminal ileum during right colectomy or subtotal colectomy for a single tumor in the absence of underlying risk) has not been shown.

Extended resection may be indicated in certain clinical situations. For example, patients who present with synchronous cancers may be treated with two separate resections based on arterial supply (e.g., right colectomy and anterior resection for synchronous tumors of the cecum and sigmoid colon) or with a single resection that incorporates both tumors (e.g., subtotal colectomy for synchronous tumors of the hepatic flexure and descending colon).[2] A subtotal colectomy may be indicated in

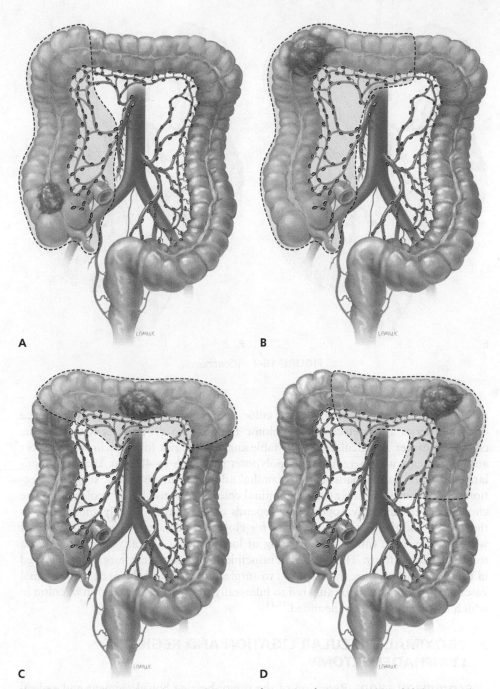

FIGURE 16-7 Illustrations showing the extent of resection for tumors within **(A)** the ascending colon, **(B)** the hepatic flexure, **(C)** the transverse colon, **(D)** the splenic flexure, **(E)** the descending colon, and **(F)** the sigmoid colon.

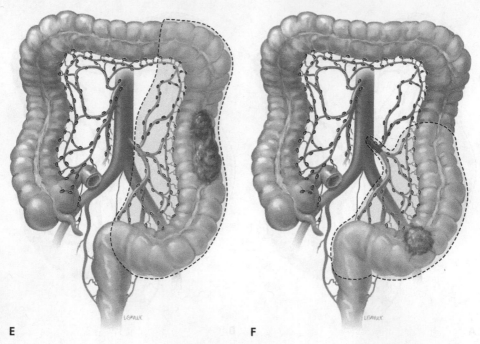

E   F

FIGURE 16-7   *(Continued).*

patients with hereditary nonpolyposis colon cancer, as they have a higher incidence of synchronous and metachronous colonic tumors than do patients with sporadic colorectal cancer. As calculated by life table analysis, the risk for metachronous cancer among patients with hereditary nonpolyposis is as high as 40% at 10 years. Similarly, for colon cancer patients with familial adenomatous polyposis, surgical resection should consist of either total abdominal colectomy or total proctocolectomy. The choice between these two operations depends on the burden of polypoid disease in the rectum and the patient's preference for close surveillance.[7,8,9] Finally, individuals who develop colon cancer in the setting of long-standing ulcerative colitis require a total proctocolectomy. The oncologic principles of colon cancer surgery as outlined in this chapter, including the attention to surgical margins and the need for proximal vascular ligation, should be adhered to bilaterally, not just for the portion of colon in which the tumor has been identified.[10,11]

3. PROXIMAL VASCULAR LIGATION AND REGIONAL LYMPHADENECTOMY

Recommendation: Resection of the tumor-bearing bowel segment and radical lymphadenectomy should be performed en bloc with proximal vascular ligation at the origin of the primary feeding vessel(s).

Type of Data: Prospective and retrospective observational studies.

Strength of Recommendation: Moderate.

Rationale

The standard of practice for the treatment of stage I to III (nonmetastatic) colon cancer is complete margin-negative resection (R0 resection) of the tumor-bearing bowel combined with en bloc resection of the intact node-bearing mesentery (i.e., regional lymphadenectomy). Regional lymphadenectomy is guided by the anatomy of the regional blood supply to the tumor-bearing bowel segment. Complete standard lymphadenectomy is facilitated by the proximal ligation of the relevant vascular pedicle of the tumor-bearing bowel segment. The pedicles that may be ligated on the basis of tumor location include the ileocolic (Fig. 16-8A–E), right colic (Fig. 16-9A,B), middle colic

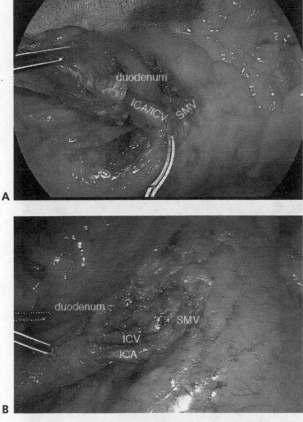

FIGURE 16-8 A–E: Intraoperative images of ileocolic vessel dissection and ligation. ICA, ileocolic artery; ICV, ileocolic vein; SMV, superior mesenteric vein.

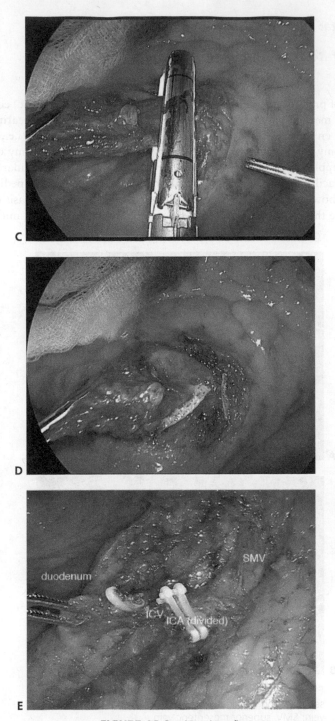

FIGURE 16-8 *(Continued).*

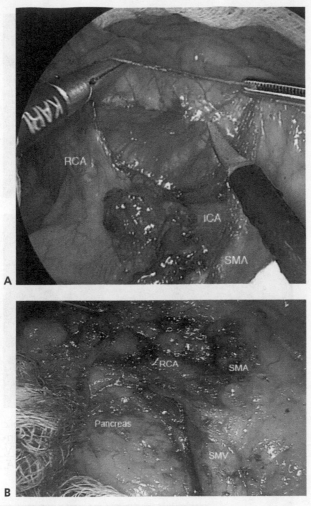

FIGURE 16-9   A,B: Intraoperative images of right colic artery dissection. ICA, ileocolic artery; RCA, right colic artery; SMA, superior mesenteric artery; SMV, superior mesenteric vein.

(Fig. 16-10A,B), left colic (Fig. 16-11), inferior mesenteric (Fig. 16-12A,B), and superior hemorrhoidal arteries and associated veins (Fig. 16-12C), which are identified centrally at the root of the colonic mesentery. Thus, the vascular anatomy of the tumor-bearing colon segment should be clearly identified, with attention to the potential anatomic variations that are commonly encountered. After the vascular ligation has been completed, the integrity of the blood supply to the remaining bowel should be carefully assessed by direct inspection of the bowel wall for adequate perfusion, visualization of pulsatile blood flow within the terminal vessels, or Doppler interrogation of the arterial supply. Although the marginal artery provides a collateral network between the primary vascular supplies, the artery may have congenital and/or acquired variations in its integrity and is subject to injury during colon mobilization.

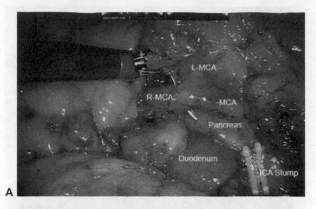

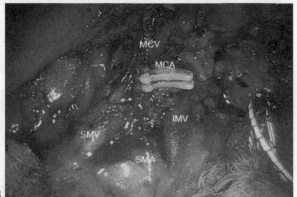

FIGURE 16-10   A,B: Intraoperative images of middle colic vessel dissection and ligation. ICA, ileocolic artery; IMV, inferior mesenteric vein; L-MCA, left middle colic artery; MCV, middle colic vein; R-MCA, right middle colic artery; SMA, superior mesenteric artery; SMV, superior mesenteric vein.

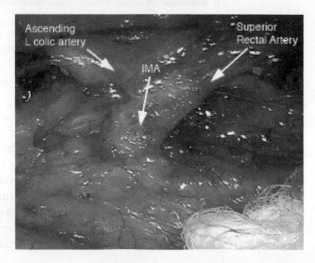

FIGURE 16-11 Intraoperative image showing the IMA giving rise to the left colic and superior rectal arteries. IMA, inferior mesenteric artery.

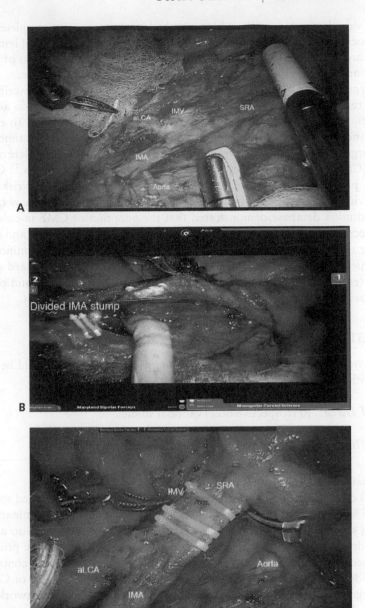

FIGURE 16-12 **A:** The inferior mesenteric artery and its branches. **B:** High ligation of the inferior mesenteric artery above left colic. **C:** Low ligation of the inferior mesenteric artery below left colic. Note complete lymphadenectomy in all cases. IMA, inferior mesenteric artery; IMV, inferior mesenteric vein; aLCA, ascending left colic artery; SRA, superior rectal artery.

Proximal vascular ligation with en bloc lymphadenectomy ensures complete resection of the associated lymph nodes for pathologic evaluation. The number of lymph nodes resected surgically and evaluated pathologically reflects the completeness of lymphadenectomy and is an indicator of surgical quality and oncologic outcome.

The term "complete mesocolic excision" (CME) has been used to describe en bloc complete resection along embryologic planes of the tumor-bearing colon and associated mesentery with its investing envelope intact and without defects. To ensure the integrity and completeness of the bowel and lymphatic excision at the time of colon cancer surgery, some groups have emphasized the practice of complete mesocolic excision (CME) and central ligation of the arteries and draining veins.[12] Observing the CME principles during resection has been associated with lower risks of margin positivity and iatrogenic tumor perforation. One retrospective review of a large, single-institution database demonstrated that the adoption of CME in colon cancer surgery decreased the 5-year local recurrence rate from 6.5% to 3.6% and improved the 5-year overall survival rate from 82.1% to 89.1%.[13] The new terminology that accompanies the adoption of CME highlights the principles of standard oncologic resection (en bloc complete resection of the associated lymph nodes) and provides a standardized method for operative technique and pathologic evaluation.

4. MULTIVISCERAL RESECTION

Recommendation: Involved adjacent organs and structures should be removed en bloc with the primary tumor.

Type of Data: Retrospective observational studies.

Strength of Recommendation: Strong.

Rationale

Colorectal cancer involving adjacent structures (T4b disease) is reported to occur in 5% to 15% of patients[3,14] and is often appreciated by history, examination, and/or staging studies (Fig. 16-13). En bloc resection of the primary tumor, associated lymph node basin, and involved adjacent structures is a key oncologic principle for colon cancer surgery and a key factor in maintaining local disease control. Consensus guidelines, National Cancer Institute (NCI), American Society of Colon and Rectal Surgeons (ASCRS), and the National Comprehensive Cancer Network (NCCN Guidelines 2014) recommend en bloc multivisceral resection of locally advanced disease when there is acceptable morbidity and curative potential.[3,15]

En bloc resection requires removal of the tumor-bearing segment of bowel and attached structures as a single unit. The dissection of a tumor off the bladder followed later by the removal of the portion of bladder to which the tumor was attached is not an en bloc resection. Similarly, the removal of the surgical specimen and subsequent, separate removal of the lymph node–bearing mesentery associated with the tumor-bearing segment is not an en bloc resection.

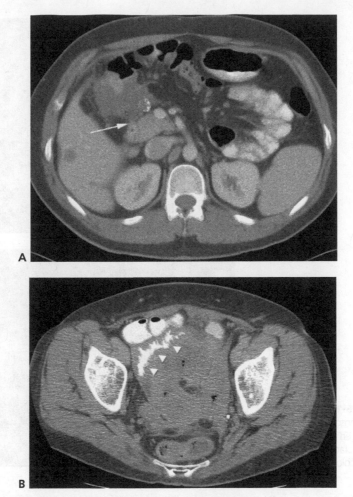

FIGURE 16-13 CT scan demonstrates **(A)** duodenal involvement (*arrow*) by a tumor of the hepatic flexure and **(B)** bladder and small bowel involvement (*arrowheads*) by a locally advanced tumor of the sigmoid colon.

At the time of surgical exploration, adherence of the tumor-bearing colon segment to adjacent structures may be due to inflammatory adhesions or to malignant invasion (Fig. 16-14A,B). Intraoperative assessment can be unreliable for distinguishing between an inflammatory or malignant adhesion; false positive rates range from 30% to 50%.[16,17] Attempting to separate planes risks incomplete oncologic resection. Therefore, gross adherence of tumor requires en bloc resection (Fig. 16-15). Determining whether a colon cancer involving adjacent organs is resectable requires a clear understanding of the anatomic boundaries required to attain negative margins, the potential for injury to adjacent structures, and the overall morbidity of the required procedure. Omitting any one of these in considering whether complete resection is a prudent

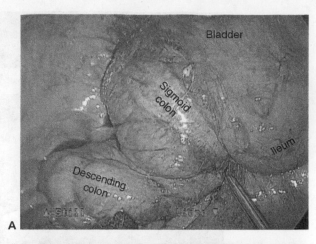

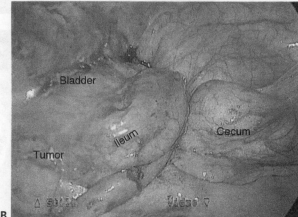

FIGURE 16-14 A,B: Intra-operative photograph of a locally advanced sigmoid colon cancer with bladder, ileum, and descending colon involvement.

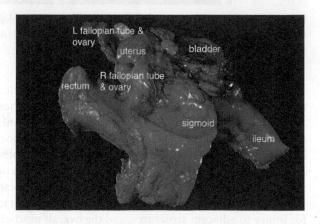

FIGURE 16-15 En bloc multi-visceral resection specimen including the sigmoid colon, rectum, terminal ileum, uterus, fallopian tubes and ovaries, and bladder.

option may result in unacceptably high morbidity. If the extent of resectability cannot be fully assessed, or if the patient and/or operative team are not adequately prepared for the extent of resection (e.g., if there is a need for multidisciplinary surgical support), the surgeon should consider performing a temporizing diversion or bypass. This should be followed by careful radiographic staging and operative planning for later definitive resection.

En bloc resection that includes structures in which removal would result in low morbidity—the small bowel, ovary, or abdominal wall, for example—should be performed in almost all situations. Major resections likely to result in high morbidity, such as pelvic exenteration, nephrectomy, pancreaticoduodenectomy, or major nerve or vascular resection, should be preceded by careful surgical preparation and preoperative patient counseling. Multivisceral resection of advanced-stage colon cancer poses many challenges to the operating surgeon and may be associated with significant morbidity. There are situations in which aggressive multivisceral en bloc resection provides the only chance for cure. Unfortunately, there are situations in which the surgery would be futile or result in unacceptably high morbidity; thus, the decision to proceed with resection should be based on a thorough preoperative evaluation and a discussion with the patient and the patient's multidisciplinary care team. Proper planning includes review of imaging to determine the plan for both resection and reconstruction and assessment of patient's functional status.

Morbidity rates following multivisceral resection range from 25% to 40% with 30-day mortality rates ranging from 4% to 9%.[3,14,18] However, these data from single-institution reports reflect careful patient selection and treatment by experienced surgeons with coordinated multidisciplinary teams and recovery units. Thus, the patient's comorbid factors and the surgeon's experience should be considered in the management of these complex tumors. The need for thorough preoperative planning to reduce morbidity, including contingency plans, cannot be overemphasized.[19] A more detailed description of some specific situations of adjacent organ involvement is outlined in the sections below.

Duodenum and pancreas. Locally advanced cancer in the right colon may extend directly into the duodenum or pancreatic head or neck. The resection of such cancer may entail en bloc pancreaticoduodenectomy or partial duodenectomy. Fortunately, only a very small proportion of locally advanced T4 colon cancers involve the pancreas (1.7% to 8%) or duodenum (0.8% to 4%). Direct tumor infiltration (pT4b disease) of the duodenum or pancreatic head suspected on the basis of tumor adhesion is pathologically confirmed in 20% to 78% of patients, which demonstrates the variability in the presentation of such tumors and the difficulty in clinically assessing whether pathologic invasion is present.[3] Depending on the series, the risk for surgical morbidity is approximately 25% and that for surgical mortality is as high as 20%. In the setting of perforation or abscess, the surgical mortality rate is particularly high. Other adverse prognostic factors include nodal and distant metastasis; in the presence of such metastasis, the rate of early recurrence approaches 50% at a median time of 15 months. Regardless of the limited published evidence guiding surgery for colon cancer invading the duodenum and/or pancreas, the fundamental principles of oncologic resection should be maintained. The tumor should never be dissected off the duodenal wall or pancreas. In healthy, well-selected patients, partial duodenal wall resection can be performed by a surgeon who has the necessary skills and experience. Pancreaticoduodenectomy can be offered only if the need for it is recognized preoperatively, but the surgery should be preceded by proper counseling and multidisciplinary discussion that includes the consideration of neoadjuvant therapy. For symptomatic high-risk scenarios, temporizing adjuncts include gastrostomy, feeding jejunostomy, and ileostomy or gastrojejunostomy bypass.

Ureters and bladder. En bloc R0 resection is often appropriate for tumors invading urologic structures in the pelvis. The bladder is the most commonly involved organ among patients with colorectal cancer, resected in 53% of cases in a large systematic literature review.[18] In a recent series in which only bladder involvement was treated with limited bladder wall resection, malignant adhesions increased the risk of local recurrence at the bladder tenfold.[20] Thus, the importance of wide, complete, and en bloc resection should be emphasized. However, following composite resection of the urinary tract for colon cancer, up to one in four patients will have urologic complications and that many of these patients (27%) will ultimately require surgical correction.[21] Thus, a multidisciplinary approach to management of patients with colon cancer involving the urologic tract should be considered.

Uterus and ovaries. Female pelvic organs may be involved in both right- and left-sided colonic malignancies. Colon cancer involvement of the ovaries can occur via direct extension, peritoneal dissemination, or hematogenous spread. Approximately 20% of multivisceral resections for colon cancer are associated with ovarian involvement.[18] The uterus and vagina may also become involved, although this is more commonly an issue in the setting of rectal cancer rather than colon cancer. Oophorectomy is advocated if there is clinical suspicion of ovarian involvement in the absence of disseminated peritoneal metastasis. Direct extension of the tumor into any female pelvic organs can be resected en bloc with curative intent and minimal morbidity.

The role of prophylactic oophorectomy in patients undergoing surgery for colorectal cancer has been a subject of some interest. The surgery can be performed with minimal morbidity, particularly among postmenopausal women. A survival benefit with prophylactic oophorectomy in patients with sporadic colorectal cancer has not been demonstrated.[22-25] Prophylactic oophorectomy should be considered and the indications preoperatively discussed for colon cancer patients who have hereditary nonpolyposis colorectal cancer syndrome, as these patients are at risk for both occult synchronous and subsequent metachronous ovarian malignancy.[26,27] Prophylactic oophorectomy not only reduces the risk for ovarian cancer but has also been shown to be cost-effective.[28]

Abdominal wall and diaphragm. Abdominal wall invasion should be resected en bloc with negative margins. Preoperative planning for colorectal cancers invading the abdominal wall and/or diaphragm should include consultation with a reconstructive surgery team. Partial-thickness abdominal wall defects resulting from such resection may not require vascularized flap-based reconstruction but may be repaired primarily or

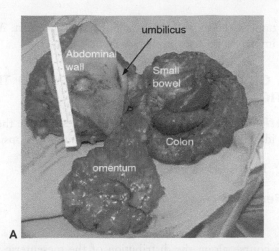

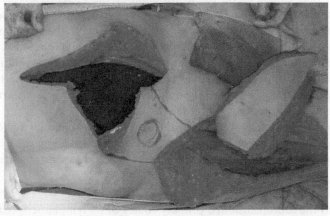

FIGURE 16-16 **A:** En bloc multivisceral resection for locally advanced ascending colon cancer with abdominal wall and small bowel involvement and **(B)** subsequent photograph demonstrating the full defect and reconstruction with an anterolateral thigh pedicle flap.

with bioprosthetic or synthetic mesh replacement of the fascia. Full-thickness abdominal wall defects and/or those with skin involvement likely require reconstruction with a vascularized flap (Fig. 16-16). There are various options for temporary and definitive abdominal wall reconstruction. Concerns about the risk for subsequent hernia should not preclude aggressive resection. However, if the need for abdominal wall resection has not been preoperatively anticipated and immediate reconstructive options are unavailable, aborting the resection with planned subsequent return to surgery with a multidisciplinary surgical team should be considered. Diaphragm involvement is not a contraindication to en bloc resection, and primary or mesh (e.g., bioprosthetic) closure in patients with diaphragm involvement may be performed. Such an approach has been performed among patients undergoing liver resection, and although associated with potentially increased morbidity, it does not increase operative mortality.[29] However, the dissemination of cancer cells into the thoracic cavity either prior to exploration or due to iatrogenic tumor seeding will limit the utility of this effort. Avoiding injury to the phrenic nerve improves postoperative respiratory recovery.

5. REMOVAL OF LYMPHADENOPATHY BEYOND THE PRIMARY DISTRIBUTION

Recommendation: Clinically positive lymph nodes outside the primary field of resection that are identified at the time of resection should be biopsied or removed.

Type of Data: Retrospective observational studies.

Strength of Recommendation: Moderate.

Rationale
Lymphatic vessels course along the distribution of the mesenteric vessels. Drainage from the intestine courses toward the root of the mesentery, along the para-aortic nodes, and ultimately into the thoracic duct. Lymphatics in the cecum and proximal ascending colon most commonly drain along the ileocolic lymph nodes, which encircle the ileocolic vascular pedicle. Metastases from tumors of the ascending colon may be present in lymph nodes along the ileocolic, right, and middle colic arteries. Lymph drainage from the transverse colon is primarily along the middle colic artery and then into the superior mesenteric lymph group.[30]

The inferior mesenteric lymph nodes, which are situated about the root of the inferior mesenteric artery, are afferent from peripheral nodes located along the marginal artery of Drummond and efferent to the lumbar nodal chain and superior mesenteric nodes.

Clinical Implications
In addition to the aforementioned primary routes of its lymphatic spread, colorectal cancer metastasis can also occur beyond the primary distribution and outside of the distribution of the primary resection along the following routes:

Para-aortic nodes. The para-aortic nodes are situated anterior to the lumbar vertebral bodies in proximity to the abdominal aorta. The para-aortic node group can be divided into three subgroups:

1. **Preaortic group:** These nodes drain the abdominal part of the gastrointestinal tract superior to the mid-rectum.
2. **Retroaortic group:** These nodes drain the lateral and preaortic regions.
3. **Lateral group:** These nodes, which drain the iliac regions, ovaries, and other pelvic organs, are located adjacent to the aorta and anterior to the spine. They extend laterally to the edge of the psoas major muscles and superiorly to the diaphragm.

Colorectal metastasis to the para-aortic nodes are uncommon but associated with poor prognosis. Metastases to the para-aortic lymph nodes most commonly occur in the preaortic or lateral groups, although multiple lymph nodes may be involved. The presence of para-aortic lymph node involvement signals the need for systemic chemotherapy and, when identified at surgery, should be removed for pathologic evaluation.

Nodes within the small bowel mesentery (SBM). The root of the SBM is contiguous with the hepatoduodenal ligament around the superior mesenteric vein and the right side of the transverse mesocolon about the gastrocolic trunk. The inferior mesenteric vein runs along the left side of the root of the SBM. Colon cancer cells can spread to the SBM by direct extension, by extension along the neural plexus or neighboring ligaments, or by way of lymphatic channels. Much like that of para-aortic nodes, colorectal cancer involvement in this node group is associated with poorer prognosis, and the clinical significance of extended dissection into this distribution remains incompletely understood.

The lymphatic spread of colon cancer from the submucosal lymphatic channels through the epi- and paracolic nodes to the intermediate nodes and then to nodes surrounding the superior mesenteric artery and/or para-aortic nodes was once considered to be an orderly and predictable process of tumor cell dissemination. Sentinel lymphatic mapping studies have shown aberrant lymphatic drainage in approximately 4% of cases (range, 0% to 10%).[31] However, these studies often do not specify the precise anatomical location(s) of the aberrant node(s). Aberrant lymphatic drainage beyond the relevant nodes in the central vascular pedicle may be identified as clinically abnormal lymph nodes by their size or other characteristics and should be resected for pathologic evaluation if it is safe to do so.

Intraoperative Assessment

The standard preoperative clinical evaluation of patients with nonmetastatic colon cancer includes CT of the chest, abdomen, and pelvis. During this evaluation, the patient should be carefully evaluated for enlarged lymph nodes along the superior mesenteric artery, superior mesenteric vein, and iliac vessels and about the abdominal aorta. Clinically suspicious lymph nodes (i.e., >1 cm) should be thoroughly evaluated and potentially resected at the time of operation (Fig. 16-17A,B). During the operation, the retroperitoneum and root of the mesentery should be carefully evaluated as part of routine exploration, and abnormal-appearing lymph nodes should be identified and resected for histologic evaluation.

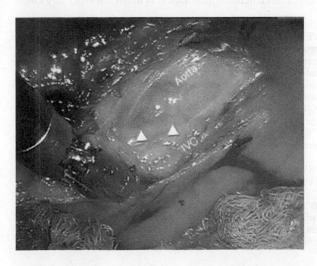

FIGURE 16-17 Intraoperative photograph showing aortocaval adenopathy. *Triangles* point to lymph node. IVC, inferior vena cava.

The vast majority of lymph nodes in colon cancer patients are small (<1 cm) and hardly visible or palpable at the time of operation. In fact, nearly 80% of nodal tumor metastases are found in lymph nodes <5 mm in maximal dimension and are easily overlooked at the time of operation or pathologic evaluation.[32–35] Nodes are generally considered to be normal if they are smaller than 1 cm^2. The consistency of nodes upon palpation may also be illustrative; for example, stony-hard nodes typically suggest cancer metastasis. Similarly, a group of mesenteric nodes that appear to be connected or move as a unit, called "matted" nodes, are consistent with lymphatic spread of disease.

Principles of Surgery for Lymphadenectomy

Traditionally, metastases in extraregional lymph node groups have been considered to be distant metastases. However, resection of isolated extraregional lymph node metastasis is associated with improved survival analogous to resection of liver metastasis.[36] At minimum, suspicious lymph nodes should be removed for diagnostic confirmation. There is insufficient data to support performing a more extended resection of the nodal basin (e.g., extended para-aortic lymph node dissection) versus targeted resection of involved lymph nodes. However, resection of isolated extraregional nodal metastasis is associated with improved survival, as has been observed following the resection of metastatic disease. Involvement of multiple lymph nodes outside of the primary distribution indicates disseminated disease, and excisional biopsy for histologic confirmation, but not routine radical lymph node dissection, should be performed when it is safe to do so. The patient should then be referred for systemic therapy.

REFERENCES

1. Nelson H, Petrelli N, Carlin A, et al. Guidelines 2000 for colon and rectal cancer surgery. *J Natl Cancer Inst* 2001;93:583–596.
2. Chang GJ, Kaiser AM, Mills S, et al. Practice parameters for the management of colon cancer. *Dis Colon Rectum* 2012;55:831–843.
3. Gezen C, Kement M, Altuntas YE, et al. Results after multivisceral resections of locally advanced colorectal cancers: an analysis on clinical and pathological t4 tumors. *World J Surg Oncol* 2012;10:39.
4. Niekel MC, Bipat S, Stoker J. Diagnostic imaging of colorectal liver metastases with CT, MR imaging, FDG PET, and/or FDG PET/CT: a meta-analysis of prospective studies including patients who have not previously undergone treatment. *Radiology* 2010;257:674–684.
5. Grossmann I, Klaase JM, Avenarius JK, et al. The strengths and limitations of routine staging before treatment with abdominal CT in colorectal cancer. *BMC Cancer* 2011;11:433.
6. Devereux DF, Deckers PJ. Contributions of pathologic margins and Dukes' stage to local recurrence in colorectal carcinoma. *Am J Surg* 1985;149:323–326.
7. Guillem JG, Wood WC, Moley JF, et al. ASCO/SSO review of current role of risk-reducing surgery in common hereditary cancer syndromes. *J Clin Oncol* 2006;24:4642–4660.
8. de Vos tot Nederveen Cappel WH, Buskens E, van Duijvendijk P, et al. Decision analysis in the surgical treatment of colorectal cancer due to a mismatch repair gene defect. *Gut* 2003;52:1752–1755.
9. Maeda T, Cannom RR, Beart RW Jr, et al. Decision model of segmental compared with total abdominal colectomy for colon cancer in hereditary nonpolyposis colorectal cancer. *J Clin Oncol* 2010;28:1175–1180.
10. Connell WR, Talbot IC, Harpaz N, et al. Clinicopathological characteristics of colorectal carcinoma complicating ulcerative colitis. *Gut* 1994;35(10):1419–1423.
11. Ullman T, Croog V, Harpaz N, et al. Progression of flat low-grade dysplasia to advanced neoplasia in patients with ulcerative colitis. *Gastroenterology* 2003;125(5):1311–1319.

12. West NP, Hohenberger W, Weber K, et al. Complete mesocolic excision with central vascular ligation produces an oncologically superior specimen compared with standard surgery for carcinoma of the colon. *J Clin Oncol* 2010;28(2):272–278.

13. Hohenberger W, Weber K, Matzel K, et al. Standardized surgery for colonic cancer: complete mesocolic excision and central ligation—technical notes and outcome. *Colorectal Dis* 2009;11(4):354–364.

14. Hoffmann M, Phillips C, Oevermann E, et al. Multivisceral and standard resections in colorectal cancer. *Langenbecks Arch Surg* 2012;397:75–84.

15. Benson AB III, Venook AP, Bekaii-Saab T, et al. Colon cancer, version 3.2014. *J Natl Compr Canc Netw* 2014;12(7):1028–1059.

16. Chen YG, Liu YL, Jiang SX, et al. Adhesion pattern and prognosis studies of T4N0M0 colorectal cancer following en bloc multivisceral resection: evaluation of T4 subclassification. *Cell Biochem Biophys* 2011;59:1–6.

17. Darakhshan A, Lin BP, Chan C, et al. Correlates and outcomes of tumor adherence in resected colonic and rectal cancers. *Ann Surg* 2008;247:650–658.

18. Mohan HM, Evans MD, Larkin JO, et al. Multivisceral resection in colorectal cancer: a systematic review. *Ann Surg Oncol* 2013;20:2929–2936.

19. Govindarajan A, Fraser N, Cranford V, et al. Predictors of multivisceral resection in patients with locally advanced colorectal cancer. *Ann Surg Oncol* 2008;15:1923–1930.

20. Luo HL, Tsai KL, Lin SE, et al. Outcome of urinary bladder recurrence after partial cystectomy for en bloc urinary bladder adherent colorectal cancer resection. *Int J Colorectal Dis* 2013;28:631–635.

21. Stotland PK, Moozar K, Cardella JA, et al. Urologic complications of composite resection following combined modality treatment of colorectal cancer. *Ann Surg Oncol* 2009;16:2759–2764.

22. Banerjee S, Kapur S, Moran BJ. The role of prophylactic oophorectomy in women undergoing surgery for colorectal cancer. *Colorectal Dis* 2005;7:214–217.

23. Sielezneff I, Salle E, Antoine K, et al. Simultaneous bilateral oophorectomy does not improve prognosis of postmenopausal women undergoing colorectal resection for cancer. *Dis Colon Rectum* 1997;40:1299–1302.

24. Tentes A, Markakidis S, Mirelis C, et al. Oophorectomy during surgery for colorectal carcinoma. *Tech Coloproctol* 2004;8(suppl 1):s214–s216.

25. Young-Fadok TM, Wolff BG, Nivatvongs S, et al. Prophylactic oophorectomy in colorectal carcinoma: preliminary results of a randomized, prospective trial. *Dis Colon Rectum* 1998;41:277–283; discussion 283–285.

26. Schmeler KM, Lynch HT, Chen LM, et al. Prophylactic surgery to reduce the risk of gynecologic cancers in the Lynch syndrome. *N Engl J Med* 2006;354:261–269.

27. Lachiewicz MP, Kravochuck SE, O'Malley MM, et al. Prevalence of occult gynecologic malignancy at the time of risk reducing and nonprophylactic surgery in patients with Lynch syndrome. *Gynecol Oncol* 2014;132:434–437.

28. Yang KY, Caughey AB, Little SE, et al. A cost-effectiveness analysis of prophylactic surgery versus gynecologic surveillance for women from hereditary non-polyposis colorectal cancer (HNPCC) families. *Fam Cancer* 2011;10:535–543.

29. Li GZ, Sloane JL, Lidsky ME, et al. Simultaneous diaphragm and liver resection: a propensity-matched analysis of postoperative morbidity. *J Am Coll Surg* 2013;216:402–411.

30. Toyota S, Ohta H, Anazawa S. Rationale for extent of lymph node dissection for right colon cancer. *Dis Colon Rectum* 1995;38:705–711.

31. Stojadinovic A, Allen PJ, Protic M, et al. Colon sentinel lymph node mapping: practical surgical applications. *J Am Coll Surg* 2005;201:297–313.

32. Herrera-Ornelas L, Justiniano J, Castillo N, et al. Metastases in small lymph nodes from colon cancer. *Arch Surg* 1987;122:1253–1256.

33. Haboubi NY, Clark P, Kaftan SM, et al. The importance of combining xylene clearance and immunohistochemistry in the accurate staging of colorectal carcinoma. *J R Soc Med* 1992;85:386–388.

34. Rodriguez-Bigas MA, Maamoun S, Weber TK, et al. Clinical significance of colorectal cancer: metastases in lymph nodes < 5 mm in size. *Ann Surg Oncol* 1996;3:124–130.

35. Ratto C, Sofo L, Ippoliti M, et al. Accurate lymph-node detection in colorectal specimens resected for cancer is of prognostic significance. *Dis Colon Rectum* 1999;42:143–154; discussion 154–158.

36. Min BS, Kim NK, Sohn SK, et al. Isolated paraaortic lymph-node recurrence after the curative resection of colorectal carcinoma. *J Surg Oncol* 2008;97:136–140.

Colon Resection: Key Question

In patients identified to have synchronous liver metastatic disease, does simultaneous curative resection (versus staged) affect survival, overall morbidity, or mortality?

INTRODUCTION

Synchronous colorectal cancer and liver metastasis presents an operative and decision-making challenge for both hepatobiliary and colorectal surgeons. Between 15% and 20% of patients presenting with colorectal cancer will harbor synchronous liver metastasis (SCRLM). Surgical resection is the only modality that potentially leads to cure, with 5-year survival rates ranging from 25% to 60%; thus, when feasible, operative resection is paramount.[1] Controversy, however, exists as to the timing of surgical resection (simultaneous versus staged) because of the potential impact on morbidity, mortality, and survival. The literature to date is composed of limited observational uncontrolled series with few meta-analyses and no randomized controlled trials. Therefore, the purpose of the review presented here is to examine the impact of timing of SCRLM on overall morbidity, mortality, and survival.

METHODOLOGY

An organized search of the MEDLINE database through PubMed was performed for the period between January 1990 and December 2013. Keyword combinations included a database search in English for the following MeSH terms: (synchronous* OR simultaneous* OR combined OR concurrent) AND (staged OR "two-stage") AND (colon OR colorectal OR rectal OR colectomy*) AND metastasis* AND (liver OR hepatectomy*). Directed searches of the embedded references from the primary articles also were performed. For studies that reported patients in more than one publication, only the most recent complete report was used. The final grade of recommendation was assigned using the Grading of Recommendations Assessment, Development, and Evaluation (GRADE) system.[2]

The initial search yielded a total of 137 studies, of which the abstracts were reviewed. Studies to be included in our systematic review focused on observational studies of staged or simultaneous operations, comparative studies of staged versus simultaneous resection, and meta-analyses of staged versus simultaneous resection. Exclusion criteria included case reports and limited single-arm series, reviews, and trials that compared issues unrelated to the primary goal of this review. Through consensus of four reviewers, 105 studies were excluded, leaving 32 studies (29 observational studies and three meta-analysis manuscripts) to be reviewed in detail. Two individual members of the group reviewed each manuscript. Each article was then assessed for inclusion and assigned a strength of evidence. This recommendation was arrived at by reviewer consensus and based on the GRADE system (Table 16-1). A total of 18 observational series

TABLE 16-1 Simultaneous versus Staged Morbidity and Mortality

First Author	Year	Number	Study Design (Meta-analysis, Observational)	Morbidity		Mortality		Grade	Conclusion
				Simultaneous	Staged	Simultaneous	Staged		
Boostrom	2011	45 simultaneous rectal with liver	Observational	80% morbidity	NA	None	None	2C	Simultaneous is feasible even in rectal resection.
Tanaka	2004	39 simultaneous	Observational	28% morbidity	NA	None	NA	2C	Simultaneous is feasible.
Lyass	2001	26 simultaneous	Observational	27% morbidity	NA	None	NA	2C	Simultaneous is feasible.
Vassiliou	2007	103 total; 25 simultaneous, 78 staged	Observational	Equal morbidity (P = NS), LOS 12 days (P <.05); transfusion rates were 2 +/−1.8, packed red blood cells (P <.05)	Equal morbidity, LOS 20 days; transfusion rates were 4 +/− 1.5, packed red blood cells	None	None	2C	Simultaneous is feasible with lower LOS and lower transfusions.
van der Pool	2010	57 total; 8 simultaneous, 20 liver first, 29 staged	Observational	Equal morbidity	Equal morbidity	None		2C	Simultaneous is feasible.
Chua	2004	96 total; 64 simultaneous, 32 staged	Observational	53% morbidity (P = NS); LOS 11 days (P = .001)	41% morbidity; LOS 22 days	None	None	2C	Simultaneous is feasible with lower LOS.

Single-arm observational series

(continued)

TABLE 16-1 Simultaneous versus Staged Morbidity and Mortality (continued)

First Author	Year	Number	Study Design (Meta-analysis, Observational)	Morbidity		Mortality		Grade	Conclusion
				Simultaneous	Staged	Simultaneous	Staged		
Abbott	2013	361,096; 3,625 simultaneous, 322,286 colon resections, 35,185 liver resections	Nationwide inpatient sample 2002–2006; patients undergoing colon or secondary liver resection	Equal morbidity; LOS 10.9 days	NA	3.50%	NA	2B	Simultaneous is feasible as long as the liver resection is not a lobectomy.
Moug	2010	32 simultaneous, 32 staged	Observational	Equal morbidity ($P = $ NS); LOS 12 days ($P = .008$)	Equal morbidity; LOS 20 days	None	None	2C	Simultaneous is feasible with lower LOS.
Nakajima	2013	86 traditional simultaneous resections vs. 59 using POT (35 simultaneous resections, 24 staged)	Observational	Using POT strategy: morbidity 44% $P < .02$, LOS 18 days ($P < .001$)	NA			2C	Using a POT strategy appears to lower risk of complications for simultaneous resection.
Martin	2003	240 total, 134 simultaneous, 106 staged	Observational	48% morbidity, 60% morbidity for major liver, LOS 10 days, 550 mL blood loss (all $< .001$)	68% morbidity, 70% morbidity for major liver only, LOS 18 days, 1100 mL blood loss	2%	2%	2C	Simultaneous is feasible with lower morbidity, LOS, and estimated blood loss.

Single-arm observational series

	Year		Study type					Grade	Conclusion
Mayo	2013	1,004 total, 329 simultaneous, 675 staged, liver first 28	Observational	Equal morbidity	Equal morbidity	2.7% (P = NS)	3.10%	2B	Simultaneous is feasible, trend in extended resection to be worse for simultaneous resection.
Yan	2007	103 total: 73 simultaneous, 30 staged	Observational	Equal morbidity; LOS 7 days (P = .001)	Equal morbidity; LOS 15 days	None	None	2C	Simultaneous is feasible with lower LOS.
Capussotti	2007	172 total; 88 simultaneous; 84 delayed; all major liver resections	Observational	33% morbidity P = .0369; transfusion 42% P = .0131, LOS 14 days P = .0001	56% morbidity; transfusion 17%; LOS 21 days			2B	Simultaneous is feasible in major liver resection with lower morbidity, LOS, and transfusion.
Luo	2010	405 total; 129 simultaneous with 276 staged	Observational	47% morbidity (P = NS); LOS 8 days (P <.0001)	54.3% morbidity; LOS 14 days	1.5% (NS)	2%	2B	Simultaneous is feasible with lower LOS.
Martin II	2009	230 total, 70 simultaneous, 160 staged	Observational	56% morbidity (P = NS), LOS 10 days (P = .001)	55% morbidity, LOS 18 days	2%	2%	2B	Simultaneous is feasible with lower LOS.
de Hass	2010	228 total: 55 simultaneous vs. 173 delayed; and 26 simultaneous vs. 26 delayed case matched	Observational	11% morbidity (P = .015); case-matched morbidity 8% P = .035	25% morbidity; case-matched morbidity 31%			2B	Simultaneous is feasible with lower morbidity.

Comparative observational series

(continued)

TABLE 16-1 Simultaneous versus Staged Morbidity and Mortality *(continued)*

First Author	Year	Number	Study Design (Meta-analysis, Observational)	Morbidity		Mortality		Grade	Conclusion
				Simultaneous	Staged	Simultaneous	Staged		
Thelen	2007	219 total: 40 simultaneous, 179 staged	Observational	NA	NA	10% (*P* = .012)	1.10%	2C	Age older than 70 years is risk for mortality after simultaneous (*P* = .029); predictor of mortality for simultaneous resection was > a lobectomy.
Reddy	2007	610 total: 135 simultaneous vs. 475 staged	Observational	14.1% morbidity for minor liver (*P* = NS), 36.1% for major liver (*P* <.05); LOS 8.5 days (*P* <.0001)	10.5% morbidity for minor liver, 17.6% for major liver; LOS 14 days (*P* <.0001)	1% for minor liver (*P* = NS); 8.3% for major (*P* <.05)	0.5% for minor liver; 1.4% for major	2B	Simultaneous is feasible with minor liver resection with lower LOS. Avoid major resections for simultaneous resections due to high levels of morbidity and mortality.

Comparative observational series

	Year							
Li	2013	1,116 simultaneous, 1,608 staged	Meta-analysis	Lower morbidity OR 0.74, P <.001, lower LOS P <.001	Higher morbidity; higher LOS	Equal	Equal	2B	Simultaneous is feasible with lower morbidity and LOS in selected patients.
Yin	2013	1,015 simultaneous, 1,865 staged	Meta-analysis	Lower morbidity OR 0.77, P <.001	Higher morbidity	Equal	Equal	2B	Simultaneous is feasible with lower morbidity in selected patients.
Chen	2010	2,204 simultaneous and staged	Meta-analysis	Lower morbidity OR 0.77, P <.002; lower LOS P <.01	Higher morbidity, higher LOS	NA	NA	2B	Simultaneous is feasible with lower morbidity and LOS in selected patients.

Meta-analysis

DFS, disease-free survival; DSS, disease-specific survival; LOS, length of stay; LR, locoregional recurrence; NA, not applicable; NS, not significant; OR, overall recurrence; OS, overall survival; POT, predicted operative time.

and three meta-analyses were included in the final analysis for this key question review. Figure 16-18 shows the CONSORT diagram summarizing study selection.

The surgical resection techniques were defined as follows. Simultaneous resection was defined as concomitant resection of both the primary colorectal lesion and the synchronous liver metastasis. Staged resection was defined as resections that involved two separate operations, including traditional (e.g., colorectal resection followed by extirpation of the liver metastasis) and reverse (e.g., liver resection followed by colorectal surgery) strategies.

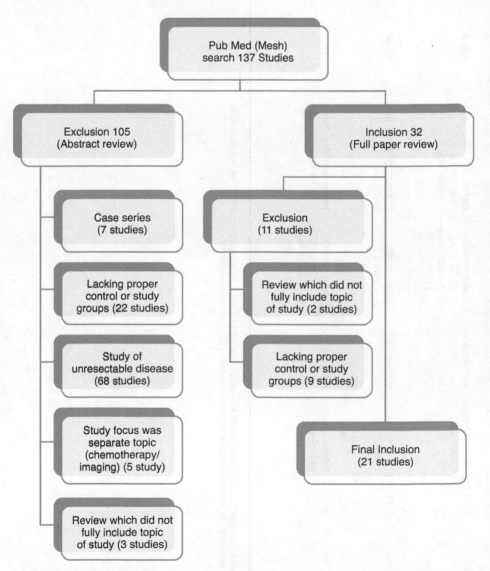

FIGURE 16-18 CONSORT diagram summarizing the literature search used for this review.

FINDINGS
Morbidity and Mortality

Recommendation: Simultaneous resection is both safe and feasible. There is growing evidence that morbidity may be improved by simultaneous resection of colon cancer and liver metastasis in well-selected patients with fewer than three segments of liver disease.

Type of Data: retrospective observational studies and three separate meta-analyses.

Strength of Recommendation: strong recommendation based on consistent findings in multiple papers of limited quality.

Rationale

Since 2001, multiple single-arm series have demonstrated the feasibility of simultaneous resection in both colon and rectal cancer.[3–5] These series, however, lack the methodology and strength of evidence to assure equal outcomes compared with a more traditional staged approach. Comparative series since 2007 have attempted to bridge this knowledge gap by addressing some of the selection bias that dominates current literature. Collectively, these series have attempted to define the impact of simultaneous resection on morbidity, mortality, and survival.

Traditionally, SCRLM resection has been avoided because of a long-held belief that the magnitude of the operation would prove excessive. In particular, concerns regarding complications and mortality, including concern about an anastomotic complication, insufficiency of the remaining liver segments, and intra-abdominal infection/abscess, have led to this historical bias. Tanaka et al[5] were one of the first groups to demonstrate that the extent of liver resection is a potential factor for increased morbidity and mortality. Several comparative studies have echoed this recommendation for caution when considering a simultaneous procedure. These series have stressed the importance of considering a staged approach in patients who require more than three liver segments resected at the time of surgery.[5–10]

Other groups have reported equivalent morbidity outcomes when limited liver resection is performed.[9–20] Nakajima et al[6] successfully mitigated the potential risks by employing criteria by which to judge the feasibility of simultaneous resection. Differentiating operative approaches by predicting operative time (planned operative time (POT) <6 hours = simultaneous resection, POT >6 hours = staged resection) allowed for the identification of a cohort of patients who reliably had improved outcomes when compared with outcomes of traditionally approached synchronous disease.[6] More recent studies have improved matching, analysis, and patient selection in further attempts to address this fundamental concern. A number of series have actually demonstrated improved complication rates for those undergoing simultaneous surgical resection.[11,14,15,18,20] Three of these series demonstrated a decreased incidence of complications for all patients, as well as patients matched for extent of hepatic resection.[11,14,18] Specifically, the study by Capussotti et al[11] controlled for the magnitude of liver resection by including only patients who had more than three liver segments resected. The authors reported an improved overall rate of total complications and an equivalent anastomotic leak rate for patients undergoing a simultaneous resection compared with a staged resection.

Only two of the 21 series demonstrated increased mortality after simultaneous resection.[7,8] Reddy et al[8] suggested that increased mortality was associated with major liver resection. Likewise, Thelen et al[7] demonstrated a high mortality rate among patients older than the age of 70 years and those who had more than a hemihepatectomy at the time of the simultaneous procedure. In general, however, the mortality rates reported by the majority of other series have not been significantly different for simultaneous and staged resection (Table 16-1).

Three meta-analyses have been published, one in 2010 and two in 2013.[1,21,22] These three studies all included over 1,000 patients who underwent a simultaneous resection and more than 2,000 operative procedures in total.[1,21,22] All three studies demonstrated improved morbidity among patients who underwent a simultaneous approach to resection of synchronous disease. It must be stated that these series were based on retrospective data and therefore are considered to be overall lower quality levels of evidence. In general, these studies concluded that simultaneous resection was both safe and efficient with the potential for decreased morbidity in properly selected patients.

Beyond the issues of morbidity and mortality, many series have commented on other aspects of care that often affect both quality and cost. The majority of series to date have demonstrated shorter total length of stay (LOS) for patients treated with a simultaneous approach.[8,11–17,20] In addition, two of the three meta-analyses reported that simultaneous resection resulted in shorter LOS.[1,21]

Survival

Recommendation: Overall survival and disease-free survival are not affected by timing of resection.

Type of Data: Retrospective observational studies and three separate meta-analyses.

Strength of Recommendation: Strong recommendation based on consistent findings in multiple papers of limited quality.

Rationale

Survival data are complicated by selection bias and the use of chemotherapy, which was rarely discussed in most of the published series (Table 16-2). In general, overall survival and disease-free survival rates have been shown to be similar after simultaneous versus staged resection in all series.[6,7,12,16,17,20] A single series noted longer disease-free survival and progression-free survival items among patients treated with a delayed or staged operative approach.[18] Overall survival rates, however, remained the same between groups in this series.[18] In the 21 studies examined, 5-year survival rates ranged from 21% to 53%. All three meta-analyses found no difference in survival between a staged or simultaneous approach for synchronous disease[1,21,22]

TABLE 16-2   Simultaneous versus Staged Survival

First Author	Year	Number	Study Design (Meta-analysis, Observational)	Survival		Grade	Conclusion	Comments
				Simultaneous	Staged			
Boostrom	2011	45 simultaneous, rectal with liver	Observational	5-yr survival 32%, LR free survival 80%; DFS 28%	NA	2C	Simultaneous is feasible.	All rectal cancers; complexity of liver and rectal surgery did not affect outcomes
Tanaka	2004	39 simultaneous	Observational	5-yr survival 53%	NA	2C	Simultaneous is feasible.	Based on low-quality evidence
Lyass	2001	26 simultaneous	Observational	5-yr survival 28%	NA	2C	Simultaneous is feasible.	Based on low-quality evidence
Vassiliou	2007	103 total; 25 simultaneous, 78 staged	Observational	5-yr survival 31% (P = NS)	5-yr survival 28%	2C	Simultaneous is feasible.	Small series but well matched with liver disease; however, more right-sided colons in simultaneous cases
Chua	2004	96 total; 64 simultaneous, 32 staged	Observational	5-yr survival 27 months (P = NS); DFS 13 months (P = NS)	5-yr survival 34 months; DFS 13 months	2C	Simultaneous is feasible.	Based on low-quality evidence
Moug	2010	32 simultaneous, 32 staged	Observational	5-yr survival 21% (P = NS); DFS 10 months (P = NS)	5-yr survival 24%; DFS 14 months	2C	Simultaneous is feasible.	Based on low-quality evidence

Single-arm observational series

(continued)

TABLE 16-2 Simultaneous versus Staged Survival *(continued)*

First Author	Year	Number	Study Design (Meta-analysis, Observational)	Survival		Grade	Conclusion	Comments
				Simultaneous	Staged			
Nakajima	2013	86 traditional simultaneous resections vs. 59 using POT (35 simultaneous resections, 24 staged)	Observational	3-yr survival 71% (P = NS)	3-yr survival 54%	2C	Simultaneous is feasible.	Assess the efficacy of the POT in SCLM by comparing POT <6 hours (simultaneous) vs. >6 hours (staged) vs. traditional simultaneous SCLM.
Mayo	2013	1,004 total; 329 simultaneous, 675 staged, liver first 28	Observational	5-yr survival 42% P = .688; recurrence 59.6% (P = .171)	5-yr survival 44%; recurrence 57.2%	2B	Simultaneous is feasible.	Based on low-quality evidence
Yan	2007	103 total; 73 simultaneous, 30 staged	Observational	5-yr survival 37% (P = NS); 5-yr DFS 14% (P = NS)	5-yr survival 36% (P = NS); 5-yr DFS 14% (P = NS)	2C	Simultaneous is feasible.	In spite of worse clinical characteristics, simultaneous resection patients had similar DFS and OS compared to staged resection.

Comparative observational series

First author	Year	Study population	Study type	Outcome	Outcome	Conclusion	Level of evidence	Comments
de Hass	2010	228 total; 55 simultaneous vs. 173 delayed; 26 simultaneous vs. 26 delayed case matched	Observational	3-yr survival 74% (P = .871); recurrence 3-yr 85% (P = .002)	3-yr survival 64%; recurrence 3-yr 70%	Simultaneous is feasible; no difference in survival with possible increased recurrence	2B	Bias led to less chemotherapy in simultaneous and some dropout of liver in delayed cases due to progression of disease.
Thelen	2007	219 total; 40 simultaneous, 179 staged	Observational	5-yr survival 53% (P = NS)	5-yr survival 39%	Simultaneous is feasible.	2C	Liver resection was determined to be simultaneous if done within 12 months of primary colon; poorly matched groups with lesser operations in simultaneous operations
Li	2013	1,116 simultaneous, 1,608 staged	Meta-analysis	Equal 5-yr survival and DFS	Equal 5-yr survival and DFS	Simultaneous is feasible.	2B	Based on low-quality evidence
Yin	2013	1,015 simultaneous, 1,865 staged	Meta-analysis	Equal 5-yr survival and DFS	Equal 5-yr survival HR 0.96 (P = .64) and DFS HR 1.04 (P = .79)	Simultaneous is feasible.	2B	Based on low-quality evidence
Chen	2010	2,204 simultaneous and staged	Meta-analysis	Equal 5-yr survival		Simultaneous is feasible.	2B	Based on low-quality evidence

(Li, Yin, and Chen rows grouped under the margin label "Meta-analysis")

DFS, disease-free survival; DSS, disease-specific survival; HR, hazard ratio; LR, locoregional recurrence; NS, not significant; OR, overall recurrence; OS, overall survival; POT, predicted operative time; SCLM, synchronous colorectal liver metastases.

Limitation

The main limitation of this review is the underlying primary data quality with a lack of well-controlled series with appropriate matching or complete statistical analyses. These observational series are therefore subject to significant selection bias that could lead to inappropriate conclusions. Moreover, the volume of data is heavily weighted toward simultaneous and traditionally staged operations, with limited data regarding other approaches such as the reverse-staged strategy. In addition, the use of neoadjuvant chemotherapy and the details of postoperative chemotherapy are largely omitted from most series. Finally, there seems little doubt that most published series are presented by centers of excellence, especially in liver surgery, which makes generalization of conclusions somewhat hazardous. In spite of the limitations mentioned, the majority of published data are consistent with less morbidity in well-selected patients undergoing simultaneous liver resection of three or fewer segments.

CONCLUSION

Simultaneous resection for patients identified with SCRLM appears to be both safe and feasible if performed by expert surgeons, especially for patients who require only a minor liver resection (≤3 segments). There is also good evidence that timing of the operation does not adversely affect overall survival or disease-free survival rates. Moreover, there is increasing evidence that overall morbidity and length of hospital stay may be lessened by a simultaneous approach. While studies of patients requiring a larger liver resection suggest that a simultaneous approach is feasible and safe, the data for such cases are more limited and do not allow for definitive recommendations. As such, for patients who require a major hepatic resection, the historical paradigm of a staged approach may be more prudent. An adequately powered randomized-controlled study in the setting of modern chemotherapy regimens would be needed to address this question more definitively.

Current evidence supports the feasibility and safety of simultaneous curative resection of colorectal cancer with liver metastasis. Simultaneous resection results in equivalent mortality and survival and potential improved morbidity in patients with fewer than three liver segments of disease.

REFERENCES

1. Yin Z, Liu C, Chen Y, et al. Timing of hepatectomy in resectable synchronous colorectal liver metastases (SCRLM): simultaneous or delayed? *Hepatology* 2013;57(6):2346–2357.
2. Terracciano L, Brozek J, Compalati E, et al. GRADE system: new paradigm. *Curr Opin Allergy Clin Immunol* 2010;10(4):377–383.
3. Lyass S, Zamir G, Matot I, et al. Combined colon and hepatic resection for synchronous colorectal liver metastases. *J Surg Oncol* 2001;78(1):17–21.
4. Boostrom SY, Vassiliki LT, Nagorney DM, et al. Synchronous rectal and hepatic resection of rectal metastatic disease. *J Gastrointest Surg* 2011;15(9):1583–1588.
5. Tanaka K, Shimada H, Matsuo K, et al. Outcome after simultaneous colorectal and hepatic resection for colorectal cancer with synchronous metastases. *Surgery* 2004;136(3):650–659.
6. Nakajima K, Takahashi S, Saito N, et al. Predictive factors for anastomotic leakage after simultaneous resection of synchronous colorectal liver metastasis. *J Gastrointest Surg* 2012;16(4):821–827.
7. Thelen A, Jonas S, Benckert C, et al. Simultaneous versus staged liver resection of synchronous liver metastases from colorectal cancer. *Int J Colorectal Dis* 2007;22(10):1269–1276.

8. Reddy SK, Pawlik TM, Zorzi D, et al. Simultaneous resections of colorectal cancer and synchronous liver metastases: a multi-institutional analysis. *Ann Surg Oncol* 2007;14(12):3481–3491.
9. Abbott AM, Parsons HM, Tuttle TM, et al. Short-term outcomes after combined colon and liver resection for synchronous colon cancer liver metastases: a population study. *Ann Surg Oncol* 2013;20(1):139–147.
10. Mayo SC, Heckman JE, Shore AD, et al. Shifting trends in liver-directed management of patients with colorectal liver metastasis: a population-based analysis. *Surgery* 2011;150(2):204–216.
11. Capussotti L, Ferrero A, Vigano L, et al. Major liver resections synchronous with colorectal surgery. *Ann Surg Oncol* 2007;14(1):195–201.
12. Yan TD, Chu F, Black D, et al. Synchronous resection of colorectal primary cancer and liver metastases. *World J Surg* 2007;31(7):1496–1501.
13. Luo Y, Wang L, Chen C, et al. Simultaneous liver and colorectal resections are safe for synchronous colorectal liver metastases. *J Gastrointest Surg* 2010;14(12):1974–1980.
14. Martin R, Paty P, Fong Y, et al. Simultaneous liver and colorectal resections are safe for synchronous colorectal liver metastases. *J Am Coll Surg* 2003;197(2):233–241; discussion 241–242.
15. Martin RC II, Augenstein V, Reuter NP, et al. Simultaneous versus staged resection for synchronous colorectal cancer liver metastases. *J Am Coll Surg* 2009;208(5):842–850; discussion 850–852.
16. Moug SJ, Smith D, Leen E, et al. Evidence for a synchronous operative approach in the treatment of colorectal cancer with hepatic metastases: a case matched study. *Eur J Surg Oncol* 2010;36(4):365–370.
17. Chua HK, Sondenaa K, Tsiotos GG, et al. Concurrent vs. staged colectomy and hepatectomy for primary colorectal cancer with synchronous hepatic metastases. *Dis Colon Rectum* 2004;47(8):1310–1316.
18. de Haas RJ, Adam R, Wicherts DA, et al. Comparison of simultaneous or delayed liver surgery for limited synchronous colorectal metastases. *Br J Surg* 2010;97(8):1279–1289.
19. van der Pool AE, de Wilt JH, Lalmahomed ZS, et al. Optimizing the outcome of surgery in patients with rectal cancer and synchronous liver metastases. *Br J Surg* 2010;97(3):383–390.
20. Vassiliou I, Arkadopoulos N, Theodosopoulos T, et al. Surgical approaches of resectable synchronous colorectal liver metastases: timing considerations. *World J Gasterenterol* 2007;13(9):1431–1434.
21. Chen J, Zhao G. Timing of resection for colorectal primary cancer and synchronous liver metastases. *Dig Dis Sci* 2010;55(12):3634–3635.
22. Li ZQ, Liu K, Duan JC, et al. Meta-analysis of simultaneous versus staged resection for synchronous colorectal liver metastases. *Hepatol Res* 2013;43(1):72–83.

Colon Resection: Key Question 2

In patients with colon cancer, does high central vascular ligation (D3 ligation) affect patient survival?

INTRODUCTION

In an effort to optimize surgical management of colon cancer, many groups have advocated extended lymphadenectomy as a strategy to improve completeness of resection and lymph node harvest. The goal of this treatment is to decrease cancer recurrence and increase cancer-specific survival in patients with nonmetastatic colon cancer. The literature on this topic contains multiple definitions of extended lymphadenectomy, as well as varied clinical methodology. The purpose of this key question is to examine the role for extended lymphadenectomy using a complete literature review.

METHODOLOGY

An organized search of MEDLINE/PubMed, EMBASE, and the Cochrane Database of Systematic Reviews was performed for the period between January 1990 and August 2013. Keyword combinations included "colon cancer," "D3 resection," "high ligation," "high-tie," and "complete mesocolic excision." Directed searches of the embedded references from the primary articles also were performed.

Our initial search yielded 141 unique articles in the English literature from 1990 to 2013. Of these, 70 were excluded based on review of the title and abstract; they discussed rectal cancer only or represented case reports or cadaver studies of the technique and thus did not meet inclusion criteria. The remaining 71 abstracts were reviewed in detail by three independent reviewers. An additional 52 were excluded because they did not address the clinical question of interest. A total of 19 manuscripts were reviewed in detail by the group members, and a final 11 manuscripts were selected for complete review of the data. Figure 16-19 shows the CONSORT diagram summarizing study selection. Each manuscript was then reviewed by at least two members of the group and assigned a strength of recommendation based on the Grading of Recommendations Assessment, Development, and Evaluation (GRADE) system[1] (Table 16-3).

For the purpose of this review, standard ligation was defined as proximal ligation of the feeding vessel with complete harvest of all pericolic nodes, as well as the main pedicle to the given segment of bowel (ileocolic, middle colic, left colic, or superior hemorrhoidal artery), while central or high ligation implies extended lymphadenectomy to include vessel ligation at the most proximal origin from the central vessel with inclusion of associated lymph nodes. It should be noted that standard ligation does not imply leaving a segment of the primary vessel, rather a complete resection that includes the lymph nodes at the primary feeding vessel (e.g., origin of the superior rectal artery just below takeoff of the left colic for sigmoid tumors or origin of the ileocolic artery at the superior mesentery artery for right colon tumors). In contrast, high

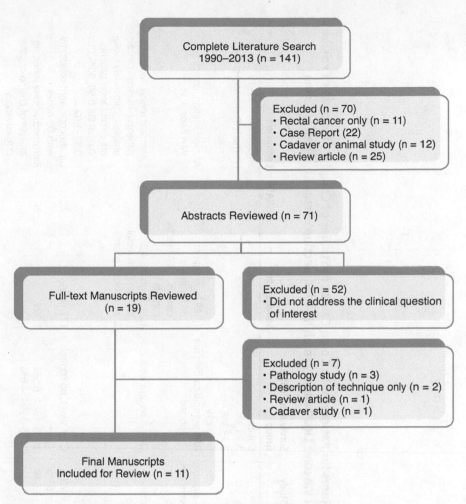

FIGURE 16-19 CONSORT diagram for the systematic review.

vessel ligation or central vascular ligation or extended lymph node dissection includes lymph nodes at the inferior mesenteric artery (IMA) ligation flush with the aorta for left-sided lesions and resection of gastroepiploic and peripancreatic nodes for right-sided or transverse colon lesions.[2] For articles in the literature that used the Japanese system, extended lymphadenectomy was classified as D3 resection (according to the Japanese Society for Cancer of the Colon and Rectum guidelines).

FINDINGS

Evidence Summary

Whether one uses the European or Japanese definition of central ligation, it is clear that involvement of the central-most nodal basin is an uncommon event. Metastasis

TABLE 16-3 Comparison of Survival Rates for Patients with Colon Cancer in Studies of Complete Mesocolic Excision with High Mesenteric Ligation/Central Vascular Ligation/D3 Lymph Node Dissection versus Standard Ligation

Author, Year	Outcomes	Survival in Study Group	Survival in Control Group	Sample Size	GRADE	Comments
Slanetz, 1997	DSS	Dukes A 95% B 83.9% C 52.5%	Dukes A 95.3% B 73.9% C 45.2%	1,027	2C	Study from 1957–1975 No modern chemotherapy
Chin, 2008	5-year DFS	7/14 IMA + sigmoid cancers were alive at 5 years	IMA sigmoid cancers not reported	1,389 high ligation; 387 sigmoid cancers, 1,002 rectal cancers	2C	All high ligation; compares IMA node + vs. –
Cirocchi, 2012	5-year OS and OR	Overall recurrence 4.9%	Overall recurrence 8.2%	4,281 high tie, 4,385 low tie; both rectal and colon cancer	2C	Systematic review. Most patients had rectal cancer; unable to separately evaluate colon cancer patients. Overall OR 0.58, 95% CI 0.32–1.07
Han, 2013	OS	60 months = 70% 72 months = 69%	Case series, no controls	177 cases	2C	Laparoscopic right colectomy with D3 nodes
Hohenberger, 2008	5-year LR	1995–2002: 3.6%	1978–1984: 6.5% 1985–1994: 4.6%	1,329	2C	Retrospective case series; no analysis of chemo or other care advances

Kawamura, 2000	10-year DFS	Nodal involvement: Limited 50% Intermediate 90% High 41%	Nodal involvement: Limited 89% Intermediate 51% High 0%	564	Retrospective, all colon cancer and node positive Only 6 patients had high nodal involvement.	2C
Adamina, 2012	OS DR	14/52 node positive OS 38 months	None	52	Prospective laparoscopic right colectomy	2C
Kanemitsu, 2013	OS	Stage I 94.5% Stage II 87.6% Stage III 79.2%	None	370 Stage I 73; Stage II 155; Stage III 142	Standardized open operation D3 resection of right-sided colon cancer	2C
Kanemitsu, 2006	5 and 10-year OS	High ligation Station 252 involved 50% OS Station 253 involved 40% OS	None	1188 N = 90 for station 252 positive; N = 20 for station 253 positive	Retrospective review of sigmoid and rectal cancer	2C
Okuna, 2007	5-year OS	Open (1991–1994) Stage I 91% Stage II 84% Stage IIIa 76% Stage IIIb 62%	Laparoscopic (1993–2001) Stage I 96.6% Stage II 94.8%; Stage III 79.6%	Open: Stage I 1,905; Stage II 3,037; Stage III 2,903 Lapar: 1,495 (not separated by stage)	Japanese registry, retrospective comparison of open vs. laparoscopic resection with standard D3 dissection	2C

CI, confidence interval; DR, distant recurrence; DSS, disease-specific survival; DFS, disease-free survival; OS, overall survival; IMA, inferior mesenteric artery; OR, overall recurrence; LR, locoregional recurrence.

to the central vasculature has been observed to occur approximately 1.7% to 5% of the time.[2-4] A study by Chin et al,[3] which included rectal and sigmoid colon cancer patients, indicated that station 252 (intermediate level) was involved in 8.3% of cases, while station 253 (central level) was involved in only 1.7% of cases. There was no clear evidence of the pattern of spread along the middle colic vessels in transverse colon cancers.

These studies' data are further limited by not assessing the completeness of mesocolic excision. In at least one study, colon cancer resected with an intact mesocolic fascia was associated with a 15% higher survival rate at 5 years compared to cases with mesocolic defects. This difference increased to 27% in stage III cases.[5] However, it is notable that these data are not based on randomized comparison nor do they consider individual surgeon skill or other patient and provider factors. There may be other important factors related to surgical resection that are not routinely measured. A study by West and colleagues[6] indicated similar rates of central vascular ligation between D3 resection cases from Japan and complete mesocolic excision/central vascular ligation cases from Germany; however, specimens from Germany encompassed far larger segments of large bowel and mesenteric surface area compared to specimens from Japan. Whether this difference in extent of resection reflects differences in patient characteristics or surgical approach or a combination of both factors is not clear. As a further limitation, some studies failed to separate colon cancer versus rectal cancer,[4,7] and some of these series are limited by the time period of the study. Slanetz et al[8] studied patients from 1957 to 1975, while Hohenberger et al[2] studied patients from three distinct time periods during 1978 to 2002. Survival analysis during the earlier time periods may have been affected by the absence of modern imaging and staging and by less effective adjuvant chemotherapy regimens.

Survival

The majority of published survival data are related to survival of patients with or without central node positivity in the setting of a central vascular ligation. Chin et al[3] reported on a series of 1,389 patients treated with central vascular ligation for sigmoid (n = 387) or rectal (n = 1,002) cancer. Rates of IMA metastasis based on T stage were 0% (pT1), 1% (pT2), 2.6% (pT3), and 4.3% (pT4). The authors concluded that central ligation of the IMA provided a theoretical benefit over intermediate ligation in 0.8% of cases. Although the authors concluded that disease-free survival was shorter in patients with central node metastasis, this group contained only 14 patients with sigmoid colon cancer, and there was no comparison to a group with intermediate ligation.

A study by Kamemitsu et al[9] from Japan examined 370 consecutive patients who had a right colectomy with D3 lymphadenectomy for right-sided colon cancer. Eleven (3%) had central node involvement, while 13.2% had intermediate node involvement. The 5-year disease-specific survival rate was 36.4% in patients with central node involvement versus 83.5% in patients with intermediate node involvement. Central node involvement was seen only in T3 and T4 tumors.[9]

Survival of patients with central node positivity in the setting of sigmoid colon or rectal cancer has also been examined.[4] This series included 1,188 consecutive patients, all of whom underwent a high ligation. A total of 1.7% of patients had involvement of central nodes (station 253), with a 5-year survival rate of 40%, while 8.3% of patients had intermediate node metastasis (station 252), with a 5-year survival rate of 50%. Only six of these patients had sigmoid colon cancer; the remainder had rectal cancer. No comparison was made to a control group receiving standard ligation. These studies imply that the impact of central node resection may be improved staging but are not informative regarding potential for improved survival. It should be noted that the performance of standard ligation would not have identified the involved central lymph node; thus, direct comparison cannot be performed.

Only three studies in the available literature compared survival in patients with colon cancer treated with intermediate-level ligation versus central ligation. Hohenberger et al[2] presented a large retrospective case series of 1,329 consecutive patients who underwent curative resection for colon cancer in Erlangen, Germany. The authors compared patients treated during three periods (1978 to 1984, 1985 to 1994, and 1995 to 2002). Although the authors reported that department policy regarding surgical approach changed in 1985 to one of central ligation and complete mesocolic excision, there were no pathology data to confirm the extent of nodal dissection before and after 1985. The authors observed 6.5% local recurrence rate and 82% 5-year survival rate in the earliest period versus 3.6% local recurrence and 89.1% 5-year survival rates in the most recent period. The data do not account for changes in other processes of care, such as chemotherapy regimens, over time. They also did not account for any effect of "stage migration" as an effect of the central ligation.

Kawamura et al[10] examined the effect of high ligation on disease-free survival in colon cancer. A total of 567 patients with an intermediate or high ligation from 1963 to 1999 were selected. In patients with limited nodal involvement, high ligation offered no survival benefit over intermediate ligation ($P = .29$). There was also no difference in survival in patients with intermediate and central node positivity. However, the numbers of patients in these groups were very small: only 47 patients with positive intermediate nodes and six patients with positive central nodes. This study was underpowered to detect any survival benefit of central ligation.

A single study from the Columbia–Presbyterian Department of Surgery showed benefit associated with high ligation.[8] This single-institution case series included 2,409 consecutive patients who had curative resection of colon or rectal cancer from 1957 to 1975. The outcomes of colon cancer patients were not distinguished from those of rectal cancer patients. The 5-year survival rate of patients with Dukes B cancer increased from 73.9% to 84% with central ligation, while the survival rate of those with Dukes C1 cancer increased from 49% to 58.6%. The level of mesenteric resection only influenced outcomes in patients with moderately or well-differentiated cancers with intermediate-level nodal involvement. Patients with >4 positive lymph nodes or poorly differentiated tumors had lower 5-year survival regardless of mesenteric ligation. This study's utility is limited by its outdated nature. No modern chemotherapy regimens were available. Additionally, no pathologic audit was performed to determine the extent of nodal harvest, and the decision about the level of mesenteric division was at the discretion of the surgeon.

CONCLUSION

Metastasis to central lymph nodes is a rare event in colon cancer. Current literature does not support the routine use of extended lymphadenectomy in patients with nonmetastatic colonic adenocarcinoma. However, metastases to central lymph nodes, when present, may often be identified clinically either during the preoperative evaluation or during surgery and should be removed to achieve a complete resection in these patients. An adequately powered randomized controlled study in the setting of modern chemotherapy regimens would be needed to address this question in a more definitive manner.

Current evidence does not support the *routine* use of extended lymphadenectomy (D3) resection as a means of improving survival in colon cancer.

REFERENCES

1. Atkins D, Best D, Briss PA, et al. Grading quality of evidence and strength of recommendations. *BMJ* 2004;328(7454):1490.
2. Hohenberger W, Weber K, Matzel K, et al. Standardized surgery for colonic cancer: complete mesocolic excision and central ligation–technical notes and outcome. *Colorectal Dis* 2009;11(4):354–364; discussion 355–364.
3. Chin CC, Yeh CY, Tang R, et al. The oncologic benefit of high ligation of the inferior mesenteric artery in the surgical treatment of rectal or sigmoid colon cancer. *Int J Colorectal Dis* 2008;23(8):783–788.
4. Li GZ, Turley RS, Lidsky ME, et al. Impact of simultaneous diaphragm resection during hepatectomy for treatment of metastatic colorectal cancer. *J Gastrointest Surg* 2012;16(8):1508–1515.
5. West NP, Morris EJ, Rotimi O, et al. Pathology grading of colon cancer surgical resection and its association with survival: a retrospective observational study. *Lancet Oncol* 2008;9(9):857–865.
6. West NP, Kobayashi H, Takahashi K, et al. Understanding optimal colonic cancer surgery: comparison of Japanese D3 resection and European complete mesocolic excision with central vascular ligation. *J Clin Oncol* 2012;30(15):1763–1769.
7. Cirocchi R, Trastulli S, Farinella E, et al. High tie versus low tie of the inferior mesenteric artery in colorectal cancer: a RCT is needed. *Surg Oncol* 2012;21(3):e111–e123.
8. Slanetz CA Jr, Grimson R. Effect of high and intermediate ligation on survival and recurrence rates following curative resection of colorectal cancer. *Dis Colon Rectum* 1997;40(10):1205–1218; discussion 1218–1209.
9. Kanemitsu Y, Komori K, Kimura K, et al. D3 Lymph node dissection in right hemicolectomy with a no-touch isolation technique in patients with colon cancer. *Dis Colon Rectum* 2013;56(7):815–824.
10. Kawamura YJ, Umetani N, Sunami E, et al. Effect of high ligation on the long-term result of patients with operable colon cancer, particularly those with limited nodal involvement. *Eur J Surg* 2000;166(10):803–807.

This joint venture between the American College of Surgeons and the Alliance for Clinical Trials in Oncology to set forth surgical standards for different types of oncologic resections is indeed a laudable effort. The portion of the work here is the surgical standards for manual colon resection and two key controversies (questions) which follow. Importantly, the format in presenting surgical standards first, followed by two controversial points, is an excellent one and thus amenable to a broad readership including general surgeons, specialists, oncologic surgeons, and colon and rectal surgeons, as well as general surgical trainees and colon and rectal surgical trainees. The critical elements in the procedures for colon resection are well-chosen, well-illustrated, nicely discussed, and completely referenced. Certainly, anytime there is a discussion of technique, multiple opinions are the norm, but interestingly, with this presentation, there is little to argue. Perhaps the only point that is of uncertain importance to this discussion of techniques is the statement "The number of lymph nodes resected surgically and evaluated pathologically reflects the completeness of lymphadenectomy and is an indicator of surgical quality and oncologic outcome," which is surely controversial, perhaps even quite controversial. There are multiple references in the literature illustrating no correlation between these quality measures and outcomes. Thus, I am unsure if it should be stated so definitively in this portion of the text. Similarly, the concept of complete mesocolic excision and central dissection is extremely controversial and should probably be best left to the key question areas and is in fact covered in the first key question. Other than these two "gray" areas, the surgical standards portion of this effort is well presented, is complete, reads nicely, and can be relied upon to be definitive.

Key question number one is important. The authors do a good job of presenting the data set and the concept of central vascular ligation is ripe for a trial. The problem of course, with any surgical trial, is generalizability of the findings obtained in specialist centers to the general population of surgeons.

Key question number two is, again, very important and controversial. The authors do an excellent job of presenting all sides of the argument and rightly note how difficult it would be to construct and conduct a good clinical trial. Indeed, I am unsure if one could actually be structured at all.

In summary, then, these efforts at establishing an oncologic surgical standard for colon resection are laudable. It is in keeping with the American College of Surgeons' commitment to try to standardize surgical practices around well-established clinical and academically sound principles. Attempts to standardize any surgical approach are tricky; the primary question being how does innovation occur if standards are rigid? The authors of this section are mindful of this potential problem and present their approaches carefully, in such a way that, as stated previously, there is little with which to argue.

John H. Pemberton, MD, FACS
Professor of Surgery
Consultant, Division of Colon and Rectal Surgery
Mayo Clinic College of Medicine
Mayo Clinic
Rochester, Minnesota

Oncologic Elements of the Operative Record—Colon

Clinical Information			
Operative Intent	Curative	Palliative	
Urgency/indication	Elective/urgent/emergent	Bleeding, obstruction, perforation	
Intraoperative Findings			
Tumor	Gross extension through colon wall	Adherence to adjacent organ or abdominal side wall structure	
Lymph nodes	Gross lymphadenopathy (Y/N)	Central or retroperitoneal lymphadenopathy (Y/N), e.g., SMV/SMA or periaortic/aortocaval	Extraregional adenopathy (Y/N)
Metastases	Liver: Describe number, size, and location, whether biopsy was performed.	Peritoneal implantation: Describe number, size, and location.	Adnexa (women)
Synchronous pathology			
Intraoperative frozen section biopsy	Y/N, result, alteration in procedure based on result		
Procedure Summary			
Operative approach	Started: laparoscopic/ hand-assisted laparoscopic/ robotic/open	Finished: laparoscopic/hand-assisted laparoscopic/ robotic/open (ESSENTIAL to define which portions of the procedure were done with or without a hand in the abdomen or as extracorporeal procedures: adhesiolysis, mobilization, vascular ligation, bowel transection, anastomosis)	
Type of resection with description of proximal and distal extent of resection	• Right hemicolectomy, distal margin proximal to middle colic artery • Extended right hemicolectomy, distal margin distal to middle colic artery • Extended right hemicolectomy, distal margin distal to splenic flexure • Transverse colectomy • Left hemicolectomy, proximal margin____, distal margin____ • Sigmoid colon resection, proximal margin____, distal margin at rectum • Total abdominal colectomy		
Level of vascular ligation	Names(s) of primary feeding vessel(s) and level(s) of ligation		
Clinical assessment of completeness of resection	R0	R1	R2
Adjacent organ resection: (Y/N)	Name the organs resected. Adjacent organ resection en bloc: (Y/N)		

Note: Pages numbers followed by *f* denote figures, those followed by a *t* denote tables.